Creating Infrastructures for Latino Mental Health

Lydia P. Buki • Lissette M. Piedra
Editors

Creating Infrastructures for Latino Mental Health

Foreword by Melba J. T. Vasquez

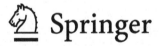 Springer

Editors
Lydia P. Buki
Department of Kinesiology &
   Community Health
University of Illinois at Urbana-Champaign
127 Huff Hall, 1206 S. Fourth St.
Champaign, IL 61820, USA
buki@illinois.edu

Lissette M. Piedra
School of Social Work
University of Illinois at Urbana-Champaign
1010 W. Nevada St.
Urbana, IL 61801, USA
lmpiedra@illinois.edu

ISBN 978-1-4419-9451-6   (hardcover)   ISBN 978-1-4419-9452-3 (e-book)
ISBN 978-1-4614-6069-5   (softcover)
DOI 10.1007/978-1-4419-9452-3
Springer New York Dordrecht Heidelberg London

Library of Congress Control Number: 2011932788

Springer is part of Springer Science+Business Media (www.springer.com)

For all those who tirelessly work toward better mental health for Latinos: In gratitude for the creation of new pathways and the inspiration you provide along the way.

Al andar se hace camino
y al volver la vista atrás
se ve la senda que nunca
se ha de volver a pisar.

Caminante no hay camino sino estelas en la mar ...

by Antonio Machado, Spain, 1912

While on a journey, one carves the path
And glancing backward
One sees the footpath never
To be traveled again.

Wayfarer, no apparent path exists, only ripples in the sea ...

Translation by Lydia P. Buki and
Lissette M. Piedra, 2011

Foreword

The problems that Latinos face in this millennium go beyond the scope of any one discipline. Many of these challenges require thoughtful interventions and policies that reach across multiple disciplines to create change that will truly transform the status quo. In Creating Infrastructures for Latino Mental Health, Drs. Buki and Piedra show the synergy that can emerge when different mental health disciplines talk to each other. The editors, a psychologist and a social worker, present the first interdisciplinary book that seeks to answer seemingly straightforward, yet deeply complex questions: "What mental health service needs will Latinos encounter in the twenty-first century?" and "How can we build infrastructures so that we can be prepared to serve those needs?"

In this volume, Drs. Buki and Piedra bring together experts from multiple disciplines and specialty areas (developmental, clinical, and counseling psychology; law; medicine; public health; social work; sociology; and Spanish) to consider the ways in which society must change to meet Latinos' emerging needs. Thus, the book provides a foundation for the creation of innovative pathways to fulfill the mental health needs of Latinos in this country. Chapter contributors take pains to move beyond what is currently known in the literature to envision the creation of mechanisms, policies, strategies, and understandings that will facilitate the provision of much-needed services to the Latino population.

The importance of this book is underscored by the fact that as the largest minority group in the United States, Latinos face formidable economic and social barriers in their quest to thrive in this country (Mendelson et al. 2008). The limited information we have about their mental health needs is quite disturbing. For example, suicide rates are alarmingly high: Suicide attempts by Latina girls are 60% higher than for their non-Latina White counterparts. In any given year, 19% of Latinas in high school will attempt suicide at least once (Centers for Disease Control and Prevention [CDC] 2000). Across gender lines, approximately 13% of Latino high school students have attempted suicide, compared with 7.3% of Blacks and 6.7% of non-Latino Whites (CDC 2000).

Consider, too, that the wars in Afghanistan and Iraq have disproportionately affected Latino communities. Because a disproportionately high number of Latinos are on active duty, their chilling experiences have a ripple effect that is detrimental for their families and communities. Thirty-nine percent of Latino veterans suffer lifetime post-traumatic stress disorder (PTSD) (Hyde 2010). Or, consider the fact that Latinos are incarcerated at rates two to three times higher than non-Latino White youth (Villarruel and Walker 2002); once imprisoned, they have the longest average length of incarceration of any racial or ethnic group (Walker et al. 2004).

Dr. Michenbaum (2009) noted that the discovery that 70% of juvenile delinquents were illiterate spurred a project to ensure that every child could read by the third grade. He noted that in a literate society like the United States, having reading skills propels a child onto a particular path filled with opportunity, whereas illiteracy stymies a child's development and relegates that child to a different path away from the mainstream. Indeed, the link between what society can do to advance the well-being of individuals, families, and communities and how this contributes to mental health outcomes must become a central part of our current discourse. Herein lies the incisive contribution made by this book. It provides answers to questions such as: "What structures can facilitate good educational outcomes for Latino children?"; "What policies can increase the number of Latino high school students who can envision a future in college?"; and "What services can provide critical assistance to families who care for a loved one with mental illness?". These are timely topics given the changing demographics and related challenges that we are facing, the need to promote a democratic society, and the imperative to facilitate psychological health and well-being in the fastest growing population in this country. Ultimately, the nation stands to benefit from a well-educated and high functioning population.

Of course, these questions evoke other concerns. Even when Latinos seek help, they do not always get the help they need. Among those who access mental health services, 60–75% do not return after one session (Carrasco 2010). Thus, we also need to ask: "What are the organizational infrastructures that promote access to health care for Latinos?", and "How do we take issues of acculturation and assimilation into account when developing relevant services for the population?". Although this book provides some answers to these formidable questions, it is the questions raised by this volume that have the lasting potential to change the status quo.

Thus, this book goes far in identifying the mechanisms, policies, strategies, and understandings that mental health professionals and administrators must adopt to meet the needs of the Latino community. This invaluable resource is a major contribution and provides exemplary leadership in promoting the complex levels of services needed at this juncture in our country. Above all, it provides a watershed for those of us who yearn for a just society.

Melba J. T. Vasquez

Preface

We are at the crossroads in Latino mental health. The future well-being of our nation rests in our ability to promote the mental and physical health in this population. In many ways, the task before us is daunting, yet history reminds us of the endless possibility of human ingenuity to use the tools at hand and realize the most seemingly impossible goals.

As scholars, practitioners, and policymakers, we can foresee a world with ample facilities, resources, and personnel—key aspects of infrastructure—to provide effective mental health services. Moreover, within that world, we can envision service access regardless of ancestry, citizenship status, language preference, or cultural belief. However, to reach our destination, we need to know where we are, where we want to go, and what obstacles we can anticipate along the way. The scholarly advances of our disciplines, the shifting demographic landscape, public policies, and the like guide us. Taking stock of where we are, we recognize that there is a growing literature on culturally responsive interventions, but a dearth of scholarship on ways to connect these interventions to our existing service systems. In many cases, we must chart new courses and build new infrastructures to deliver these interventions. In the chapters that follow, this book shows how an interdisciplinary group of scholars used their expertise to document where we are, propose future pathways, and illuminate potential obstacles along the way.

Throughout the book, one overarching theme emerged: Achieving a service structure that meets the mental health needs of Latinos will entail a radical change in the status quo. Without a concerted and coordinated effort to change our course, we can foresee a nation in which its largest ethnic minority—expected to comprise nearly a quarter of the future workforce—is unnecessarily hampered by mental health morbidity.

To reach our destination, we must navigate complex and uncertain terrain, recognizing the need to take stock of our surroundings by surveying interdisciplinary perspectives to move the mental health field forward. As co-editors from two different disciplines (psychology and social work), we sought to bring together authors from a wide range of disciplines, writing from diverse geographic locations, and reflecting insights from established and new scholars. In the process, we felt challenged by the constraints of disciplinary perspective and discourse. For many of our authors, the writing process necessitated many revisions, but was punctuated by the exhilaration of thinking of their work in new, innovative ways. Thus, the final products are pioneering, and we look forward to our readers benefiting from the authors' insights.

We have grouped 14 chapters into four parts. The first part contains three chapters that provide an overview of the forces shaping service provision and the implications of those forces. In the first chapter, Andrade and Viruell-Fuentes offer a window into the future: How the current demographic trends drive the ongoing population transformation and ultimately affect service provision. Their analysis includes a discussion of panethnic labels, which serve a methodical purpose but often mask the diversity of the population. By delineating the diversity within the Latino population and then contrasting broad population trends with those of non-Latino Whites, they build an argument for the development of infrastructures aimed at specific dimensions of structural inequality, such as education, income, access to health insurance, immigrant status, and English language proficiency. Andrade and Viruell-Fuentes argue that federal, state, and local governments have a role in infrastructure development, and contend that there is a great need for infrastructures built at the local level attuned to the specific needs of those communities.

In Chap. 2, Perez draws a similar conclusion about the role of government in addressing acculturation issues. In her discussion of acculturation and assimilation, Perez underscores the range of contextual and individual-level factors that interact in ways unique to each immigrant. She argues that because the contemporary sociopolitical context complicates Latino immigrants' incorporation into US life, their nuanced realities challenge contemporary notions of service provision and institutional arrangements. Simply put, a "one-size-fits-all" approach to mental health services is inadequate for Latino immigrants. Moreover, Perez argues that because the federal government regulates immigration policy, it must direct attention to the full incorporation of immigrants within its borders, seriously consider its role in protecting them, and regulate the admission of new immigrants and refugees. The current approach leaves much to the individual immigrants and the local communities in which they reside. Neglect fuels community tensions, marginalizes immigrants, and ultimately affects Latinos' mental health and well-being.

In Chap. 3, Piedra, Andrade, and Larrison point to a confluence of factors that undermine linguistically accessible services. The increasing number of people who need these services and the lack of a bilingual workforce contribute to the problem. Shifting settlement patterns into nontraditional immigrant communities further compound the situation. In this context, the authors argue for staff- and agency-level solutions that improve the quality of interpretation and enhance its effect on the professional relationship between provider and client. Consistent with the arguments advanced by Andrade and Viruell-Fuentes (Chap. 1), and Perez (Chap. 2), the authors conclude that solutions for building infrastructure must be multifaceted, responsive to current demographic trends, reflect sound social policy, and be grounded within the institutional, cultural, and social context of the existing mental health and health care delivery system. Even so, the authors in this first part of the book unanimously indicate that infrastructure building must extend beyond the borders of the mental health and health care sectors, a theme more fully explored in Part 2.

In the second part of the book, four chapters discuss the need for organizational change and for infrastructure-building across service sectors. In Chap. 4, Acevedo-Polakovich, Crider, Kassab, and Gerhart present a conceptual model for enhancing the availability, accessibility, and utilization of mental health services for Latinos by focusing on organizational cultural competence—the compatibility between service environments and local conceptions of behavioral health. According to their model, service disparities arise from a fundamental incompatibility in how service providers and ethnic-minority communities conceive of behavioral health and useful interventions. Because existing interventions reflect the conceptualization of service providers, the authors argue that reducing service disparities requires organizations to align their interventions with how local communities understand behavioral health. The authors argue that without organizational change to bridge this gap, efforts to develop a culturally competent workforce and implement culturally competent practices will be undermined.

In Chap. 5, Delgado-Romero, Espino, Werther, and González tackle the challenge of building infrastructure through training and interdisciplinary collaboration. They draw attention to structural issues present in mental health training and the specific challenges related to training a bilingual and bicultural workforce. By highlighting exemplary bilingual and bicultural mental health training programs, the authors illustrate the need to create an infrastructure that promotes interdisciplinary collaborations and that makes use of untapped resources such as students, faculty, and staff at Hispanic-serving institutions; international Latino mental health workers; and non-Latino mental health workers.

In Chap. 6, Piedra, Schiffner, and Reynaga-Abiko tackle the factors that contribute to a leaky educational pipeline. They reason that in a technologically advanced society such as the United States, access to higher education is arguably the *sine qua non* for a high quality of life, and therefore is a cornerstone of Latino mental health. The authors posit that because so many current and future Latino college students are the first in their families to attend college, increasing the number of college graduates among Latinos entails prioritizing the academic and psychological needs of first-generation college students. They propose three foundational strategies to facilitate recruitment, retention, and successful degree completion for this population, such as engaging multiple levels of government and creating institutionally based programs that meet both the instrumental and psychological needs of first-generation college students.

In Chap. 7, Abbott offers another important cornerstone of a culturally and linguistically responsive infrastructure: university–community partnerships that create opportunities for university Spanish students to act as brokers, navigators, and advocates for Latinos with limited English proficiency. First, Abbott calls attention to the fact that the rapid increase of Spanish speakers in the United States has created parallel shifts in human service infrastructure needs and the curricular design of university Spanish studies. In this context of heightened need, Spanish community service learning (CSL) holds much promise by taking students out of the classroom and placing them in the community. Abbott shows how students with language skills but no mental health background can still play an important, supportive role to direct service providers. Because language barriers complicate even the most mundane tasks, in the absence of these Spanish CSL students, many of the tasks would fall to an overburdened service provider or completely through the cracks. Thus, these Spanish CSL programs can help reduce mental health disparities among Spanish speakers.

In the third part of the book, four chapters highlight priority contexts for infrastructure development. Although it would be impossible to address the needs of all the especially vulnerable Latino populations, the chapters reflect a synergy of research, practice, and policy to promote greater social inclusion and social justice for populations easily overlooked.

In Chap. 8, Barrio, Hernández, and Barragán discuss how many Latino families compensate for service disparities by providing essential care to family members diagnosed with serious mental disorders. Because these families represent a critical and often unrecognized resource in the care of Latinos living with mental illness, the authors argue that engaging and supporting family caregivers must be a central component of any mental health infrastructure for Latinos. Toward this end, the authors examine the sociocultural issues that program managers and practitioners need to consider in supporting these families. Drawing from the research and practice literature, as well as from their own experiences as scientists and practitioners, Barrio, Hernández, and Barragán discuss the need for family involvement in services during the early stages of illness and promising theory-based psychoeducational programs known to help Latino families. The authors make a compelling argument that, given the strong role played by families in the care of Latinos with serious mental disorders, existing billing mechanisms that fail to reimburse family services actually harm Latinos. Therefore, they conclude that if we are to build a mental health services infrastructure that effectively meets the needs of Latinos, service reimbursement requires further consideration.

Weemhoff and Villarruel also draw from their research and practice experiences to tackle the plight of youth in the juvenile justice system. They provide evidence that Latino youth are disproportionately represented at each of the critical intervention points in the system, which eventually results in them suffering harsher treatment for the same offenses than non-Latino White youth. They explore ways in which trauma and mental health issues contribute to Latino youths' overrepresentation, and argue that court decisions must hinge upon early identification of mental health needs through culturally appropriate screening and assessment. Further, they contend that courts must rely on evidence-based diversion programs, and that the multiple needs of youth require a coordinated plan to ensure that they are referred to services relevant to their needs.

In Chap. 10, Aldarondo and Becker broach a topic we seldom hear about: the well-being of thousands of minors who immigrate to the United States without a legal guardian. Putting their lives at risk, these children leave their home countries to escape poverty, abuse, and exploitation, or to join relatives in the United States, among other reasons. The authors place this phenomenon in a global context, and point to the ways in which immigration policies and the journey to the United States itself affect these young migrants' health and well-being. To meet the needs of these youth, they discuss an ongoing, innovative academic–community partnership that promotes youths' rights and well-being. Through the partnership's efforts, the service infrastructure has been enhanced by strengthening local detention facilities' ability to serve these youth in an equitable manner.

In Chap. 11, Cristancho, Garcés, and Peters draw from their community-based research in the Upper Midwest in their discussion of ways to enhance access to mental health services for Latinos in rural areas. The authors point to the clash of cultures that occurs as newly arrived immigrants in rural areas encounter a service infrastructure ill prepared to serve their needs. Based on a multisite study involving several rural communities, Cristancho, Garcés, and Peters present data showing that mental health issues are quite prevalent in rural communities, and illustrate ways in which existing community resources can be mobilized to enhance service capacity while empowering community members to become active agents of change. The authors argue that to be effective, programs must emerge from an empirical approach based on assessment, planned action, implementation, evaluation, and dissemination; moreover, these programs must be easily accessible, offered through several sites, and be responsive to the social and environmental challenges facing the rural Latino population.

The fourth and last part of the book comprises three chapters that reflect on service opportunities in Latino mental health. These chapters illustrate the various forms and models through which effective practice can enhance the mental health of Latino populations.

In Chap. 12, Mayfield and Buki argue that with the expected increase in the number of Latinas in the United States, more women will be diagnosed with breast cancer. Yet, despite evidence that Latinas with breast cancer experience physical and mental health disparities, we are ill prepared to serve the support needs of this population. As an illustration, the authors use a comprehensive service model from a community-based organization dedicated to enhancing the mental health and well-being of Latinas with breast cancer. Mayfield and Buki argue that for such programs to be optimally effective, services must be provided by bilingual staff well versed in women's cultural backgrounds, and must provide not only mental health services, but also support in accessing health care and successfully navigating the complicated US health care system.

In Chap. 13, Morales reflects on another health disparity: The disproportionate number of Latinos diagnosed with HIV/AIDS, particularly gay and bisexual men, and men who have sex with men. He contends that with the greater attention currently paid to behavioral aspects of prevention, advocacy is needed to increase the resources devoted to this area. Moreover, given the challenges in reaching this population, he argues that one way to enhance infrastructure is through social capital development. Morales provides an overview of ways in which social capital may be harnessed, and illustrates these strategies through the work of two community-based programs in which he has been actively involved.

Comas-Díaz closes the part with Chap. 14, in which she discusses lessons she has learned from her "niche" group private practice with Latino clients. Her writing will inspire those who aspire to develop such a niche as practitioners. The chapter begins with Comas-Díaz's personal reflections on how to build a group private practice with Latino clients and how she came to develop that practice. In particular, she shares how she increased her visibility in the Latino community and the profession at large, and ways in which she conceptualizes her work with Latinos. She closes her brief reflection with a series of concrete and aspirational suggestions for building a successful private practice.

The book concludes with an epilogue by Toro, who invites us to consider that politics and mental health are inextricably related. She begins by reviewing various efforts to promote mental health at the policy level, pointing out ways in which recent health care and immigration legislation may affect our ability to provide adequate mental health services for Latino populations. She contends that as a society, we have a responsibility to ensure that health care, and specifically mental health, does not become an item of choice for those who need services but cannot afford them. Thus, she urges us to become politically involved and advocate for the types of policies that will foster greater infrastructure development.

We are delighted to present this book to you, and do so with the hope and expectation that it will inspire you to envision and forge new, fruitful paths in your quest to promote mental health among Latinos.

Lydia P. Buki
Lissette M. Piedra

Acknowledgements

Every project has its genesis in an idea, an idea that grows from a series of observations. The seeds of this project were first sown the fall of 2005, when a frantic e-mail went out to Latino faculty at the University of Illinois seeking crisis services for a severely depressed Spanish-speaking woman. Unable to locate bilingual services in Champaign-Urbana, mental health workers reached out to former interim Director Rosalinda Barrera from the University of Illinois Center for Democracy in a Multiracial Society (CDMS) for help. She, in turn, sent an e-mail seeking the assistance of bilingual faculty with mental health expertise at the University. After some brainstorming and cage-rattling, the woman in distress obtained assistance. However, this experience served to illustrate a troubling reality: There was clearly an unmet need for bilingual mental health services in Champaign County. Like many communities with rapidly growing Latino populations, Champaign County found itself ill-equipped to respond to these individuals' mental health needs. In this context, Dr. Barrera recognized the special role that universities could play through partnerships with local service providers. Long before she left the University of Illinois, she endeavored to build interdisciplinary bridges by bringing together faculty with complementary interests and putting them in touch with the service community. Her efforts reflect a belief in the unique ability of academic institutions to facilitate social change through academic collaborations that seek to improve the well-being of the larger community. We remain beholden to Dr. Barrera's insight and her legacy.

The next interim CDMS Director, Kent Ono, and his successor, Director Jorge Chapa, both provided seed money to support the fledging efforts of an interdisciplinary team working to expand mental health services for Latino immigrants in Champaign-Urbana. Our early experiences as members of this group demonstrated the challenges confronting the social service sector in this area, as well as the limited amount of scholarship available on how to address the growing population's needs. CDMS inspired us to pursue a line of inquiry that we have found both challenging and rewarding. We are forever indebted to Drs. Ono and Chapa and to CDMS for opening this door.

Family, friends, and colleagues offered support and guidance during the complex process of editing this book. Lydia P. Buki thanks Jack Ikeda and Helen Neville for their ongoing support throughout this project. She also thanks Norman Anderson, who generously shared his thoughts and suggested important avenues of inquiry. Lastly, she is especially grateful to Wojtek Chodzo-Zajko, Head of the Department of Kinesiology and Community Health, for providing a stimulating intellectual space that supports this scholarship. Lissette M. Piedra is grateful for the ongoing support of the School of Social Work and Dean Wynne Korr for advancing a vision of social justice that requires a steadfast commitment to use the tools of research, teaching, practice, and policy to meet the needs of vulnerable populations. In particular, she thanks Jan Carter-Black, Rob Kiely, Janet Liechty, and Chi-Fang Wu for their ongoing support, their courage to pursue difficult questions, and their passion for scholarship and teaching.

The copyediting skill of Brooke Graves greatly improved the book and we are grateful that her magic graces these pages. We also wish to acknowledge the staff at Springer, especially Anna Tobias, for her effort to make this book a reality.

Finally, we acknowledge the intellectual climate fostered by the University of Illinois at Urbana-Champaign. As land-grant University with a strong mission for community engagement, the University of Illinois facilitates our ability to make a difference locally through service and research, and lays the groundwork for us to have an enhanced impact at the local, state, and national levels. We are grateful to be part of this book and part of a growing community of scholars and practitioners dedicated to eradicating mental health service disparities for linguistic minorities.

Contents

About the Authors

Annie R. Abbott is an associate professor in the Department of Spanish, Italian, and Portuguese at the University of Illinois at Urbana-Champaign. In addition to her research and teaching on Spanish community service learning and transcultural competence, she earned the campus *Distinguished Teacher/Scholar Award* for her work on building a series of community-campus summits. She is also a faculty fellow with the Academy for Entrepreneurial Leadership, where she teaches courses on social entrepreneurship and business Spanish. Abbott is the author of the textbook *Comunidades: Más allá del aula* (Pearson/Prentice Hall).

I. David Acevedo-Polakovich is a faculty member at Central Michigan University, where he is assistant professor in the Clinical Psychology Doctoral Program and director of the Center for Community-Academic Initiatives for Development. His research and professional work focus on developing effective health and human services for historically underserved youth and families, with a particular emphasis on prevention and applied development programs targeted at adolescents. He is also actively involved in scholarship examining the development of successful community-academic initiatives and approaches to the development of practice-based evidence. More information on Dr. Acevedo-Polakovich and his work is available at: http://www.cmich.edu/chsbs/x23916.xml.

Etiony Aldarondo is associate dean for research and director of the Dunspaugh-Dalton Community and Educational Well-Being Research Center in the School of Education at the University of Miami. The recipient of various recognitions for academic excellence and community involvement, his scholarship focuses on positive development of ethnic minority and immigrant youth, domestic violence, and social justice-oriented clinical practices. His publications include the books *Advancing Social Justice through Clinical Practice*, *Programs for Men who Batter: Intervention and Prevention Strategies in a Diverse Society* (with Fernando Mederos, Ed.D.), and *Neurociencias, Salud y Bienestar Comunitario* (with Enrique Saforcada and Mauro Mañas).

Flavia C. D. Andrade is an assistant professor at the University of Illinois at Urbana-Champaign. She received her doctorate from the University of Wisconsin-

Madison. Dr. Andrade's research focuses on demography of health and aging. Her work has been published in books and various academic journals, including *The Journals of Gerontology, Population Studies*, and the *Journal of Adolescent Health*. Her current projects focus on the social, behavioral, economic, and biological determinants of population health over the life course, with a focus on Latin American and Caribbean populations.

Armando Barragán is a doctoral student at the School of Social Work at the University of Southern California. His research interests are in the area of Latino mental health, specifically in the area of severe mental illness. His current work focuses on pathways to mental health treatment among Latinos, recruitment and retention of Latinos in mental health services research, and culturally adapted interventions. He received his BA from the University of California, Los Angeles, and his master's in social welfare from the University of California, Berkeley.

Concepción Barrio is associate professor of social work at the University of Southern California. She brings over 20 years of practice experience with multicultural populations to her research focus on ethnocultural factors in severe mental illness and the cultural relevance of psychosocial rehabilitation services. Her recent research contributions address culturally based intervention development for Latino families dealing with schizophrenia, as well as culturally based factors that affect the early illness experience and concurrent pathways to care. Her record of productive research has been funded by the National Institute of Mental Health and is complemented by extensive interdisciplinary collaborations.

Rachel Becker is a doctoral student at the University of Miami Counseling Psychology Program. Her research, clinical, and academic interests converge around work with immigrant children and families. Her role as the university partnership coordinator at the Dunspaugh-Dalton Community and Educational Well-Being Research Center has led to her involvement in ICAN, an intervention to promote resilience in unaccompanied immigrant youth, as well as in an arts-based initiative to reduce stereotyping and prejudice in adolescent youth, and a community-based intervention in San Luis, Argentina. She also serves as member-at-large, Diversity Focus for the American Psychological Association of Graduate Students.

Lydia P. Buki is an associate professor in the Department of Kinesiology and Community Health at the University of Illinois at Urbana-Champaign. Her research interests include the psychosocial, cultural, individual, and institutional factors that contribute to health disparities in medically underserved Latino populations. She is a founding member of the DHHS Office on Women's Health, Minority Women's Health Panel of Experts, has served on the editorial board of various journals, and is associate editor of *Cultural Diversity and Ethnic Minority Psychology*. She recently completed a health literacy study with funding from the National Institutes of Health. Dr. Buki is a fellow of the American Psychological Association.

Lillian Comas-Díaz is a private practitioner in Washington, DC, executive director of the Transcultural Mental Health Institute, and a clinical professor at the George

Washington University Medical School. She directed the Hispanic Clinic at Yale University's Psychiatry Department as well as the Office of Ethnic Minority Affairs of the American Psychological Association (APA). Dr. Comas-Díaz has written extensively on the interaction between culture, gender, ethnicity, race, class, and mental health. She serves on several editorial boards, is an associate editor of the *American Psychologist*, and is a past president of the APA Division of Psychologists in Independent Practice.

Elizabeth A. Crider is a doctoral student in the Industrial/Organizational Psychology Department at Central Michigan University. Her research focuses on workplace cross-cultural training for employees who are placed abroad, and on evaluations of organizationally relevant outcomes. Prior to coming to graduate school, she worked as a research assistant at the University of Michigan, where she contributed to multiple projects on culture-based psychological differences in values and attitudes.

Sergio Cristancho is research assistant professor in the Department of Family and Community Medicine and the National Center for Rural Health Professions, University of Illinois College of Medicine at Rockford. He is now visiting faculty and mental health research coordinator at the National School of Public Health, Universidad de Antioquia, Colombia. Dr. Cristancho earned his doctoral degree at the University of Illinois at Urbana-Champaign and his undergraduate degree at the Universidad de Los Andes, Colombia. His main research interests lay at the intersection of psychology, culture and health, particularly related to underserved Latino immigrants in the United States and indigenous groups in Latin America.

Edward A. Delgado-Romero is professor in the Counseling Psychology Doctoral Program at the University of Georgia in the College of Education. He received his doctoral degree in psychology from the University of Notre Dame and has held faculty positions at the University of Florida (clinical professor) and Indiana University. He is president of the National Latina/o Psychological Association and a fellow of the American Psychological Association. His research interests include Latino psychology, the training of linguistically and culturally competent psychologists, and the use of race and ethnicity in psychological research.

Michelle M. Espino is an assistant professor in the College Student Affairs Administration Program at the University of Georgia. She earned a doctorate in higher education from the University of Arizona with funding from the Ford Foundation. Her research interests include Latino educational pathways to the doctorate, intersections of race, gender, and social class in accessing college and graduate school, and student engagement at minority-serving institutions such as Historically Black Colleges and Universities, and Hispanic-serving institutions. She is currently working on a grant focusing on institutional responses to the influx of potential Latino college students within the state of Georgia.

D. Marcela Garcés is an assistant professor in the Department of Preventive Medicine and Public Health at the School of Medicine, Universidad de Antioquia.

She has also been affiliated with the National Center for Rural Health Professions, University of Illinois College of Medicine at Rockford, since 2004. Dr. Garcés earned her master of science in public health at the University of Illinois at Urbana-Champaign and her medical degree at the Universidad CES in Colombia. Her main research interests are related to health disparities in vulnerable indigenous, immigrant, and displaced populations living in rural areas.

James I. Gerhart is a doctoral candidate in clinical psychology at Central Michigan University. His research focuses on therapeutic processes in violence reduction training, social problem solving, and positive outcomes of bicultural involvement. He is currently conducting research on the associations among emotional avoidance, anger, and aggression. His clinical interests include community-based interventions for at-risk youth and behavior therapies for aggression and trauma.

Marta J. González is a doctoral student in counseling psychology at the University of Georgia. She earned her master's degree in educational psychology and counseling with an emphasis in marriage and family therapy, and her bachelor's degree in psychology and child and adolescent development from California State University Northridge. Her research interests focus on Latino mental health and on factors that influence the pursuit of higher education in Latinos.

Mercedes Hernández is a doctoral student at the School of Social Work at the University of Southern California. Her research interests include Latino mental health disparities, intervention development for individuals diagnosed with severe mental illness, and community-based, culturally competent, and evidence-based practice. Prior to her doctoral studies, she worked as a psychiatric social worker for the Los Angeles County Department of Mental Health and the Los Angeles Unified School District. Her extensive clinical background has served to inform many of the issues she is interested in addressing in her research.

Veronica A. Kassab is a doctoral student in the Clinical Psychology Program at Central Michigan University (CMU). She is currently a research associate at the Center for Community-Academic Initiatives for Development at CMU, where she coordinates a project focused on the development and evaluation of anti-violence and sexuality education interventions for at-risk Latino youth. She has worked as a program coordinator for the Chaldean American Ladies of Charity in Farmington Hills, MI, where she provided services for Chaldean youth and newly arrived refugees. She received her bachelor's degree from the University of Detroit Mercy and is a provisionally certified family life educator.

Christopher R. Larrison is an associate professor at the School of Social Work, University of Illinois at Urbana-Champaign. His research is focused on the organizational and staff factors that shape client outcomes at community-based agencies. Dr. Larrison has studied community mental health services in the United States, community development in rural Mexico, and the impact of welfare reform in Georgia using multilevel primary data and mixed methods.

Jennifer B. Mayfield is a doctoral student in the Counseling Psychology Division at the University of Illinois at Urbana-Champaign. Her research interests focus on cultural and psychosocial determinants of health among racial and ethnic minority women, including the role of health literacy in cancer screening behaviors of African-American women. She received her bachelor's degree in psychology from Xavier University of Louisiana and her master's in educational psychology from the University of Illinois. She is currently working on her dissertation.

Eduardo Morales is distinguished professor in the Clinical Psychology Doctoral Program at the California School of Professional Psychology, San Francisco (CSPP-SF), Alliant international University. He is also an executive director of AGUILAS, an HIV prevention program for Latino gay and bisexual men. Dr. Morales has received many awards, including the 2009 *American Psychological Association Award for Distinguished Contributions to Institutional Practice*, the 2009 *Latino Business Leadership Award* by the San Francisco Hispanic Chamber of Commerce, and the National Latino Psychological Association 2006 *Star Vega Distinguished Service Award*. His areas of expertise include health prevention and promotion, HIV, substance abuse, community interventions, program evaluation, and strategic planning and policy development in communities and organizations.

Rose M. Perez, an assistant professor in the Graduate School of Social Service at Fordham University, migrated from Cuba as a child. Influenced by her entrepreneurial family, she obtained an MBA from the University of Michigan and marketed products to diverse populations. This work and her own migration experience inspired her to seek further studies focusing on Latino acculturation. Dr. Perez holds a master's degree in Latin American studies and a master's and doctorate in social work from the University of Chicago. She strives to teach students how to think critically about immigrant and refugee adaptation to the United States—the same topics that drive her research.

Karen E. Peters is an assistant professor of community health sciences at the School of Public Health of the University of Illinois at Chicago, and holds a joint faculty appointment in the National Center for Rural Health Professions in the UIC College of Medicine at Rockford. She received her Dr. P.H. from UIC and currently serves as co-director for public health practice and director of research dissemination in the Center for Research on Health and Aging. Her current research, teaching, and practice interests include community-based participatory action research, global public health, chronic disease prevention, evaluation, health workforce development, inter-professional education, and health policy analysis.

Lissette M. Piedra is an assistant professor at the University of Illinois at Urbana-Champaign in the School of Social Work. She is a licensed clinical social worker who received her doctorate from the School of Social Service Administration at the University of Chicago. Her research explores how the language and culture of immigrants affect their access to and their use of social and health services. Dr. Piedra's work has appeared in *Social Work, Administration in Social Work,* and *Journal of Social Service Review*. In addition, she co-edited *Our Diverse Society:*

Race and Ethnicity—Implications for 21st Century American Society (NASW Press 2006).

Geneva Reynaga-Abiko is a licensed clinical psychologist who works as assistant director and director of training at the University of California, Merced Counseling and Psychological Services. She earned her doctorate in clinical psychology from Pepperdine University in Los Angeles and completed pre- and post-doctoral training in neuropsychological assessment at the Department of Mental Health in Vacaville, CA. Dr. Reynaga-Abiko has worked in higher education since 2005 as a clinician, faculty member, and administrator. Her areas of interest include the Latino educational pipeline, training multiculturally competent mental health professionals, intersectionality and borderlands theory, and psychological assessment with Latinos.

Tiffany A. Schiffner is a staff psychologist at the Counseling Center at the University of Central Florida. She is the chair of the Diversity Committee and the liaison to Latino students. She received her doctorate in counseling psychology from the University of Illinois at Urbana-Champaign, and completed her internship and a postdoctoral fellowship at Duke University Counseling and Psychological Services. Her clinical interests include diversity and multicultural issues, relationship difficulties, and women's issues. Her primary research interests are sexual health issues of Latino young adults, health disparities within the Latino community, and educational pursuits of Latino students.

Annie G. Toro is governmental affairs manager of Population Services International. Previously, she was associate executive director for government relations at the American Psychological Association, where she provided overall direction, developed, managed, and coordinated the association's legislative and regulatory policy agenda impacting vulnerable populations. In addition, she has been senior legislative counsel to U.S. Representative Luis Gutierrez, and minority staff director for the House Financial Services Committee Subcommittee on Oversight and Investigations. She earned a Juris Doctor from Syracuse University and a master's in public health from The George Washington University.

Melba J. T. Vasquez is a psychologist in independent practice in Austin, Texas. She was elected as the 2011 president of the American Psychological Association. She has also served as president of the Texas Psychological Association, APA Division 17 (Society of Counseling Psychology), and APA Division 35 (Society for the Psychology of Women). She is a cofounder of APA Division 45 (Society for the Psychological Study of Ethnic Minority Issues) and of the National Multicultural Conference and Summit. She publishes in the areas of ethics, multicultural psychology, psychology of women, psychotherapy, and supervision. She is an APA fellow and holds the diploma of the American Board of Professional Psychology.

Francisco A. Villarruel received his doctorate in human development from the University of Wisconsin. He is a University Outreach and Engagement Senior Fellow and a professor of human development and family studies at Michigan State University. His research focuses on Latino youth and youth who are in conflict with the law. He sits on the National Board for the Campaign for Youth Justice, the Michigan Council on Crime and Delinquency, and is a consultant to the Office of Juvenile Justice and Delinquency Prevention.

Edna A. Viruell-Fuentes is an assistant professor in the Department of Latina/ Latino Studies at the University of Illinois at Urbana-Champaign. She is the author of several publications examining the roles of discrimination, ethnic identity, and social ties in shaping Latino and immigrant health outcomes. Previously, she was a joint Yerby and Kellogg scholar in health disparities at the Harvard School of Public Health. She holds an MPH degree from the School of Public Health at the University of North Carolina in Chapel Hill and a doctorate from the School of Public Health at the University of Michigan.

Michelle M. Weemhoff is senior policy associate at the Michigan Council on Crime and Delinquency, where she plans, develops, and implements juvenile justice programs. Using a research-based approach to advocacy and public policy development, she has worked on juvenile justice campaigns dealing with adjudication and sentencing, mental health treatment, and conditions of confinement. She is the co-chair of the Michigan Juvenile Justice Collaborative, co-chair of the Michigan Youth Reentry Workgroup, and has worked with state departments, juvenile facilities, and local communities to implement re-entry infrastructures for youth in prisons and juvenile justice placements. She received her master's of social work degree from the University of Michigan.

Eckart Werther is a doctoral candidate in the Counseling Psychology Program at the University of Georgia. He is a licensed clinical social worker and has worked with the Latino population in a variety of clinical, community, and educational settings. His interests include anxiety-related issues, multidisciplinary collaboration, multicultural psychology, domestic violence, and adjustment difficulties.

Contributors

Annie R. Abbott University of Illinois at Urbana-Champaign, Urbana, IL, USA
e-mail: arabbott@illinois.edu

I. David Acevedo-Polakovich Central Michigan University, Mount Pleasant, MI, USA
e-mail: david.acevedo@cmich.edu

Etiony Aldarondo School of Education, University of Miami, Miami, FL, USA
e-mail: etiony@miami.edu

Flavia C. D. Andrade University of Illinois at Urbana-Champaign, Champaign, IL, USA
e-mail: fandrade@illinois.edu

Armando Barragán School of Social Work, University of Southern California, Los Angeles, CA, USA

Concepción Barrio University of Southern California, Los Angeles, CA, USA
e-mail: cbarrio@usc.edu

Rachel Becker University of Miami, Miami, FL, USA

Lydia P. Buki University of Illinois at Urbana-Champaign, Champaign, IL, USA
e-mail: buki@illinois.edu

Lillian Comas-Díaz The George Washington University, Washington, DC, USA
e-mail: lilliancomasdiaz@gmail.com

Elizabeth A. Crider Central Michigan University, Mount Pleasant, MI, USA

Sergio Cristancho College of Medicine, University of Illinois, IL, USA

Facultad Nacional de Salud Pública, Universidad de Antioquia, Medellín, Colombia
e-mail: scrista@uic.edu

Edward A. Delgado-Romero College of Education, University of Georgia, Athens, GA, USA
e-mail: edelgado@uga.edu

Michelle M. Espino University of Georgia, Athens, GA, USA

D. Marcela Garcés School of Medicine, Universidad de Antioquia, Antioquia, Colombia

James I. Gerhart Central Michigan University, Mount Pleasant, MI, USA

Marta J. González University of Georgia, Athens, GA, USA

Mercedes Hernández School of Social Work, University of Southern California, Los Angeles, CA, USA

Veronica A. Kassab Central Michigan University, Mount Pleasant, MI, USA

Christopher R. Larrison School of Social Work, University of Illinois at Urbana-Champaign, Urbana, IL, USA

Jennifer B. Mayfield University of Illinois at Urbana-Champaign, 127 Huff Hall, 1206 S. Fourth St., Champaign, IL 61820, USA
e-mail: jaymay03@gmail.com

Eduardo Morales Alliant International University, San Francisco, CA, USA
e-mail: dremorales@aol.com

Rose M. Perez Fordham University, New York, NY, USA
e-mail: roseperez2@gmail.com

Karen E. Peters School of Public Health, University of Illinois at Chicago, Chicago, IL, USA

Lissette M. Piedra School of Social Work, University of Illinois at Urbana-Champaign, Urbana, IL, USA

Geneva Reynaga-Abiko University of California, Merced, CA, USA

Tiffany A. Schiffner University of Central Florida, Orlando, FL, USA

Annie G. Toro Population Services International, Washington, DC, USA
e-mail: annietoro@yahoo.es

Melba J. T. Vasquez Private Practice, Austin, TX, USA

Francisco A. Villarruel Michigan State University, East Lansing, MI, USA

Edna A. Viruell-Fuentes University of Illinois at Urbana-Champaign, Champaign, IL, USA

Michelle M. Weemhoff Michigan Council on Crime and Delinquency, Lansing, MI, USA
e-mail: mweemhoff@miccd.org

Eckart Werther University of Georgia, Athens, GA, USA

Part I
Forces Shaping Service Provision

Chapter 1
Latinos and the Changing Demographic Landscape: Key Dimensions for Infrastructure Building

Flavia C. D. Andrade and Edna A. Viruell-Fuentes

Abstract By 2050, close to one in four US residents will be of Latino origin. Given this fact, the welfare of the nation as a whole will largely depend on the economic and social well-being of this population. This chapter presents the demographic and social trends that are driving this transformation. It first discusses the creation of pan-ethnic labels, which mask the diversity of the Latino population and provides brief overview of the historical origins of the major Latino groups in the United States. The chapter, then, examines the demographic and socioeconomic profiles of this heterogeneous population and shows that, despite the prominent role that Latinos play in the economy and demographics of the US economy, troubling socio-economic trends indicate an urgent need to reexamine current service infrastructures. For instance, the social and economic disparities Latinos experience are reflected in their limited access to health care, and overall physical and mental health status disadvantages. In the mental health service sector, access to quality care remains a persistent problem. The chapter concludes by discussing the implications of the major Latino demographic trends for building infrastructures capable of meeting their physical and mental health care needs. The heterogeneity and the growing geographic dispersion of the Latino population also call for the development of infrastructures attuned to the needs and characteristics of the specific Latino communities to be served. We suggest that the development of viable infrastructures and programs aimed at improving the health, and mental health outcomes of Latinos should include addressing structural inequalities, such as those related to education, income, access to health insurance, and citizenship status.

The authors are listed alphabetically. Both authors contributed equally to this chapter.

F. C. D. Andrade (✉)
Department of Latina/Latino Studies, University of Illinois at Urbana-Champaign, Champaign, IL, USA
e-mail: fandrade@illinois.edu

National demographic trends signal the need for an increased focus on the unprecedented growth in the Latino[1] population that shows little sign of declining. In 1960,
about 4% of the US population was of Latino origin (Bean and Tienda 1987; Tienda
and Mitchell 2006). Estimates from 2008 indicate that about 47 million, or 15.4% of
the residents in the United States, were Latinos (Pew Hispanic Center 2010). Conservative estimates project that, by 2050, approximately one out of five residents in
the United States will be of Latino descent.

Despite the prominent role that Latinos play in the US economy, troubling social
trends indicate an urgent need to reexamine current service infrastructures. In comparison to the average population, the Latino population is younger, poorer, less educated,
and has less access to health care. In addition, the limited availability of linguistically
and culturally competent providers renders many services inaccessible to Latinos,
especially immigrants and older adults (Rumbaut 2006). Moreover, whereas Latino
immigrants continue to be geographically concentrated in a few states and cities, they
are increasingly relocating to new destination areas. This new migratory pattern has
profound implications for host communities, many of which lack the services and
community infrastructures found in traditional immigrant destinations that facilitate
adaptation and promote health. In these new destinations, providing adequate health
and mental health care to Latinos poses particular challenges, especially as Spanish-
speaking service providers are not uniformly distributed across the United States.

In this chapter, we present the demographic trends that are driving the current
population transformation. We first discuss the creation of pan-ethnic labels, which
serve an analytic purpose but also mask the diversity of the population. We then
provide a brief overview of the historical origins of the major Latino groups in the
United States, followed by the demographic and socioeconomic profiles of this heterogeneous population. In addition, we compare Latinos with the general US population along demographic and socioeconomic factors that influence health and mental health disparities. We present an overview of the Latino population's access to
health care as well as their health status. We conclude by discussing the implications
of the major demographic trends observed among this richly heterogeneous Latino
population for building the types of infrastructures capable of meeting their needs.

The Construction of the Latino Pan-Ethnic Category

Efforts to document the social, demographic, and economic characteristics of Latinos
date back to 1850, when the first efforts to account for Mexicans in the census were
made by inquiring about place of birth (Rodríguez 2000; Rumbaut 2006). These efforts eventually resulted in the creation of a pan-ethnic category to classify a highly
diverse population under the umbrella term *Hispanic*. The term was first introduced
in the context of the post–Civil Rights era by the Office of Management and Budget
in 1977. Beginning with the 1980 Census, the Hispanic category has been used, with

---

[1] The terms *Latino* and *Hispanic* are used interchangeably in this chapter, as are the terms *foreign-
born* and *immigrant*.

minor variations, in the collection of federal and other administrative data on people with origins in any of the 19 different Spanish-speaking Latin American countries and Spain (Rodríguez 2000; Rumbaut 2006). Following earlier trends of defining Latinos on the basis of sociocultural criteria, the Hispanic construct is intended to denote ethnicity. Thus, Latinos are the only ethnic group that, by law, is counted in the census (Rodríguez 2000; Rumbaut 2006). However, even though the Latino category was introduced to designate ethnicity rather than race, the term *Latino* "is used routinely and equivalently alongside 'racial' categories such as Asian, black, and non-Hispanic white, effecting a de facto racialization of the former" (Rumbaut 2006, pp. 22–23). In other words, in practice, the Latino category is used as an ethnoracial one.

The term *Latino*, though used extensively, has been debated widely, with many scholars and advocates acknowledging both the utility and drawbacks of this pan-ethnic category. On the one hand, critics have pointed out that, in its day-to-day use, this category homogenizes the experiences and histories of a hugely diverse population (Etzioni 2002; Oboler 1995; Rumbaut 2006). In other words, this ethnic identifier renders invisible the varied historical, political, and economic processes that have shaped the peoples of Latin-American origin who are present in the United States. Indeed, Latinos have resisted their undifferentiated classification, choosing to identify by and large with their specific countries of origin (Etzioni 2002; Rumbaut 2006). Furthermore, as defined by the Census Bureau, the Hispanic category includes people from Spain, whose social and historical experiences in the United States differ significantly from those of individuals of Latin-American ancestry. On the other hand, the use of the Latino construct has some utility, in that "the main unifying factor among the peoples of Latin-American descent in the United States is political" (Oboler 1995, p. 4). Thus, in strategic and specific contexts, the Latino pan-ethnic category can help facilitate the mobilization of communities that share a common experience of inequality (Oboler 1995).

Addressing social inequities, including those related to access to care for Latinos, requires paying attention to the heterogeneity within this population. To this end, in the next section we provide a brief overview of the historical, political, and economic forces that have shaped the distinct groups of people of Latin-American origin who are present in the United States. Rather than being exhaustive, our discussion merely highlights key processes that have shaped the context of reception for these groups and their incorporation into the broader US society.

Latino Origins

The presence of Latinos in the United States is closely tied to the country's foreign political and economic policies, dating back to the 1800s and continuing into the present. Although each Latino group has its unique history, they all share a history of US interventionism, whether political, military, and/or economic. Our historical overview begins with the three largest and oldest Latino groups in the United States: Mexicans, Puerto Ricans, and Cubans. We then present information on Dominicans, Central Americans, and South Americans. We are aware that our discussion of the latter two groups is by necessity extremely brief and, therefore, does not do justice to the histories of individual nationality groups. Nevertheless, our discussion provides a point of departure for understanding both the diversity within the Latino population and the experiences of dislocation and inequality that they share.

Mexicans

Mexicans became part of the US demographic landscape in the nineteenth century as a result of the US territorial expansionist efforts that culminated in the Mexican-American War. When that war ended, in 1848, nearly half of Mexico's territory was annexed to the United States. Upon annexation of what is now the Southwest, Mexicans living in the region instantly became US citizens; however, "within two decades of the American conquest it had become clear that, with few exceptions, Mexican Americans had been relegated to a stigmatized, subordinate position in the social and economic hierarchies" (Gutiérrez 1995, p. 21).

In the early 1900s, US labor contractors actively recruited Mexicans to alleviate labor shortages in mining, agriculture, and the construction of the railroads, among others. The US efforts to recruit laborers from Mexico, combined with the political and economic upheaval Mexicans experienced prior to and during the Mexican Revolution, contributed to the first wave of Mexican immigration to the United States. This first wave, however, suffered severe disruptions during the depression of 1920–1921 and the Great Depression of the 1930s, when indiscriminate deportations of both foreign- and US-born Mexicans took place (Durand and Massey 2002; Valdés 2000).

As industrial production resumed at the onset of World War II, the second stage of Mexican immigration began. Again, the United States turned to Mexico to meet its wartime labor needs through the Bracero Program of 1942 (Durand and Massey 2002). In the period surrounding World War II, the Mexican population in the United States grew significantly. Although the closing of the Bracero Program in 1964 officially ended labor recruitment from Mexico, the structural demand for Mexican labor remained in place. To meet this ongoing demand for labor, the United States unofficially implemented a de facto guest worker program that came to rely on undocumented immigrant labor (Durand and Massey 2002).

In the last decades of the twentieth century, the United States experienced major economic restructuring. In addition, the introduction of the North American Free Trade Agreement exacerbated the lack of viable employment alternatives in Mexico. These factors, combined with an historic reliance on Mexican immigrant labor and the growing wage differentials between the two countries, spurred a surge of Mexican migration in the 1990s. Given the long historical presence of Mexicans in the United States, both through annexation and the ongoing US reliance on Mexican immigrant labor, it is not surprising that Mexicans are the oldest and the largest Latino group in the United States. Indeed, estimates for 2008 indicate that 31 million individuals, or 66% of the Latino population, are of Mexican origin (Pew Hispanic Center 2010).

As in the previous periods, in the late twentieth and early twenty-first centuries, US-born and immigrant Mexicans faced the growing anti-immigrant sentiments and actions that have historically accompanied economic downturns. In the first decade of the twenty-first century, nativist sentiments have intensified, resulting in the escalation of border control, the militarization of the border, the criminalization of immigrants, and the introduction of a growing number of state- and local-level anti-immigrant policies (Chávez 2008; DeGenova 2004). Anti-immigrant sentiments are often framed around issues of undocumented migration. However, in the popular imagination, all Latinos are portrayed as being Mexican, all Mexicans are represented as being immigrant, and all immigrants are characterized as being undocumented. This conflation of ethnic and immigrant categories suggests that nativist sentiments are primarily aimed against Latinos, and against Mexicans in particular (Chávez 2008; DeGenova 2004).

Puerto Ricans

The United States acquired Puerto Rico as part of the final settlement of the Spanish–American War in 1898, and declared it an official part of its territory through the Foraker Act of 1900. The annexation of the island made it possible for US sugar companies to appropriate the lands of thousands of independent farmers, thus displacing growers from their lands and creating a growing class of unemployed agricultural workers (González 2000; Oboler 1995; Rumbaut 2006). As a newly acquired colony, Puerto Rico was disenfranchised politically and economically. Puerto Rican leaders actively challenged the provisions of the Foraker Act; however, none of their efforts, either at gaining US statehood or at becoming an independent nation, were successful. Instead, the Jones Act of 1917 granted Puerto Ricans US citizenship; this made them eligible to be drafted into military service during World War I, but left their status as economically exploited and politically disenfranchised citizens unchanged (González 2000; Oboler 1995; Rumbaut 2006). Puerto Rico acquired official commonwealth status in 1952, which (along with some policies introduced in the late 1940s) slightly altered the island's power to self-rule. At present, as a US commonwealth, Puerto Rico may elect its own governor and local legislators, so Puerto Ricans at least have control over the island's internal affairs. However, Puerto Ricans continue to lack voting representation in the US Congress, and those living on the island are unable to vote in the US presidential elections (González 2000; Oboler 1995; Rumbaut 2006).

Against this historical backdrop of economic and political inequalities, migration to the mainland began in earnest in the 1940s and 1950s. As was the case with Mexicans, labor recruitment of Puerto Ricans began in the 1900s but grew remarkably during and after World War II (Engstrom 2001; Rodríguez 1997; Rumbaut 2006). In addition, Operation Bootstrap—a set of economic policies designed to spur economic growth through industrialization, first introduced in the late 1940s— "failed to solve the urban employment and population growth problems, intensifying internal economic pressures for migration to the mainland" (Rumbaut 2006, p. 31). Although present net migration to the mainland is far lower than it was in the 1950s, the combination of ongoing economic disparities between the island and the mainland, ease of air travel, and citizenship by birth have made circular migration commonplace for many Puerto Ricans.

That Puerto Ricans are US citizens distinguishes them from other Latino immigrants. However, in most other respects, the experiences of Puerto Ricans in the mainland have historically been similar to those of other Latino immigrants, especially Mexicans (i.e., whose presence in the United States was initially forced by the annexation of Mexican territory). Puerto Ricans share with many other Latinos the experiences of social and geographic displacements, limited opportunities for economic advancement, residential segregation, and discriminatory treatment based on their ascribed racialized status (González 2000; Oboler 1995; Rodríguez 1997). Although New York City has been the primary settlement destination for Puerto Ricans in the mainland, Puerto Rican communities are also present in the suburbs of New York, in other Northeastern cities, and in states such as California, Florida, and Illinois, among others (Rodríguez 1997). At present, Puerto Ricans are the second largest Latino subgroup. With 4.2 million Puerto Ricans in the mainland as of 2008, they represent 9% of the Latino population (Pew Hispanic Center 2010).

Cubans

The presence of Cubans in the United States dates back to the early nineteenth century (González 2000; Rumbaut 2006). However, formal Cuban immigration to the United States began in 1960 and has unfolded in four different waves, each with distinct characteristics. The first wave was composed of the middle and upper classes that fled the country when the Cuban revolution overturned the existing economic and political structures, establishing a communist regime. In the midst of the Cold War with the Soviet Union, the presence of a communist government in the Western hemisphere (only 90 miles from Florida) garnered national concern and created a unique context for Cuban exiles (Pedraza 1996; Rumbaut 2006; Stepick and Stepick 2002). The second wave of migration took place from the mid-1960s through the 1970s, when the US and Cuban governments coordinated a set of orderly airlifts of would-be refugees. This second wave was composed mostly of small business owners and skilled workers (Pedraza 1996). Cubans who arrived in the United States during these first two waves were admitted as political refugees under the Cuban Refugee Program (Henken 2005; Pedraza 1996). Various government agencies actively helped Cubans find jobs and locate housing. In addition, the US federal government funded bilingual education and college loan programs that greatly facilitated the economic integration of Cubans, particularly in Miami. The federal aid provided for the resettlement of the Cuban refugees was unprecedented and completely absent in the incorporation of other Latino immigrant groups. Although it proved beneficial to both the refugees and the host communities, the federal response also reflected the connection between foreign policy and domestic immigration policy (Stepick and Stepick 2002).

The third wave of migration, which began with the Mariel boatlifts of 1980, differed significantly from the two previous waves in that it included a higher proportion of young, unaccompanied males and Blacks, mostly of working-class backgrounds (Pedraza 1996). Following the Mariel boatlifts, a fourth wave was composed of Cuban immigrants fleeing the growing economic crisis following the collapse of the Soviet Union (Pedraza 1996). This wave was characterized by "increasingly desperate crossing[s] of *balseros* (rafters) in the 1980s and early 1990s," who were largely undocumented (Rumbaut 2006, p. 32).

Cubans who arrived in these last two waves entered a climate that had begun to turn hostile against them. Those who came during the Mariel boatlifts were no longer officially considered refugees under new policies, and were "initially ineligible for most of the special assistance given to previous Cuban refugees" (Henken 2005, p. 397), though they eventually became eligible for refugee-type benefits through various shifts in policy. Cuban immigrants from the fourth wave were clearly treated differently from those who had arrived in the previous waves. The *balseros,* or rafters (named after the fragile rafts and makeshift boats that many used to travel the 90-mile stretch between Cuba and Florida), were at first rescued at sea by the US Coast Guard and welcomed in Florida, but by 1994 another turn in Cuban immigration policy was enacted by then-President Clinton. Under this new policy, the US Coast Guard was ordered to intercept *balseros* and redirect them to Guantánamo Bay Naval Station. Additional changes in Cuban refugee policy enacted in the mid-1990s provided for a limited number of US visas to Cuban refugees (Henken 2005; Pedraza 1996).

With 1.6 million Cubans residing in the United States, per 2008 estimates, they represent 3.5% of the Latino population and are the third largest Latino subgroup. Their class standing and refugee status, especially for those who arrived in the first two waves of migration, have made it possible for Cubans to enjoy higher rates of citizenship (75%), college graduation (25%), and home ownership (60%) than most Latinos in the United States (Pew Hispanic Center 2010).

Dominicans

Immigration from the Dominican Republic to the United States has its roots in the political and economic contexts of the 1800s (Levitt 2001). However, the first significant wave of Dominican migration took place in the early 1960s, with people fleeing the political upheavals that ensued due to the military coup of 1963, the subsequent US military occupation, and the civil war of 1965 (Grasmuck and Pessar 1991; Hernández 2002; Levitt 2001). From the mid-1960s through the 1970s, out-migration from the Dominican Republic intensified as the political and economic policies of a repressive government resulted in a pattern of rampant social and economic inequalities. Under these conditions, the Dominican Republic's government instituted an unofficial policy of encouraging people to leave the country (Hernández 2002). Immigrants from the Dominican Republic to the United States during this period were mostly blue-collar workers (Hernández 2002). In the context of the Cold War, the United States feared that social unrest would lead to a left-leaning revolution in the island, particularly after the assassination of Rafael L. Trujillo, the island's dictator. Thus, at critical moments, US policy facilitated outmigration by streamlining the visa application process and making visas more readily available to Dominicans (Mitchell 1992b; Hernández 2002; Engstrom 2001).

In the 1980s, immigration from the island increased. This time, however, working-class immigrants were joined by professional and technical workers who were negatively affected by the economic restructuring that resulted, in part, from policies imposed on the country by the International Monetary Fund (IMF). Following the passage of increasingly restrictive immigration policies in the United States, migration from the Dominican Republic decreased in the 1990s. Nevertheless, the need and desire to migrate remain for many Dominicans (Hernández 2002; Levitt 2001).

Dominican migration coincided with widespread economic restructuring in the United States. Many low-skilled jobs were disappearing, particularly in the New York City area where many had settled (Hernández 2002). Furthermore, Dominicans arrived "into a racially stratified society, where blacks and other dark people were marginalized, and where, since the very beginning, poor Dominicans were not needed nor wanted as workers" (Hernández 2002, p. 85). Thus, although a thriving Dominican entrepreneurial class has emerged in the New York City area, most Dominican immigrants have encountered few opportunities for economic integration (Grasmuck and Pessar 1991; Guarnizo 1997; Hernández 2002). By 2008, 1.3 million Dominicans resided in the United States (Pew Hispanic Center 2010).

Central Americans

As Hamilton and Chinchilla (1991) pointed out, immigration to the United States from Spanish-speaking Central American countries—that is, Costa Rica, El Salvador, Guatemala, Honduras, Nicaragua, and Panama—has been shaped by the interaction of economic and political factors, and "in many cases it is difficult to separate the two" (p. 75). Central American migration dates back to the late nineteenth century, and although it increased during the first half of the twentieth century, it remained limited until the early 1960s. In the 1960s and 1970s, industrialization, the modernization of agriculture, political upheavals, and growing US and other foreign interventions resulted in increased displacement of farmers and workers who migrated to urban areas, to other countries in the region, and to the United States (Hamilton and Chinchilla 1991). Central Americans who immigrated to the United States during this period were mostly economic migrants from middle to upper socioeconomic backgrounds. By the mid-1970s, however, the reasons for migration had shifted, as growing numbers of refugees fled persecution and violence, particularly in El Salvador, Guatemala, and Nicaragua (Engstrom and Piedra 2005; Hamilton and Chinchilla 1991). These trends further intensified during the 1980s, as many more Central Americans were displaced and fled the US-backed civil wars in their countries. As Engstrom and Piedra noted, "the brutalities of civil war, political violence, egregious human rights abuses, oppression, and poverty" (2005, p. 173) have been the primary factors forcing the northward migration of Central Americans. The increasingly segmented US labor market, which required low-skilled workers, combined with the political and social instability in the Central America region, shaped the demographic makeup of immigrants during those years. As a result, immigrants from Central America tended to come from rural areas and to have lower levels of education than the previous migrants (Hamilton and Chinchilla 1991). Yet, although Central Americans immigrated to the United States for political reasons, refugee and asylum policies were largely not applied to them. Thus, they were denied assistance that would have facilitated their reception and incorporation into the United States.

Altogether, Central Americans represent a significant component of the Latino population, at 8.2%. Specifically, according to 2008 estimates, 1.6 million Salvadorans, close to 1 million Guatemalans, 610,000 Hondurans, 350,000 Nicaraguans, 150,000 Panamanians, 120,000 Costa Ricans, and 40,000 other Central Americans reside in the United States (Pew Hispanic Center 2010).

South Americans

Although South American migration can be traced back to the late eighteenth century, the first major wave from this region began in earnest in the period following World War II, with nearly half a million South Americans entering the United States as immigrants between 1951 and 1977 (Oboler 2005). As was the case with other Latin American and Caribbean countries, each period of immigration from the nine Spanish-speaking South American countries (Argentina, Bolivia, Chile, Colombia, Ecuador, Paraguay, Peru, Uruguay, and Venezuela) has been shaped by US foreign and economic policies (Mitchell 1992a). Indeed, the economic policies instituted by the United States in the 1960s—in the context of the Cold War and the fear of communist satellite states in the Western hemisphere—set the stage for economic and political instability in the region that led to the international migration of professionals to the United States from the 1960s through the mid-1970s. A subsequent period of South American migration ensued, from the mid-1970s through the 1980s, as political exiles fled the US-backed dictatorships in Argentina, Chile, Paraguay, and Uruguay (Oboler 2005).

Even though these dictatorships had collapsed by the end of the twentieth century, immigration from South America to the United States continued in the 1980s and 1990s. In this latter period, however, it was the economic policies that the IMF instituted in South America that generated outmigration flows. South American immigrants to the United States in the late twentieth century were economic migrants fleeing widespread poverty and unemployment in their countries. By 2008, 2.7 million South Americans lived in the United States, representing altogether 5.8% of the total Latino population. Among South Americans, the three largest groups are Colombians, Ecuadorians, and Peruvians, accounting for 33%, 22%, and 19%, respectively, of the South American population in the United States (Pew Hispanic Center 2010).

Summary

As these overviews suggest, Latinos have very different historical experiences, even as they share common experiences of US political interventions and economic expansion in their sending communities. Each group's specific immigrant history has had implications for its reception and its subsequent economic and social integration (or lack thereof) into the United States. These histories are reflected in each group's current social and economic position, as well as in the group's access to resources, including health care. We now turn to an examination of the present sociodemographic characteristics of Latinos in the United States.

The Demographic Growth of the Latino Population in the United States

In 1970, 9.6 million Latinos lived in the United States, a number that represented 4.7% of the US population (U.S. Census Bureau 2008a). Between 1970 and 2000, the US Latino population increased by 368%, in contrast to a growth of 138% in the general population. By 2000, the US Latino population had grown to 35 million, representing 13% of the US population (U.S. Census Bureau 2008a). This fast growth of the US Latino population has continued over recent years. Between 2000 and 2008, the growth in the Latino population represented about half (51%) of the total US population growth, which increased by 22.6 million individuals, with 11.6 million being of Latino origin. Conservative estimates forecast an increase of the Latino population to 68 million, or 21% of the US population, by 2050 (U.S. Census Bureau 2009c). Less conservative estimates indicate that by 2050, the Latino population may grow to 102 million, or 24% of the total population (U.S. Census Bureau 2008a). In both scenarios, the Latino population will be the major element driving US population growth in the next four decades.

Age Composition

As a whole, the US-Latino population is considerably younger than the general population (Fig. 1.1). In 2008, the median age of the Latino population was 27 years, which is considerably lower than that of the general population at 36 years. However, the age distributions of the native- and foreign-born Latino populations are quite different. Native-born Latinos are much younger than foreign-born Latinos. In 2008, approximately 44% of the native-born Latino population was younger than 15 years of age, compared to only 6% of foreign-born Latinos and 17% of non-Latino Whites (Pew Hispanic Center 2010).

Even though the Latino population is characterized by its youthfulness, the older adult Latino population will grow at a faster pace than younger age groups in the next decades. By 2050, the share of older Latino adults will grow from the current 6% to 15%, whereas the relative sizes of the young and working-age populations are expected to decrease (U.S. Census Bureau 2004). With a larger share of older adults in the Latino population, the next decades will confront challenges to provide bilingual and culturally competent health care services, caregiving, and long-term care for this growing aging population. The current health care system has been inadequate in promoting preventive services that could avert or delay some of the health decline usually associated with aging. Currently, Latinos have a higher life expectancy than would be expected given their socioeconomic conditions, but they are more exposed to certain health conditions, such as obesity, diabetes, and some mental health conditions (for reviews, see Argeseanu Cunningham et al. 2008; Vega et al. 2009). These factors will certainly influence their health status and quality of life as they grow older. Social and health disparities

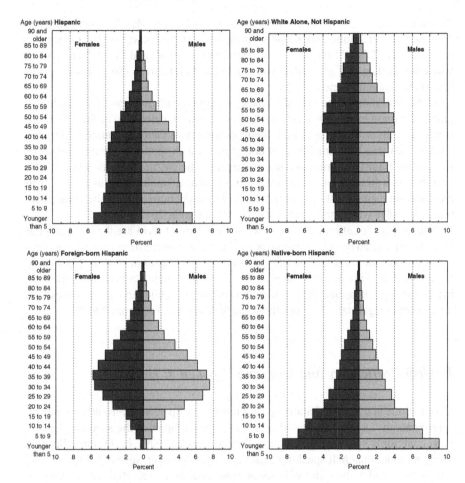

Fig. 1.1 Age and gender composition of foreign-born, native-born, and non-Latino White US populations, 2008. (Source: © 2010. Pew Research Center, Pew Hispanic Center project. *Statistical Portrait of Hispanics in the United States*, 2008. http://pewhispanic.org/factsheets/factsheet.php?FactsheetID=58)

experienced by Latinos throughout their life course (e.g., limited financial resources, inadequate health care access, and higher exposure to unhealthy environments) will undoubtedly have effects on their health statuses in old age (Vega et al. 2009).

Nativity and Citizenship

Contrary to representations of Latinos as newcomers, most Latinos are US-born and are US citizens (Pew Hispanic Center 2010). In 2008, 73% of Latinos, including

Puerto Ricans, were citizens (Pew Hispanic Center 2010). Besides Puerto Ricans, the other largest Latino subgroups with the highest percentage of US citizenship were Cubans (75%), Mexicans (71%), Dominicans (70%), and Colombians (66%), whereas less than half of Guatemalans (47%) and Hondurans (46%) have citizenship (Pew Hispanic Center 2010).

In the past, most of the growth in the US Latino population was driven by immigration (Durand et al. 2006). However, natural growth, calculated as the difference between births and deaths, is now the most important factor in Latino population growth. Between 2000 and 2008, natural growth was responsible for approximately 62% of the total US Latino population growth, whereas net migration (the difference between immigration and emigration) played a smaller role in total growth rates. Recent estimates show that 62% of Latinos were born in the United States; the remaining 38% were immigrants (Pew Hispanic Center 2010).

Although most Latino children are US-born, many of them are the children of at least one immigrant parent. Engstrom pointed out that "more than one in seven families in the United States is headed by a foreign-born adult" (Engstrom 2006, p. 27). Among Latino children, 58% live in immigrant families. Quite often, US-born children living in these immigrant families have difficulty in accessing public services, because of the differences in legal status between them and their parents (Engstrom 2006).

English Proficiency and Language Spoken at Home

Most Latinos in the United States speak English, but Spanish is currently spoken by approximately 35 million individuals, which makes Spanish the second language most commonly spoken at home (U.S. Census Bureau 2009a, b). Of these Spanish speakers, more than half speak English very well. However, approximately 47% of individuals aged 5 and older who speak Spanish at home reported limited English proficiency (LEP), measured as speaking English "less than very well" (U.S. Census Bureau 2009b). In addition, according to the 2000 census, 2.8 million Spanish speakers were unable to speak English (Shin and Bruno 2003).

As expected, LEP is much more prevalent among immigrants. Among adults, 72% of foreign-born Latinos have LEP. However, by the second and third generations, most Latinos speak English well and only 13% of the native-born report having LEP (Pew Hispanic Center 2010). That a large share of the adult Latino population has LEP is of concern because English language proficiency is a key determinant of access to and quality of health care services (Yu and Singh 2009). Although access to health care for LEP populations continues to be a challenge in states with large Latino populations, the recent spatial dispersion of the Latino population signals additional difficulties for Latinos in new destination states. The high prevalence of LEP among certain Latino groups calls for health care infrastructures with adequately trained health care professionals to provide services for this culturally diverse and Spanish-speaking population.

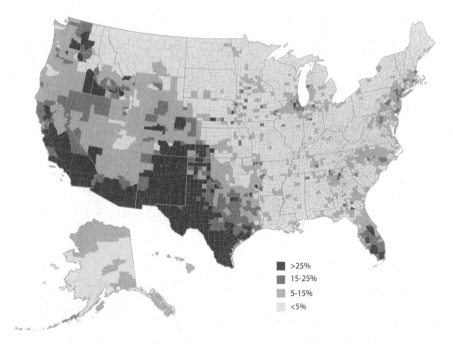

Fig. 1.2 The Hispanic share of population by county. (Source: © 2009. Pew Research Center, Pew Hispanic Center project. *Latinos by Geography.* http://pewhispanic.org/states/population/)

Spatial Dispersion of the Latino Population in the United States

The Latino population is largely concentrated in a few states and cities along the Southern border with Mexico, the Northeast, Illinois, and Florida. California and Texas are historically the two states with the largest populations of Latinos. In 2008, there were more than 13 million Latinos residing in California and almost 9 million in Texas. In relative terms, New Mexico is the state with the largest percentage of Latinos (45%), followed by California (37%) and Texas (36%) (Pew Hispanic Center 2010). Figure 1.2 highlights the share of the Latino population by county.

Despite their concentration in certain states and urban areas, Latinos are increasingly settling in more diverse locations across the US territory than in the previous decade, particularly in the South and the West (Lichter and Johnson 2006). During the 1980s, this geographic dispersion into areas previously dominated by non-Latino Whites was already underway, but it accelerated with remarkable speed during the 1990s (Fisher and Tienda 2006). Georgia, Nevada, and North Carolina each experienced more than a three-fold increase in their Latino populations during the 1990s; Oregon, Virginia, and Washington state each more than doubled their Latino populations (Durand et al. 2006). The growth of the Latino population in non-traditional areas has continued into the first decade of the twenty-first century (see

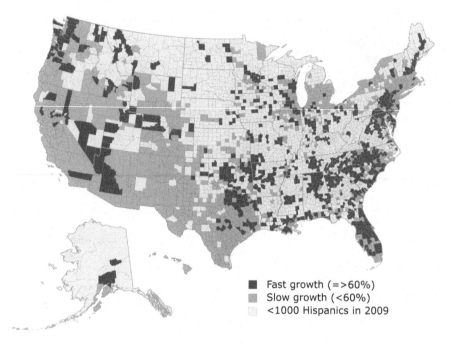

Fig. 1.3 Growth of the Hispanic population by county, 2000–2008. (Source: © 2009. Pew Research Center, Pew Hispanic Center project. *Latinos by Geography.* http://pewhispanic.org/states/population/)

Fig. 1.3). During the period 2000–2008, the Latino population more than doubled in Arkansas, Minnesota, Nebraska, New Hampshire, North Dakota, South Carolina, South Dakota, and West Virginia; some of these states experienced growth of more than 80% in their Latino populations (Pew Hispanic Center 2010). The rapid growth of the Latino population in these areas has changed the demographic profiles of these communities and has challenged the way services are provided.

Demographic changes in traditional destination states are also evident, although trends are in the opposite direction. Traditional recipient areas such as California and New York experienced growth in their Latino populations, but because this growth was slower than in other areas, the relative share of their Latino populations actually declined. The proportion of the total Latino population that resided in California declined from 31% in 2000 to 28.7% in 2008. Likewise, in 2008, 6.9% of all Latinos in the United States resided in New York, in contrast with 8.1% in 2000. The Latino population grew in Texas during the period 2000–2008, but its relative share remained around 19% (Pew Hispanic Center 2010).

The Latino population has traditionally settled in urban areas, but their latest geographic dispersion has resulted in a significant increase in Latino population growth in rural areas. By 2000, 5.5% of the non-metropolitan US population was of Latino origin, in contrast with only 3% in 1980. Indeed, during the 1990s, Latinos were responsible for 25% of the population growth in rural areas (Kandel and Cromartie 2004); in 2000, approximately 3.2 million Latinos resided in rural areas in the United States (Kandel and Cromartie 2004).

The growth in the rural Latino population is partly due to relocation of manufacturing, particularly food industries, to rural areas (Blewett et al. 2005). As a result, many of the Latinos who have settled in rural areas with fast growth have low levels of education and LEP (Kandel and Cromartie 2004). The presence of larger contingents of Latinos—often young, undocumented men who have recently immigrated—in rural areas that have historically been dominated by non-Latino Whites have many times been marked by anti-immigrant sentiments (Kandel and Cromartie 2004). Most service providers and local governments in these small rural communities are unprepared to deal with the new members of their communities, who are likely to be immigrant with LEP. Beyond differences in nativity, ancestry, citizenship, and spatial dispersion, Latinos are also a diverse group in terms of educational, social, and economic background. A mental health services infrastructure has to address these aspects of diversity.

Socioeconomic Conditions

On average, Latinos, particularly immigrant Latinos, have lower levels of education, are more likely to work in low-wage jobs, and are more likely to lack health insurance than the general population (Pew Hispanic Center 2010). These socioeconomic disadvantages translate into higher exposure to occupational and environmental hazards, and lower levels of access to adequate health care across the life course (for a detailed review, see Vega et al. 2009). In this section, we discuss the disparities that Latinos face in education, employment, occupation, and income.

Educational Disadvantage

Latinos, on average, lag behind the general population in educational attainment. A staggering 39% of the Latino population aged 25 and over has less than a high school education, compared to 10% of non-Latino Whites and 19% of African-Americans. Among individuals who have dropped out of high school, Latinos have lower rates (9%) of obtaining a General Educational Development (GED) credential than African-Americans (20%) (Fry 2010). With a smaller percentage of Latinos possessing the necessary credentials to attend college, it is not surprising that Latinos also have lower rates (13%) of college degree attainment than Asians (50%), non-Latino Whites (31%), and African-Americans (18%) (Pew Hispanic Center 2010). In addition, Latinos are more likely to be enrolled in two-year colleges than non-Latino Whites and Blacks. Given the fast growth of Latinos predicted in the next decades, one of the biggest challenges for the US educational system will be to reduce the inequalities in educational achievement (Gándara and Contreras 2009).

Fig. 1.4 Educational attainment of the 2008 Latino population aged 25 and older. (Source: © 2010. Pew Research Center, Pew Hispanic Center project. *Statistical Portrait of Hispanics in the United States,* 2008. http://pewhispanic.org/factsheets/factsheet.php?FactsheetID=58)

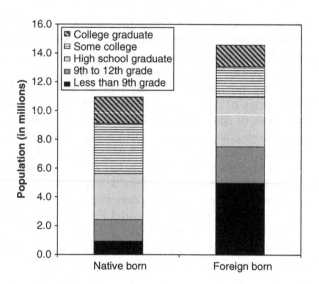

Comparisons by Latino subgroup and nativity status reveal important differences in educational disparities, especially in the attainment of higher education. Among the three largest Latino groups, only 9% of Mexicans have a college degree, compared to 16% of Puerto Ricans and 25% of Cubans. These differences in college attainment are a consequence of the varying historical, economic, and political contexts of reception and incorporation that these Latino groups have experienced in the United States. Still, even the higher rates of college degree completion among Cubans and Puerto Ricans are lower than those of the general population (28%).

Differences in educational attainment are also evident by nativity status. Foreign-born Latinos have lower levels of formal education than native-born Latinos. As Fig. 1.4 shows, in 2008 the proportion of the foreign-born Latino population 25 years of age or older that had not completed high school (52%) was double that of native-born Latinos (23%) (Pew Hispanic Center 2010). Among high school dropouts, native-born Latinos are more likely to obtain a GED than foreign-born Latinos (Fry 2010). A higher percentage of native-born Latinos (29%) have completed high school than foreign-born Latinos (24%). Native-born Latinos are also more likely to have some college education (32%) or a college degree (17%) than are the foreign-born (15% and 10%, respectively). The lower educational achievement of foreign-born Latinos may be due to both educational disadvantages that preceded migration and/or little or no contact with the US educational system. Yet, Latino immigrants from Cuba, the Dominican Republic, El Salvador, Guatemala, and Mexico tend to have higher rates of formal education attainment than those who remain in their home countries (Feliciano 2005b). The only exception is Puerto Rico, where migrants have lower education than those who remain in their sending communities (Feliciano 2005b). The lower costs of transportation from Puerto Rico to the mainland, combined with their status as US citizens, may explain why Puerto Ricans are the least selective group in terms of education (Feliciano 2005b). Other Latino groups have to bear higher costs to migrate to the United States, which may increase their selectivity. Nevertheless, even though immigrants from Latin America and the Caribbean tend to be more educated than the average population in their countries of origin, their levels of formal education are lower than those of the general US population and other immigrant groups (for a fuller examination of these patterns and the factors that may explain them, see Feliciano 2005a, 2005b).

Although educational disadvantage among Latino children can be partially attributed to the educational disparities their parents have experienced (Feliciano 2005a), Latinos face additional barriers throughout their school years. Immigrant-Latino parents are more likely to be unfamiliar with the educational system. In addition, as a result of socioeconomic inequalities, many Latino families live in neighborhoods where schools have fewer resources available to them, which translates into fewer societal investments in the education of young Latinos (Gándara and Contreras 2009). In these educational environments, Latino students do not always receive the educational resources that are necessary to promote their academic development, and are more likely to have teachers who lack adequate training. There is also evidence that teachers hold lower expectations for their Latino students (Cammarota 2004). With so many structural barriers, it is not surprising that Latino students have lower academic performance than the average population.

Employment and Occupation

Low levels of education and LEP lead to worse employment prospects for Latino immigrants and their native-born children. Latinos are disproportionately employed in unstable, low-wage jobs, and they also face worse working conditions, with many of them employed in positions that offer few or no benefits (Blewett et al. 2005; Pew Hispanic Center 2010; Queneau 2009). As with other demographic indicators, there are important differences in employment and occupation by Latino subgroup and nativity status. These variations reflect differences in human capital; historical, economic, and political contexts of reception and incorporation in the United States; geographic location; and labor market concentrations. Such differences, particularly those by nativity status, have important implications for access and use of health care services in the United States.

Between 1983 and 2002, the restructuring of the US economy resulted in highly segmented labor markets and substantial increases in job segregation between Latinos and non-Latinos in the United States (Queneau 2009). During this period, the representation of Latinos in low-skill jobs (e.g., farming, production, food preparation, repair and maintenance, domestic services, and other service occupations) increased, with negative consequences for Latino wages (Pew Hispanic Center 2010; Queneau 2009). During the 1990s, male Latino immigrants contributed to about half of the employment growth in low-skill jobs in the United States (Bean et al. 2004). In 2008, the five main occupational groups in which Latinos were employed were office and administrative support (13%), followed by maintenance and repair work (12%), construction and extraction (11%), sales (10%), and cleaning and maintenance (9%) (Pew Hispanic Center 2010). Transportation and material moving employed 8.5% of the Latino population, whereas food preparation and service industries occupied 8.2% (Pew Hispanic Center 2010). Among these occupations, Latinos were overrepresented in the cleaning and maintenance of buildings and grounds, food preparation, transportation, maintenance, and construction. In addition, Latinos are three times more likely to work in farming than the general US population: 2.4% and 0.8%, respectively (Pew Hispanic Center 2010).

Although this is not exclusively so, Latinos in low-skill jobs are more likely to be immigrant rather than US-born, which reflects US employers' historical reliance on immigrant labor. For instance, in 2008, 16% of the foreign-born worked in construction, compared to only 6% of the native-born (Pew Hispanic Center 2010). About 15% of foreign-born Latinos were employed in repair and maintenance work, whereas 9% of the native-born worked in similar occupations (Pew Hispanic Center 2010). Even more striking, 13% of the foreign-born worked in cleaning and building maintenance, but only 4% of the native-born had similar jobs (Pew Hispanic Center 2010). Work on farms was five times more frequent among the foreign-born (4%) than among the native-born (0.8%) (Pew Hispanic Center 2010).

That many Latinos occupy low-skill positions has significant health consequences, as these jobs offer few to no benefits. For instance, nearly a third of Latinos working in the meatpacking industry and more than half of the Latinos working in construction and food service are uninsured (Blewett et al. 2005). Those working in farming are the most disadvantaged, with 79% of those in rural areas having no health insurance (Blewett et al. 2005). In addition, the current economic recession has been particularly difficult for Latinos in low-skill jobs. Between 2007 and 2008, the increase in unemployment was higher among the foreign-born than among native-born Latinos (Kochhar 2009). Although Blacks have been particularly hard-hit by the recession, with unemployment rates reaching 12% in 2008, the unemployment rates among foreign-born (8%) and US-born (10%) Latinos were also substantially higher than those of non-Latino Whites (6%) (Kochhar 2009).

In contrast to the overrepresentation of Latinos in low-skill jobs, Latinos (especially the foreign-born) are underrepresented in middle-tier jobs such as office and administrative support, education, sports, media, and health care (Pew Hispanic Center 2010). Middle-tier occupations are more prevalent among native-born Latinos, as the improvement in education from first to second generations translates into better employment and earning opportunities. Finally, Latinos represent a small percentage of individuals in high-tier jobs, such as management (5%) and business operations (1.2%); less than 3% are engaged in the areas of computers and mathematics, architecture and engineering, and legal services (Pew Hispanic Center 2010).

Income/Poverty

Facing worse labor market placement and lower education, it is not surprising that median household income is lower among Latinos (US $ 41,041) than the national average (US $ 51,938) (Pew Hispanic Center 2010). In addition, household size is larger in the Latino population than in the general population. Therefore, more limited resources have to be distributed among a larger number of individuals at home. Similarly, the median personal income is lower among Latinos (US $ 21,488) than among non-Latino Whites (US $ 31,570) and non-Latino Blacks (US $ 24,951). Individual earnings, however, vary across generations and Latino subgroup. Among native-born Latinos, median individual earnings are higher (US $ 24,441) than among foreign-born Latinos (US $ 20,368) (Pew Hispanic Center 2010).

With lower earnings and larger households, Latinos are overrepresented among the poor. In 2008, more than 10 million Latinos in the United States lived in poverty (U.S. Census Bureau 2008b). The poverty rate among Latinos (20%) is more than twice as high as that for non-Latino Whites (8%), but lower than among non-Latino Blacks (22%) (Pew Hispanic Center 2010). Latinos born in the United States have a poverty rate comparable to that of Latino immigrants (20% versus 19%, respectively) (Pew Hispanic Center 2010). Among Latinos of various origins, those of Dominican, Puerto Rican, and Mexican descent have higher poverty rates than those of Cuban descent.

Latinos not only face higher poverty rates than the general US population, but they are also overrepresented among the severely poor (Woolf et al. 2006). Poverty is particularly serious among Latino children. Timberlake (2007) showed that 42% of Latino children in 2000 resided in neighborhoods classified as "high poverty" and "extreme poverty," which contrasts with approximately 10% of non-Latino White children. Compared with non-Latino White children, Latino children are expected to spend a higher proportion of their childhood in poor neighborhoods, which may have detrimental consequences for their educational, occupational, and health outcomes. Given that individuals at the bottom of the income-distribution curve face higher morbidity, worse mental health, and earlier mortality (for a review, see Holzer et al. 2007; Woolf et al. 2006), the sharp increase in severe poverty in the last few years and the continued recession may have deleterious effects on the health of Latinos in the United States.

Health Status and Access to Health Care

The heterogeneity of the Latino population in the United States is reflected in the diversity of health patterns observed within this population. There are important differences in health status within the Latino population, which depend not only on the health indicator under consideration, but also on the Latino subgroup, generational status, and, for immigrants, length of time in the United States (Acevedo-García et al. 2007; Cacari-Stone et al. 2007; Palloni and Morenoff 2001; Williams and Mohammed 2008). Despite evidence that Latinos experience some positive health outcomes, as a whole Latinos experience health disadvantages that are likely to increase in light of their limited access to health care (Escarce et al. 2006; Vega and Amaro 1994; Vega et al. 2009).

For some outcomes, Latinos seem to have better health than would be expected, given their average low socioeconomic standing (Escarce et al. 2006; Vega and

Amaro 1994; Vega et al. 2009). This apparent health advantage is particularly evident among immigrants vis-à-vis their US-born co-ethnics. Despite worse socioeconomic conditions, foreign-born Latinos have lower infant mortality (Mathews et al. 2003), fewer low-birth-weight babies (Acevedo-García et al. 2005), and lower all-cause mortality (Singh and Siahpush 2001; Vega et al. 2009) than US-born Latinos (for a review of health disparities in the Latino population, see Vega et al. 2009). Although this epidemiological paradox is a complex phenomenon that is not necessarily generalizable across Latino subgroups and health outcomes, it suggests that in some cases Latino immigrants tend to be healthier than US-born Latinos. The evidence regarding the mechanisms underlying these effects remains inconclusive, though some factors that have been examined include selectivity, cultural practices, social ties, neighborhood environments, discrimination, and racialization processes (Jasso et al. 2004; Palloni and Arias 2004; Palloni and Morenoff 2001; Viruell-Fuentes 2007; Viruell-Fuentes and Schulz 2009).

Although some Latino groups experience a health advantage with respect to certain health outcomes, they also experience health disadvantages vis-à-vis non-Latino Whites (Cacari-Stone et al. 2007; Vega et al. 2009). Most notably, Latinos have a higher prevalence of chronic diseases such as type 2 diabetes and obesity (Harris et al. 1998), asthma (Lara et al. 2006), HIV (Centers for Disease Control and Prevention [CDC] 2007), tuberculosis (Sumaya 1991), and cervical and stomach cancer (American Cancer Society 2009; Ramirez and Suarez 2001). In fact, as a whole, Latinos "bear a disproportionate burden of disease, injury and disability when compared with non-Hispanic Whites" (CDC 2004, p. 935).

In the mental health service sector, access to quality care remains a persistent problem (Alegría et al. 2008; Cardemil et al. 2007). In one study, based on a nationally representative sample of 8762 persons, researchers found differences in access to and quality of depression treatment between racial-ethnic minority groups and non-Latino Whites (Alegría et al. 2008). These findings indicate that in the absence of efforts to address the unique barriers to care confronting minority populations, their reluctance to seek mental health care might reflect an accurate perception of the limited quality of usual care (Alegría et al. 2008). In fact, the authors argue that their findings call for the development of policy, practice, and community solutions to address the barriers that generate these disparities.

That Latinos are experiencing growing health and mental health disparities is of particular concern, given that their access to health care is decreasing, even as access appears to be increasing for other US minority groups (Agency for Healthcare Research and Quality 2005). Latinos, for instance, are more likely to be uninsured than the general population, with almost 15 million Latinos in the United States lacking health insurance. This means that about one-third of Latinos do not have health insurance, compared to 11% of non-Latino Whites and 19% of non-Latino Blacks (Pew Hispanic Center 2010). Uninsured rates are particularly high among immigrants; one in every two foreign-born Latinos lacks health insurance, compared to one out of four native-born Latinos (Pew Hispanic Center 2010). There are also important disparities across Latino groups, with health care access being better for Cubans and Puerto Ricans, but worse for Mexicans and Central and South

Americans. The lower rates of insurance coverage among Latinos is closely related to their higher representation in lower-skilled and lower-paid jobs that do not offer health insurance benefits (McCollister et al. 2010).

Age and nativity differences in access to health insurance signal differential access to care for Latinos along several demographic indicators. In 2008, Latinos of working age (18 to 64 years old) had higher uninsured rates (42%) than individuals in any other age group (Pew Hispanic Center 2010). Uninsurance rates among those younger than 18 and among older adults reached 19% and 7%, respectively (Pew Hispanic Center 2010). Great disparities also exist between first and second generations. Among first-generation adults of working age, uninsured rates reached 54%, compared to 28% among the second generation (Pew Hispanic Center 2010). Even more dramatic, more than half (52%) of first-generation Latinos under age 18 lack health insurance. This is in stark contrast to the much lower rates of uninsurance among second-generation Latinos less than 18 years of age (15%) (Pew Hispanic Center 2010). At older ages, there are also important disparities, as elderly Latinos are most likely to have worked at jobs that did not offer benefits. Indeed, uninsured rates among older adult (age 65 years and older) non-Latino Whites is less than 1%, yet it reaches 11% among foreign-born Latinos and 2% among US-born Latinos (Pew Hispanic Center 2010). The consequences of lack of insurance are many, as it imposes severe limitations on Latinos' ability to receive optimal health care. Of particular interest to readers of this book, the lack of health insurance makes Latinos with mental health problems more likely not to receive treatment or to receive inadequate treatment (González et al. 2010).

Recommendations

Given the heterogeneity of the Latino population in the United States, we believe that development of viable infrastructures and programs aimed at improving the health and mental health outcomes of Latinos should include addressing specific dimensions of structural inequality such as education, income, access to health insurance, immigrant status, and English language proficiency. At the macro level, this would involve investing in policies and programs intended to improve educational outcomes for Latinos at all levels, such as those that "prepare children early in life for school success and continue to support [their] academic achievement" from elementary school to secondary and higher education (Cacari-Stone et al. 2007, p. 93). Enhancing educational outcomes would, in turn, yield improvements in employment and income. Expanding employment opportunities would help increase access to health-promoting resources—especially to health insurance, as access to health insurance in the United States is still largely employment-based.

To address inequalities by immigrant status, policies that facilitate immigrants' access to health services are necessary. Repealing restrictions on federally funded health care for lawful permanent immigrants who have resided in the United States for five years or less—as currently mandated under the Personal Responsibility and

Work Opportunity Reconciliation Act of 1996—would be a step in the right direction. The role of federal policies in improving the well-being of Latinos cannot be underestimated. Without federal support, it is unlikely that state and local governments will be able to meet the health care needs of the fastest growing ethnic group in the nation.

A key demographic shift highlighted in this chapter is the growing geographic dispersion of Latinos across the country. This dispersion has led to substantial growth of the Latino population in new destinations—that is, regions, including rural areas, with limited to no history of a Latino presence. Latinos in new destinations face particular challenges because these locales lack the infrastructure to provide culturally and linguistically competent services. To address the varied needs of Latinos in both new and traditional Latino destinations, "resources and mechanisms must be developed for enlarging the pool of Latino health professionals to provide culturally competent care, particularly in underserved areas" (Cacari-Stone et al. 2007, p. 94) and particularly to individuals with LEP.

The heterogeneity of the Latino population and its geographic dispersion call also for the development of local-level health and mental health infrastructures attuned to the specific needs and characteristics of the Latino communities to be served. We believe that the details of such infrastructures are best developed in partnership with local Latino communities, and that community-based participatory strategies are the most promising vehicles for doing so. At their core, community-based participatory strategies seek to identify and build on the strengths of a community and develop collaborative and equitable relationships with the communities and populations to be served. Through equitable collaboration, these strategies can enable the creation of programs that address locally relevant health and mental health issues and that attend to the contextual factors giving rise to such issues (Israel et al. 2005).

In recent years, policies aimed at restricting immigrant rights have proliferated, including those that attempt to restrict access to services. These policies reflect and fuel anti-immigrant sentiments, and their effects are widespread not only for immigrant populations but also for US-born Latinos, given the conflation of immigrant status and Latino identity. Against this backdrop, Latinos are likely to experience increased levels of emotional distress (Lauderdale 2006; Williams and Mohammed 2008). In addition, anti-immigrant sentiments also have the effect of discouraging service utilization. Through the community-based strategies previously outlined, local-level providers can play a key role in addressing the chilling effect that such policies have on care-seeking behaviors of Latinos and immigrants.

Summary and Conclusion

The Latino population in the United States will continue to grow independently of new waves of immigration. By 2050, close to one in four US residents will be of Latino origin. Given this fact, the welfare of the nation as a whole will largely depend on the economic and social well-being of this population. Latinos are a richly heterogeneous group, and the specific historical and contextual factors that have shaped their presence and experiences in the United States vary by subgroup. Nevertheless, Latinos share long-standing histories of inequality that are reflected in their current (on average) disadvantaged socioeconomic position. As providers and policy makers move to develop viable health and mental health care infrastructures to address health and service inequities, attending to the diversity of the Latino population becomes imperative, because, as Cafferty and McCready proposed, programs designed for a broad Latino population are likely to "help some and harm others because there are, in one sense, no generic Hispanics" (Cafferty and Mc-Cready 1985, p. 253).

Several important sociodemographic domains require attention in the development of effective health care infrastructures. As a whole, for instance, Latinos are younger than the overall US population, though the proportion of older Latinos is growing quickly. Contrary to representations of Latinos as newcomers, most Latinos are US-born, hold US citizenship, and are proficient in English. In fact, the growth of the Latino population in the United States has been driven primarily by natural growth rather than immigration. Yet, despite the benefits that US citizenship and English language proficiency should confer, the historical inequalities that Latinos in the United States share are evident in their lower levels of educational attainment, worse socioeconomic conditions, and higher poverty rates. This is particularly the case for Latinos who lack the benefits of citizenship and legalized immigrant status.

Given the evidence that socioeconomic status is a key determinant of health and access to health care, policies that aim to reduce social inequalities are likely to have a positive effect on the health of marginalized populations as a whole, including Latinos. Indeed, as Vega, Rodríguez, and Gruskin pointed out, the "essential drivers for trends in health disparities are demographic and are rooted in population structure and social inequalities" (Vega et al. 2009, p. 106). Latinos, especially those who are poor, are less likely to have access to mental health services, for instance (Alegría et al. 2002).

Although a growing Latino presence in the United States signifies the need for improved policies and service infrastructures, it also highlights the economic and social contributions that Latinos have made and continue to make to the betterment of the nation. For instance, as young Latinos enter the labor market, they are likely to strengthen the economy. However, these and other contributions will not be realized unless adequate policies are in place to remedy historical inequalities in the educational, health care, and other systems. In the coming decades, the health status and health care needs of the Latino population, and that of the nation as a whole, will be dependent on the health of young Latinos today. Allocating resources to the health and well-being of the Latino population should therefore not be seen as a burden, but rather as an opportunity to invest in the future well-being of the nation. Some promising investments include programs to improve the educational opportunities of Latinos from early childhood to postsecondary education; policies that remove restrictions on access to care for legal immigrants; federal allocation of resources to help alleviate fiscal pressures on state and local governments; and programs to increase the number of Latino health professionals. Health and mental health infrastructures designed in partnership with local Latino communities are also more likely to be effective in meeting the needs of these communities. Policies and infrastructures that address intersecting dimensions of inequality will help meet not only the needs of Latinos, but also the needs of other groups that share similar experiences of marginalization.

Acknowledgments Short excerpts from Cacari-Stone, Viruell-Fuentes, and Acevedo-García (2007) are republished here with copyright permission from the Californian Journal of Health. This project was partially supported by the Network for Multicultural Research on Health and Healthcare, Dept. of Family Medicine, David Geffen School of Medicine, U.C.L.A., funded by the Robert Wood Johnson Foundation [to EAVF].

References

Acevedo-García, D., Soobader, M. J., & Berkman, L. F. (2005). The differential effect of foreign-born status on low birth weight by race/ethnicity and education. *Pediatrics, 115*(1), e20–e30. doi:10.1542/peds.2004-1306

Acevedo-García, D., Soobader, M. J., & Berkman, L. F. (2007). Low birthweight among US Hispanic/Latino subgroups: The effect of maternal foreign-born status and education. *Social Science & Medicine (1982), 65*(12), 2503–2516. doi:10.1016/j.socscimed.2007.06.033

Agency for Healthcare Research and Quality. (2005). *National healthcare disparities report.* Rockville, MD: U.S. Department of Health and Human Services.

Alegría, M., Canino, G., Rios, R., Vera, M., Calderon, J., Rusch, D., & Ortega, A. N. (2002). Mental health care for Latinos: Inequalities in use of specialty mental health services among Latinos, African Americans, and non-Latino whites. *Psychiatric Services, 53*(12), 1547–1555. doi:10.1176/appi.ps.53.12.1547

Alegría, M., Chatterji, P., Wells, K., Cao, Z., Chen, C., Takeuchi, D. (2008). Disparity in depression treatment among racial and ethnic minority populations in the United States. *Psychiatric Services, 59*, 1264–1272.

American Cancer Society. (2009). *Cancer facts & figures for Hispanics/Latinos 2009–2011.* Retrieved from http://www.cancer.org/acs/groups/content/@nho/documents/document/ffhispanicslatinos20092011.pdf

Argeseanu Cunningham, S., Ruben, J. D., & Venkat Narayan, K. M. (2008). Health of foreign-born people in the United States: A review. *Health & Place, 14*(4), 623–635. doi:10.1016/j.healthplace.2007.12.002

Bean, F. D., & Tienda, M. (1987). *The Hispanic population of the United States.* New York, NY: Russell Sage Foundation.

Bean, F. D., Leach, M., & Lowell, B. L. (2004). Immigrant job quality and mobility in the United States. *Work & Occupations, 31*(4), 499–518. doi:10.1177/0730888404268902

Blewett, L. A., Davern, M., & Rodin, H. (2005). Employment and health insurance coverage for rural Latino populations. *Journal of Community Health, 30*(3), 181–195. doi:10.1007/s10900-004-1957-z

Cacari-Stone, L., Viruell-Fuentes, E. A., & Acevedo-García, D. (2007). Understanding the socioeconomic, health systems & policy threats to Latino health: Gaining new perspectives for the future. *Californian Journal of Health Promotion, 5* (Special Issue on Health Disparities & Social Justice), 82–104.

Cafferty, P. S. J., & McCready, W. C. (1985). *Hispanics in the United States: A new social agenda.* New Brunswick, NJ: Transaction.

Cammarota, J. (2004). The gendered and racialized pathways of Latina and Latino youth: Different struggles, different resistances in the urban context. *Anthropology & Education Quarterly, 35*(1), 53–74.

Cardemil, E. V., Adams, S. T., Calista, J. L., Connell, J., Encarnación, J., Esparza, N. K. (2007). The Latino mental health project: A local mental health needs assessment. *Adm Policy Ment Health, 34*(4), 331-341. doi:.1007/s10488-007-0113-3

Centers for Disease Control and Prevention (CDC). (2004). Health disparities experienced by Hispanics—United States. *Morbidity & Mortality Weekly Report 53*(40), 935–937.

Centers for Disease Control and Prevention (CDC). (2007). HIV/AIDS among Hispanics in the U.S. 2001–2005. *Morbidity & Mortality Weekly Report, 56*(40), 1052–1057.

Chávez, L. (2008). *The Latino threat: Constructing immigrants, citizens, and the nation.* Stanford, CA: Stanford University Press.

DeGenova, N. (2004). The legal production of Mexican/migrant "illegality". *Latino Studies, 2*(2), 160–185.

Durand, J., & Massey, D. S. (2002). *Beyond smoke and mirrors: Mexican immigration in an age of economic integration.* New York, NY: Russell Sage Foundation.

Durand, J., Telles, E., & Flashman, J. (2006). The demographic foundations of the Latino population. In M. Tienda & F. Mitchell (Eds.), *Hispanics and the future of America* (1st ed., pp. 66–99). Washington, DC: National Academies Press.

Engstrom, D. W. (2001). Hispanic immigration in the new millennium. In P. S. J. Cafferty & D. W. Engstrom (Eds.), *Hispanics in the United States: An agenda for the twenty-first century* (pp. 31–68). New Brunswick, NJ: Transaction Publishers.

Engstrom, D. W. (2006). Outsiders and exclusion: Immigrants in the United States. In D. W. Engstrom & L. M. Piedra (Eds.), *Our diverse society: Race and ethnicity—Implications for 21st century American society* (1st ed., pp. 19–36). Washington, DC:NASW Press.

Engstrom, D. W., & Piedra, L. M. (2005). Central American survivors of political violence: An examination of contextual factors and practice issues. *Journal of Immigrant & Refugee Services, 3*(1/2), 171–190.

Escarce, J. J., Morales, L. S., & Rumbaut, R. G. (2006). The health status and health behaviors of Hispanics. In M. Tienda & F. Mitchell (Eds.), *Hispanics and the future of America* (pp. 362–409). Washington, DC: National Academies Press.

Etzioni, A. (2002). Inventing Hispanics: A diverse minority resists being labeled. *Brookings Review, 20*(1), 10–13.

Feliciano, C. (2005a). Does selective migration matter? Explaining ethnic disparities in educational attainment among immigrants' children. *International Migration Review, 39*(4), 841–871.

Feliciano, C. (2005b). Educational selectivity in U.S. immigration: How do immigrants compare to those left behind? *Demography, 42*(1), 131–152.

Fisher, M. J., & Tienda, M. (2006). Redrawing spatial color lines: Hispanic metropolitan dispersal, segregation, and economic opportunity. In M. Tienda & F. Mitchell (Eds.), *Hispanics and the future of America* (1st ed., pp. 100–137). Washington, DC:National Academies Press.

Fry, R. (2010). *Hispanics, high school dropouts and the GED.* Washington, DC: Pew Hispanic Center.

Gándara, P., & Contreras, F. (2009). *The Latino education crisis: The consequences of failed social policies.* Cambridge, MA: Harvard University Press.

González, H. M., Vega, W. A., Williams, D. R., Tarraf, W., West, B. T., & Neighbors, H. W. (2010). Depression care in the United States: Too little for too few. *Archives of General Psychiatry, 67*(1), 37–46. doi:10.1001/archgenpsychiatry.2009.168

González, J. (2000). *Harvest of empire: A history of Latinos in America.* New York, NY: Viking Press.

Grasmuck, S., & Pessar, P. R. (1991). *Between two islands: Dominican international migration.* Berkeley: University of California Press.

Guarnizo, L. E. (1997). Los dominicanyorks: The making of a binational society. In M. Romero, P. Hondagneu-Sotelo, & V. Ortiz (Eds.), *Challenging fronteras: Structuring Latina and Latino lives in the U.S.* (pp. 161–174). New York, NY: Routledge.

Gutiérrez, D. G. (1995). *Walls and mirrors: Mexican Americans, Mexican immigrants, and the politics of ethnicity.* Berkeley: University of California Press.

Hamilton, N., & Chinchilla, N. S. (1991). Central American migration: A framework for analysis. *Latin American Research Review, 26*(1), 75–110.

Harris, M. I., Flegal, K. M., Cowie, C. C., Eberhardt, M. S., Goldstein, D. E., Little, R. R., Byrd-Holt, D. D. (1998). Prevalence of diabetes, impaired fasting glucose, and impaired glucose tolerance in U.S. adults: The third national health and nutrition examination survey, 1988–1994. *Diabetes Care, 21*(4), 518–524.

Henken, T. (2005). *Balseros, boteros, and el bombo*: Post-1994 Cuban immigration to the United States and the persistence of special treatment. *Latino Studies 3*(3), 393–416.

Hernández, R. (2002). *The mobility of workers under advanced capitalism: Dominican migration to the United States*. New York, NY: Columbia University Press.

Holzer, H. J., Schanzenbach, D. W., & Duncan, G. J. (2007). *The economic costs of poverty in the United States: Subsequent effects of children growing up poor* (Institute for Research on Poverty Discussion Paper No. 1327). Madison: University of Wisconsin.

Israel, B. A., Eng, E., Schulz, A. J., & Parker, E. A. (2005). Introduction to methods in community-based participatory research for health. In B. A. Israel, E. Eng, A.J. Schulz, & E. A. Parker (Eds.), *Methods in community-based participatory research for health* (pp. 3–26). San Francisco, CA: Jossey-Bass.

Jasso, G., Massey, D. S., Rosenzweig, M. R., & Smith, J. P. (2004). Immigrant health: Selectivity and acculturation. In N. B. Anderson, R. A. Bulatao, & R. Cohen (Eds.), *Critical perspectives on racial and ethnic differences in health in late life* (pp. 227–266). Washington, DC: National Academies Press.

Kandel, W., & Cromartie, J. (2004). *New patterns of Hispanic settlement in rural America* (Rural Development Research Report No. 99). Washington, DC: Economic Research Service, U.S. Department of Agriculture.

Kochhar, R. (2009). *Unemployment rises sharply among Latino immigrants in 2008*. Washington, DC: Pew Hispanic Center.

Lara, M., Akinbami, L., Flores, G., & Morgenstern, H. (2006). Heterogeneity of childhood asthma among Hispanic children: Puerto Rican children bear a disproportionate burden. *Pediatrics, 117*(1), 43–53. doi:10.1542/peds.2004-1714

Lauderdale, D. S. (2006). Birth outcomes for Arabic-named women in California before and after September 11. *Demography, 43*(1), 185–201.

Levitt, P. (2001). *The transnational villagers*. Berkeley: University of California Press.

Lichter, D. T., & Johnson, K. M. (2006). Emerging rural settlement patterns and the geographic redistribution of America's new immigrants. *Rural Sociology, 71*(1), 109–131.

Mathews, T. J., Menacker, F., & MacDorman, M. F. (2003). Infant mortality statistics from the 2001 period linked birth/infant death data set. *National Vital Statistics Report, 52*(2), 1–28.

McCollister, K. E., Arheart, K. L., Lee, D. J., Fleming, L. E., Davila, E. P., LeBlanc, W. G., Erard, M. J. (2010). Declining health insurance access among US Hispanic workers: Not all jobs are created equal. *American Journal of Industrial Medicine, 53*(2),163–170. doi:10.1002/ajim.20720

Mitchell, C. (1992a). Introduction. In C. Mitchell (Ed.), *Western Hemisphere immigration and United States foreign policy*. University Park, PA: The Pennsylvania State University Press.

Mitchell, C. (1992b). U.S. foreign policy and Dominican migration to the United States. In C. Mitchell (Ed.), *Western Hemisphere immigration and United States foreign policy* (pp. 89–124). University Park, PA: The Pennsylvania State University Press.

Oboler, S. (1995). *Ethnic labels, Latino lives: Identity and the politics of (re)presentation in the United States*. Minneapolis: University of Minnesota Press.

Oboler, S. (2005). Introduction: *Los que llegaron*: 50 years of South American immigration (1950–2000)—An overview. *Latino Studies, 3*, 42–52.

Palloni, A., & Arias, E. (2004). Paradox lost: Explaining the Hispanic adult mortality advantage. *Demography, 41*(3), 385–415.

Palloni, A., & Morenoff, J. D. (2001). Interpreting the paradoxical in the Hispanic paradox: Demographic and epidemiologic approaches. *Annals of the New York Academy of Sciences, 954*, 140–174.

Pedraza, S. (1996). Cuba's refugees. In S. Pedraza & R. G. Rumbaut (Eds.), *Origins and destinies: Immigration, race, and ethnicity in America* (pp. 263–279). Belmont, CA: Wadsworth.

Pew Hispanic Center. (2010). *Statistical portrait of Hispanics in the United States, 2008*. Retrieved from http://pewhispanic.org/factsheets/factsheet.php?FactsheetID=58

Queneau, H. (2009). Trends in occupational segregation by race and ethnicity in the USA: Evidence from detailed data. *Applied Economics Letters, 16*(13), 1347.

Ramirez, A. G., & Suarez, L. (2001). The impact of cancer on Latino populations. In M. Aguirre-Molina, C. W. Molina, & R. E. Zambrana (Eds.), *Health issues in the Latino community* (pp. 211–224). San Francisco, CA: Jossey-Bass.

Rodríguez, C. E. (1997). A summary of Puerto Rican migration to the United States. In M. Romero, P. Hondagneu-Sotelo, & V. Ortiz (Eds.), *Challenging fronteras: Structuring Latina and Latino lives in the U.S.* (pp. 101–114). New York, NY: Routledge.

Rodríguez, C. E. (2000). *Changing race: Latinos, the Census, and the history of ethnicity in the United States*. New York, NY: New York University Press.

Rumbaut, R. G. (2006). The making of a people. In M. Tienda & F. Mitchell (Eds.), *Hispanics and the future of America* (1st ed., pp. 16–65). Washington, DC: National Academies Press.

Shin, H. B., & Bruno, R. (2003). *Language use and English-speaking ability: 2000* (Census 2000 Brief). Washington, DC: U.S. Census Bureau.

Singh, G. K., & Siahpush, M. (2001). All-cause and cause-specific mortality of immigrants and native born in the United States. *American Journal of Public Health, 91*(3), 392–399.

Stepick, A., & Stepick, C. D. (2002). Power and identity: Miami Cubans. In M. M. Suárez-Orozco & M. M. Páez (Eds.), *Latinos remaking America* (pp. 75–92). Berkeley: University of California Press.

Sumaya, C. V. (1991). Major infectious diseases causing excess morbidity in the Hispanic population. *Archives of Internal Medicine, 151*(8), 1513–1520.

Tienda, M., & Mitchell, F. (2006). Introduction: E pluribus plures or E pluribus unum? In M. Tienda & F. Mitchell (Eds.), *Hispanics and the future of America* (1st ed., pp. 1–15). Washington, DC: National Academies Press.

Timberlake, J. M. (2007). Racial and ethnic inequality in the duration of children's exposure to neighborhood poverty and affluence. *Social Problems, 54*(3), 319–342.

U.S. Census Bureau. (2004). *U.S. interim projections by age, sex, race, and Hispanic origin*. Retrieved from http://www.census.gov/population/www/projections/usinterimproj/

U.S. Census Bureau. (2008a). *U.S. census bureau, 1970, 1980, 1990, and 2000 decennial censuses; population projections, July 1, 2010 to July 1, 2050*. Retrieved from http://www.census.gov/population/www/socdemo/hispanic/files/Internet_Hispanic_in_US_2006.pdf

U.S. Census Bureau. (2008b). *Social and economic characteristics of the Hispanic population: 2008* (Current Population Reports, P20-545 and earlier reports). Washington, DC: Author.

U.S. Census Bureau. (2009a). *2007 American community survey: C16005. Nativity by language spoken at home by ability to speak English for the population 5 years and over using American FactFinder*. Retrieved from http://factfinder.census.gov/servlet/ACSSAFFPeople?_submenuId=people_8&_sse=on

U.S. Census Bureau. (2009b). *2008 American community survey: Language spoken at home by ability to speak English for the population 5 years and over using American FactFinder*. Retrieved from http://factfinder.census.gov/servlet/STSelectServlet?ds_name=ACS_2008_3YR_G00_&_SubjectNodeID=17560973&geo_id=01000US&_lang=en

U.S. Census Bureau. (2009c). *Table 4-Z: Projections of the population by sex, race, and Hispanic origin for the United States: 2010 to 2050 zero net international migration series* (NP2009-T4-Z). Washington, DC: U.S. Census Bureau, Population Division.

Valdés, D. N. (2000). *Barrios norteños: St. Paul and Midwestern Mexican communities in the twentieth century*. Austin: University of Texas Press.

Vega, W. A., & Amaro, H. (1994). Latino outlook: Good health, uncertain prognosis. *Annual Review of Public Health, 15*, 39–67.

Vega, W. A., Rodriguez, M. A., & Gruskin, E. (2009). Health disparities in the Latino population. *Epidemiologic Reviews, 31*(1), 99–112. doi:10.1093/epirev/mxp008

Viruell-Fuentes, E. A. (2007). Beyond acculturation: Immigration, discrimination, and health research among Mexicans in the United States. *Social Science & Medicine (1982), 65*(7), 1524–1535. doi:10.1016/j.socscimed.2007.05.010

Viruell-Fuentes, E. A., & Schulz, A. J. (2009). Toward a dynamic conceptualization of social ties and context: Implications for understanding immigrant and Latino health. *American Journal of Public Health, 99,* 2167–2175.

Williams, D. R., & Mohammed, S. A. (2008). Poverty, migration, and health. In D. R. Harris & A. C. Lin (Eds.), *The colors of poverty: Why racial and ethnic disparities persist* (pp. 135–169). New York, NY: Russell Sage.

Woolf, S. H., Johnson, R. E., & Geiger, H. J. (2006). The rising prevalence of severe poverty in America: A growing threat to public health. *American Journal of Preventive Medicine, 31*(4), 332–341.e2. doi:10.1016/j.amepre.2006.06.022

Yu, S. M., & Singh, G. K. (2009). Household language use and health care access, unmet need, and family impact among CSHCN. *Pediatrics, 124* (Suppl. 4), S414–S419. doi:10.1542/peds.2009-1255M

Chapter 2
Latino Mental Health: Acculturation Challenges in Service Provision

Rose M. Perez

Abstract Acculturation and assimilation—terms used to describe the complex processes that immigrants go through as they incorporate into a host society's culture—are important considerations for mental health providers. Acculturation and assimilation include a range of contextual and individual-level factors that interact in ways unique to each immigrant. Hence, a "one-size-fits-all" approach for access to and provision of mental health services is inadequate for Latino immigrants. This chapter focuses on explaining the complexity of the acculturation and assimilation processes as they relate to mental health, particularly in terms of macro-level structural and micro-level individual effects. The chapter illustrates the influence of acculturation and assimilation on mental health and how these processes complicate the provision of services.

According to classical assimilation theory, immigrants become fully incorporated into US life—in the sense that they completely adopt the host culture and leave behind their culture of origin—in the first generation. This theory, however, does not seem to describe the incorporation of Latino immigrants. The standard used to evaluate whether immigrants to the United States are assimilating often refers to the ability of a group to achieve economic prosperity, learn English, and lose native cultural values and norms. Arguments about how today's Latinos are assimilating are often framed as comparisons with earlier waves of European immigrants; the popular belief is that Latinos are not assimilating (Huntington 2004a, b). However, concerns about the ability of the latest group of newcomers to assimilate are similar to those of earlier times. Invidious comparisons between different waves of immigrants over the course of this nation's history resonate with ongoing issues of inclusion and exclusion in a diverse society (Engstrom and Piedra 2006).

Compared to earlier waves of immigrants, Latino newcomers have similarly low-skill levels. However, because Latinos today enter into a far more technologically advanced and globally driven labor market than did immigrants of the nineteenth

R. M. Perez (✉)
Fordham University, New York, NY, USA
e-mail: roseperez2@gmail.com

century, their path to economic success is much more difficult (Borjas 2001). Furthermore, Latinos' large group size, along with their continual population replenishment from Latin America (Jiménez 2008), and their transnational (Levitt 2003), circular (Massey 1987), and undocumented patterns of migration, contribute to Latinos retaining their native language and culture longer than other immigrant groups.

Although acculturation is now viewed as considerably more complex than it was earlier, economists and sociologists still attempt to understand Latinos in terms of general patterns—and to compare these patterns across immigrant cohorts. These analyses influence federal immigration policy, which often ignites arguments regarding the incorporation of immigrants at the local level. What is sometimes forgotten is that although many other immigrant groups were also once thought to be inassimilable, time in the United States proved naysayers wrong. In other words, immigration policy is subject to fundamental attribution errors in which personal-level factors (e.g., Latinos retaining native language and culture) are overvalued and contextual factors are undervalued (Ross 1977). Thus, before asking how the current Latino population will assimilate, we need to consider the contextual differences that help or hinder the incorporation of newcomers and that facilitate or obstruct the acculturation process. In light of the complex issues involved in acculturation, it is also worthwhile to reevaluate the standards by which groups of immigrants are compared, both across time and within the current climate.

Even though the presence of language and cultural retention rankles nativists who unwittingly support a classical—and outdated—theory of assimilation (in which the immigrant wholeheartedly adopts the host culture and abandons her or his culture of origin), it is possible that use of the native language and cultural retention are not necessarily incongruent with the social incorporation of newcomers into the host society; for some groups, in some regions, it may even aid acculturation. Latino newcomers to the United States vary in many aspects, including their demographics and reasons for migration. At the same time, the sociopolitical climate of the United States constantly changes, making it nearly impossible to predict how the current wave of Latino immigrants will acculturate. Furthermore, because most Latinos arrived in the United States after 1965, not enough time for evaluation has elapsed; full assimilation often requires several generations (Gans 1999).

The nuanced realities faced by Latinos in today's socioeconomic context complicate their incorporation into US life and challenge contemporary notions of service provision and institutional arrangements. Service providers struggle to understand and meet the needs of this heterogeneous population, who live in so many different types of regions and are at so many different levels of acculturation and social status. For the health and mental health of both immigrant families and the host society, it is critical that we understand the acculturation and assimilation processes of the many subgroups that make up the very broad "Latino" category, and devise ways to alleviate problems that arise during these processes. Thus, in this chapter I review traditional and modern theories of acculturation, elaborate on the complex nature of the acculturation process, and address ways in which the process complicates access to mental health services. I argue that although acculturation is important for understanding the mental health of immigrants, its complex, multifaceted nature does not allow for simple views or solutions to problems of service access. Rather, the evolving concept of acculturation is best seen as a process that affects both the individual and larger society. The extent to which we change our existing mental health service structures to accommodate the incorporation of immigrants will reflect the way in which US society lives up to its democratic ideals (Torres 2006). In this context, I present suggestions for building infrastructures to improve the provision of mental health services.

Theories of Second-Culture Acquisition

Although *acculturation* is sometimes confused with *assimilation*, the terms differ slightly in meaning (Gans 1999). In general, both acculturation and assimilation describe social processes through which immigrants become incorporated into the host country to which they have migrated. Classically, *acculturation* is defined as the "phenomena which result when groups of individuals having different cultures come into continuous first-hand contact, with subsequent changes in the original cultural patterns of either or both groups" (Redfield et al. 1936, p. 149). Within the parameters of this definition, both the immigrant and the host culture could conceivably change, and no particular assumptions are made as to how or at what rates these changes might occur. *Assimilation*—specifically, "straight-line" assimilation—is a more restrictive concept than acculturation in that it refers to a unidirectional process whereby the immigrant accepts and integrates into US mainstream society and renounces her or his native culture. This classical definition was once heralded as the ideal mode of incorporation (Alba and Chamlin 1983; Gordon 1964; Sowell 1981; Warner and Srole 1945). In this view, assimilation necessarily follows acculturation (Gans 1999). However, the straight-line assimilation philosophy fails to acknowledge (a) the role of dominant social groups in allowing immigrants access to institutions in their new homeland (Gans 1999), (b) the improbability of giving up one's native culture in one or even two generations, and (c) the societal changes occurring over time that help or hinder immigrant incorporation. Furthermore, there is evidence that the host society does, in fact, accommodate immigrant ways. Take, for example, the incorporation of Mexican foods (e.g., tacos, hot sauce), Latino cultural traditions (e.g., Cinco de Mayo), and appreciation for their entertainers (e.g., Jennifer Lopez, Ricky Martin, and Shakira)—all of which have been embraced by many members of US society. The impractical expectations associated with assimilation suggest that acculturation should have been the preferred term all along (Gans 1999).

It is interesting that despite these conceptual and practical problems, classical assimilation continues to signify successful acculturation (Sam and Oppedal 2002). Considering the importance placed on immigrants' adaptation to US life (Gordon 1964), even a neutral term such as *acculturation* has come to be associated with the expectation that the immigrant will change to accommodate the host society, whereas the host society itself is subject to no such expectations. As a result, acculturation, despite its neutral nature, has come to be more commonly associated with the process of second-culture acquisition, at least in the United States (Rudmin 2009).

According to LaFromboise's (1998) extensive review of the literature, newer models describing the process by which immigrants adapt give greater recognition to the

United States as a diverse, socially stratified society in which cultural retention and even bilingualism can emerge as possible outcomes in the incorporation of immigrants (Portes and Rumbaut 2001). In the "alternation" model, individuals choose the extent to which they wish to associate with their native culture or the culture of the host society (LaFromboise 1998). Immigrants' ability to choose their acculturation level elevates their sense of agency, and therefore benefits their psychological well-being. Likewise, in a "multicultural" (pluralistic) model, immigrants are thought to have the ability to maintain distinct cultural identities while also subscribing to broader cultural norms and working toward shared societal goals (LaFromboise 1998). These newer models help explain the cultural phenomenon of ethnic enclaves that emerge as immigrants assimilate into the larger landscape. For example, cities such as Miami, and communities such as Little Village or Humboldt Park in Chicago, gain political prominence through the retention of native language and culture, demonstrating that multiculturalism can be a pathway to greater social inclusion. The last model posited by LaFromboise (1998), "fusion," resonates with the older melting-pot theory. With fusion as a strategy, formerly distinct cultures "fuse" together after sharing geographic, economic, and political realms, resulting in a new, shared culture (Zane and Mak 2003). The broad range of views on how immigrants become incorporated (whether by assimilation, acculturation, alternation, multiculturalism, or fusion), have implications for how immigrants are viewed and expected to conform. Regardless of which model is most popular at a given time or in a given context, use of the term *acculturation* has become a convention when describing the process of second-culture acquisition, and will be used in this chapter to guide the discussion of these multifaceted processes.

Modern conceptions of acculturation feature a complexity missing from early theories. The paradigm shift toward systemic or ecological thinking (Bronfenbrenner 1986) has more than likely facilitated a richer contextual understanding of the ways in which the actions of immigrants, like those of individuals in any society, are clearly influenced by broader societal factors (Blau 1994). In the case of immigrants, for example, factors such as the presence of a co-ethnic population living in their vicinity; broad social tolerance for cultural differences; and the economic, social, and human capital they possess all affect their adjustment to the broader society (Portes and Rumbaut 2001). This adjustment, in turn, affects the mental health of their children. Therefore, understanding the complexity inherent in acculturative processes is critical to the formation and delivery of services for immigrants.

To understand and assess the effects of acculturation in immigrant populations, we must develop a valid and reliable measure of acculturation and employ careful research designs. Acculturation is considered necessary in studies evaluating health outcomes (Hunt et al. 2004; Rudmin 2009). However, the complexity inherent in the acculturation process renders precise measurements difficult, and scholars struggle to find such measures (Rudmin 2009). Simpler proxy measures—language and length of stay—are easily accessible. Some argue that they are useful until more complex ones can be validated scientifically (Escobar and Vega 2000), whereas others claim that they miss important contextual factors. One individual-level proxy for acculturation, language acquisition, captures a complex process that includes affective, cognitive, and behavioral components (Cuéllar et al. 1995), and has been shown to be influential in more complex acculturation measures (Rogler et al. 1991). The difficulty—indeed, the impossibility—of accurately capturing a complex and dynamic process such as acculturation with a single measure is likely to remain, considering the large number of multidirectional factors affecting the process. Also, degree of acculturation affects a society's ability to provide services, even as the conditions and circumstances of acculturation create their own mental health issues.

Factors Affecting Acculturation

As theories of acculturation have evolved and informed our understanding of the immigrant experience, our appreciation for the psychological stressors that frame the transition has deepened. In early studies, Park (1928) and Stonequist (1935) described the person undergoing the acculturation process as "the marginal man"— someone not quite acculturated to the new culture but no longer holding the values of the old. Because it was thought that the immigrant could never fully assimilate, the marginal-man condition was viewed as a permanent condition: The marginal man would never be wholly accepted by the host society and yet could not completely shed the culture of origin. The marginal-man concept, regardless of the validity of its assumptions, reveals real psychological tensions inherent in the acculturation process. It is not surprising, therefore, that many of the issues Latino immigrants present when they enter mental health services stem from tensions caused by acculturation processes (Caldwell et al. 2010). Unfortunately, the effects of acculturation on the mental health of Latinos are not well understood (Lara et al. 2004).

A higher number of variables affect the acculturation experience than had been previously acknowledged (Ward 1996). Both macro- and micro-level factors interact with each person to yield quite different behavioral, cognitive, and affective responses to acculturation across individuals (Ward 1996). Skilled or unskilled, young or old, English speaking or not, and adaptable or not, each individual experiences the process of acculturation differently. The following paragraphs discuss some of the macro- and micro-level factors thought to influence the effect of acculturation on the mental health of Latinos. The term *macro-level factors* refers to larger social structures that constrain and limit opportunities between social groups in society (Blau 1994); *micro-level factors* refer to the individual's traits such as skills, language(s) spoken, and personality.

Macro-Level Factors

At the macro level, the effect of acculturation on health outcomes can vary according to whether migration was voluntary or involuntary (Ogbu 1993), the extent to which an immigrant maintains ties to her or his home country (Drachman and Shen-Ryan 1991; Lambert and Taylor 1990; Portes and Mozo 1985; Rumbaut 1995), her or his length of time in the United States (Caplan 2007; Smokowski et al. 2009), contextual factors pertaining to the sending and receiving countries, and conditions of the migration itself (Murphy 2009). Distinct differences in immigration status— such as that between immigrants and refugees—illustrate how macro-level factors influence the acculturation process.

Context of Reception

Currently, the US government makes provisions for the health of refugee aliens (i.e., those unable to return to their country of origin because of a well-founded fear of persecution) (Pine and Drachman 2005; Weissbrodt and Danielson 2005). This stance suggests that the United States welcomes refugees but not immigrants. Refugees qualify for health services immediately, under the provisions of the Personal Responsibility and Work Opportunity Reconciliation Act (PRWORA) of 1996, by-passing the five-year minimum wait imposed on immigrants (Singer 2004). Such aid is considered meaningful for refugees, who are unable to return to their country of origin, at least in the short term. Thus, the refugee's experience of the acculturation process is thought to differ from that of the economic migrant, whose move is motivated by employment opportunities and who does not enjoy similar access to health care services (Donà and Berry 1994). Those who fled political strife in their homeland might be more susceptible to mental health problems such as depression and post-traumatic stress disorder (PTSD) (Engstrom and Okamura 2004). Resolving trauma may be a salient part of their acculturation experience and mental health treatment may be critical to that process. However, the experiences of individual immigrants making their way to the United States can be more or less severe, depending on many things. Consider that in the course of traveling through Mexico, many South and Central Americans face life-threatening challenges that may pose a threat to mental health (Nazario 2007). The policy distinction between political and economic migrants is driven by political forces and based on assumptions that do not necessarily reflect the individual realities of new entrants; hence, the policy that provides health benefits to refugees but not immigrants is not entirely justified.

For political reasons, the context of reception in the United States has been known to differ for groups with comparable reasons for migrating. For example, even when groups of people flee their home countries for political reasons, the decision as to which groups are subsequently deemed eligible for asylum is subject to current US immigration policy (Díaz Briquets 1995), and this has led to differential treatment of similar groups. The varied receptions given to Cubans and Central Americans— both groups that fled for politically motivated reasons—illustrates how the foreign policy regarding granting of asylum can affect acculturation.

Case Study: Cubans and Central Americans

Since Cubans began arriving in the United States following the 1959 revolution, they have had little difficulty gaining political asylum in the United States. In particular, a federally supported resettlement program served as a significant source of funds to assist the first wave of Cubans who relocated to Miami in their initial adaptation (Mitchell 1962). The trauma involved in fleeing the revolution could have resulted in serious health effects for many exiles (Suárez and Perez in press). However, these immigrants' ability to transcend much of their adversity can arguably be attributed to a favorable context of reception.

By comparison, Central Americans fleeing from civil wars suffered much political strife, yet initially were not granted asylum in the United States. In the decades leading up to the 1980s, increasing numbers of Central Americans came to the United States from countries with extreme political instability (Gzesh 2006). Many had witnessed atrocities such as murder, rape, and torture or were themselves victims of political violence (Engstrom and Piedra 2005). Yet, upon arrival in the United States, Nicaraguans (Portes and Stepick 1994), Guatemalans, and Salvadorians (Hernandez 2005) were not granted asylum, but remained here in a hostile atmosphere (Hernandez 2005). Because they were "undocumented," they were ineligible for the benefits accorded to those with refugee status (Hernandez 2005). More recently, though, many of these groups have been able to obtain temporary protection and refugee status. Given their immigration history, however, Central Americans have been found to experience higher levels of post-traumatic stress than Mexicans (Cervantes et al. 1989), and as a result of gender-specific terror in the contexts from which they migrated, many females experienced severe trauma (Aron et al. 1991).

For nonrefugees experiencing acculturation stresses and lacking resources, there is no choice but to wait the five years to qualify for health benefits under the PRWORA. As a result, they are forced to turn to informal sources of help at the community level, including religious institutions and support from family and peers (Skerry 2004). Understanding the macro-level factors as well as informal and formal supports at the local level has implications for infrastructure building. Collaborative agreements between formal and informal sources of support can range from disseminating relevant information and educating groups about preventative care, to providing public services that can help with various issues. Maneuvering through social structures to obtain services is difficult enough when one understands English; for those who do not, merely attempting to access services can add to the stress of acculturation.

Geographic Effects and Local Tensions

Sociologists studying groups in society posit that group size and geographic concentration patterns between societal groups can influence the relationships between them (Blau 1994), and that this, in turn, can affect immigrants' acculturation patterns and their ability to become fully incorporated and assimilated (Cabassa 2003). For example, groups of immigrants from similar sending countries who settle in densely populated ethnic enclaves (e.g., Cubans in Miami) have more opportunities for cultural and linguistic retention; many will thus feel less of a need to acculturate on these dimensions (Rumbaut 1997). However, when a group becomes sizeable and therefore visible, other social groups may feel vulnerable, and social tensions between less acculturated and more acculturated groups can develop (Sullivan 2000).

Analyzing settlement patterns can help us understand the ways in which immigrant and host society members relate to one another (Sullivan 2006) and how the quality of those relationships affects acculturation. An examination of how population differences contribute to social tensions provides interesting insights for building infrastructures for the provision of mental health services. Although immigrants are heavily concentrated in certain regions and meet local labor needs, in many communities (especially those with a large percentage of undocumented immigrants) the immigrants' contributions to the general economy are frequently overlooked (Fix 1999). Instead, the emphasis is on their use of public spaces and local resources such as schools, and this often creates tensions in the community. Local tensions can detract from the mental health of immigrants by hindering their ability to incorporate (Sullivan 2000).

Historically, sociologists have viewed living in enclaves, *barrios,* or ghettos as a form of segregation (Wilson and Portes 1980; Zhou and Logan 1989). As scholars continue to tease out the benefits and drawbacks of living in co-ethnic communities (Chiswick and Miller 2005; Chiswick et al. 2008; Jensen and Portes 1992; Portes and Jensen 1987), it is important to consider the psychological benefits to immigrants of living among fellow co-ethnics. Arguably, acculturative stressors such as the loss of homeland, family separation (Smart and Smart 1995), difficulties adjusting culturally and linguistically, and discrimination (Araújo Dawson and Panchanadeswaran 2010; Hovey 1999; Ward and Kennedy 1994) may be mitigated by living among co-ethnics who understand such stressors. By contrast, Latinos separated from others and who have little in common with other people in their new communities are more likely to experience the effects of linguistic and cultural isolation.

Take the mental health issue of loss of homeland (Ainslie 1998), which is common to many immigrant groups. The acculturation experience of mourning the loss and adaptation is different in ethnic enclaves than in places in which there are few co-ethnics. In addition to a sizable number of compatriots, established ethnic enclaves garner political, social, and economic strength in their larger community, which allows them to influence local policies and gain access to existing social or economic institutions. Frequently, the use of English is not a prerequisite for social inclusion. For example, to participate in the business sector in Miami, it is necessary to have knowledge of Spanish. Within such contexts, newcomers can easily access jobs and services in ways that allow them to continue speaking Spanish, to participate in their new society, and to gradually learn English. Living in an ethnic enclave permits immigrants to alternate between enculturation to their country of origin and acculturation to the host society (Suárez and Perez in press), a luxury not afforded to immigrants living in new settlements in the South and Midwest.

The ability of an immigrant group to create transitional spaces to facilitate the acculturation experience can hinge on geographic and regional differences and the sociopolitical context of reception. Immigrants are welcomed in some parts of the country and in some sectors of the economy more than in others. For example, in some places employers prefer immigrant workers to US-born workers (Waldinger 1999). Also, many Americans hold the perception that undocumented immigrants wrongfully benefit from public services and do not contribute anything—either not recognizing or ignoring the fact that undocumented immigrants do indeed contribute to the tax base and spend money on consumer goods and services, thereby stimulating the economy. Anti-immigrant fears stemming from public misperceptions have led to policies aimed at excluding the undocumented population. For example, early in 2010, the state of Arizona passed an initiative to allow its law enforcement agencies to question individuals' immigration status. Before that, the state of California passed Proposition 187, which attempted to bar undocumented immigrants from accessing health care. More recently, a myriad of cities across the United States have also passed or considered local ordinances influenced by anti-immigrant sentiment stemming from local tensions. These local policies are reported on the national news and send strong anti-immigrant messages that can extend far beyond their intended audience. Immigrant groups for whom these ordinances were intended—in most cases undocumented Mexicans—may feel marginalized (Jiménez 2008). Individual immigrants, upon hearing such national local news reports, can come to internalize the message that they are not wanted in US society, in sharp contrast to the expectations they had prior to migrating. Especially in areas with few co-ethnics, available supports can be virtually nonexistent. Thus, the macro-level factors of the acculturation process can contribute to, exacerbate, and even initiate mental health issues.

Micro-Level Factors Affecting Acculturation

In addition to broad macro-level effects on acculturation, individual-level factors are part and parcel of the acculturation experience (Berry et al. 1992; Ward et al. 1996). Like macro-level factors, micro-level factors can influence affective, behavioral, and cognitive responses to the situations faced during acculturation. Providers need to understand these effects so that they can better meet the needs of constituents at different levels of acculturation. For example, the ability to understand or acquire knowledge of English is typically a first step in acculturation, but many Latinos' experiences show that it is not absolutely necessary. In addition, having sufficient skills to obtain meaningful work can also greatly enhance the acculturation experience. Newcomers who do not speak English and who lack basic skills may benefit from education outreach to facilitate their incorporation along these dimensions.

Language

The ability to learn English is an especially important factor in acculturation, and is related to an individual's age and the number of co-ethnics in the community. Children are at different developmental stages than their parents and, because they participate in the US educational system, they quickly learn English, leaving their parents behind, culturally speaking. Generally, immigrant youth learn a host society's language rapidly. Older immigrants, by contrast, are less able to acquire a second language. Moreover, it is much easier to retain a language when the community has a high proportion of co-ethnics. An immigrant who settles in an immigrant enclave where her or his native language is the dominant language will probably have an experience different from that of an immigrant who settles in an English-dominant community. The former setting is likely to facilitate native-language retention, and the latter is likely to prompt a person to learn English. Those who live in a high co-ethnic enclave where they are able to retain their language and culture in a welcoming context have been reported to experience better psychological health (Cuéllar et al. 2004).

Skills

Another micro-level factor that influences the acculturation process is the immigrant's skill level. Although there are wide variations in skill level among the general immigrant population, low-skill levels and poor language ability combine to relegate an individual to the low-wage employment sector. Because the best-paying jobs require higher levels of formal education, the mismatch between the skill level needed for such work and the generally low-skill levels of today's Latino immigrants puts them at an economic disadvantage relative to other immigrant groups (Borjas 2001). Furthermore, second-generation Latinos—tomorrow's workforce—are less likely to have a high school diploma compared to other groups (Fry 2010). This has important implications for acculturation. Immigrants with higher skill levels and better-compensated employment can more effectively use resources to advance their children's social mobility (Portes and Rumbaut 2001). For instance, having a better-paying job enables a child to receive higher-quality child care and allows parents time to attend English as a second language (ESL) classes. Those without high-level skills or additional resources must weigh such tradeoffs as engaging in self-improvement or working a few extra hours.

In sum, at the level of the individual, behavioral changes occurring during acculturation do not occur uniformly for all individuals. Rather, it is believed that acculturation occurs in each person in different ways and at different rates. During the course of the acculturation process, the many contextual interactions in which immigrants' lives are embedded have significant and multifaceted effects on emotional experiences. Acculturation is inherently stressful because individuals must come to terms with different cultural norms, some of which compete with one another. Mental health ultimately depends on how the individual handles the stressors encountered. Person-level resources, including coping mechanisms, social supports, and adequate skills, greatly influence acculturation outcomes. Altogether, such complex person-level factors, together with the broader macro-level factors, result in hugely varied outcomes across people. To be optimally effective, providers need to understand the growing knowledge base associating individual-level factors with different levels of acculturation.

Factors That Influence Acculturation Stress

Individual immigrants experience acculturation in different ways and have different coping styles. For example, among the personality types, neuroticism has been associated with acculturative stress (Mangold et al. 2007), and extraversion has predicted a person's ability to adapt socioculturally (Ward and Kennedy 1993). In short, who a person is and how he or she perceives the world contributes to his or her experience of acculturation. Several important factors begin to influence a person upon migration, such as the individual's (a) cultural frame of reference, (b) experiences of discrimination, (c) cultural assimilation or retention, (d) changing roles, (e) availability of family support, and (f) intergenerational status. These, in turn, can affect individual immigrants' roles, perceptions, and patterns of acculturation, as well as their experience of acculturation stress. Some of these factors, depending on how each is experienced, become risk factors, whereas others can insulate individuals from the stressors of the acculturation process. The following sections examine these factors more closely, to explain how they affect the acculturation of Latino immigrants. The last factor—intergenerational status during the process of assimilation—is discussed through the lens of segmented assimilation theory.

Cultural Frame of Reference

Depending on the level of acculturation, the type of stresses encountered will differ, as will the individual's experience of those stressors. For example, recent immigrants are more likely to face short-term linguistic and economic struggles than second- and later-generation immigrants. The recently arrived judge their well-being relative to people from their country of origin rather than to those in the host society. Assuming that recent immigrants left their home countries for a better life in the United States, this group might be optimistic regarding their future prospects in the United States and may be willing to overlook initial hardships, because the point of comparison between their current experiences and their past history relates to those in the country that they left. By contrast, the point of reference for second- and later-generation immigrants usually differs. Being further removed from the country of origin, second- and later-generation immigrants are more likely to judge their well-being by US mainstream cultural standards than by a referent group in the country of origin. Latinos who have been in the United States for generations might have experienced the effects of years of social and economic inequities common to many minority groups in this country. They may have given up on the American dream, synonymous with success through hard work, so often cherished by immigrants aspiring to a better life.

Discrimination

Some individuals attempt to blend in with the dominant societal groups in the host country. However, physical differences such as indigenous features or darker phenotypes may set them apart from others in ways they cannot control. Those separated by social inequality may feel a heightened awareness of their relatively slow advancement, and the resulting disillusionment may translate into reduced well-being. Some disparities in mental health outcomes between Latinos born in the United States and abroad are explained by protective factors associated with immigrant Latino culture (Chapman and Perreira 2005). For instance, cultural retention is considered a protective factor (Gonzales et al. 2004; LaFromboise 1998) that can mitigate the effects of stressors such as discrimination (Araújo Dawson 2009). Differences in how individuals and families experience discrimination can be attributed to variations in the places to which they migrate. For example, those migrating to areas with a large co-ethnic community may experience considerably more kinship support than those migrating to isolated communities; informal support often mediates the experience of discrimination.

Cultural Assimilation or Retention

Latino culture is frequently described as collectivist (interdependent), in contrast to US culture, which has been described as autonomist or individualist (Fuligni 1998; Kitayama 2006). In collectivist cultures, individuals derive a contextualized identity that reflects their social interdependence and how they relate to others. In contrast, people in autonomous cultures place more emphasis on their individuality than on their interrelatedness with others in the social context (Markus and Kitayama 1991). It is useful for providers to be aware of this difference in orientation, because as immigrants acculturate, family members may find some of the differences in these cultural orientations difficult to reconcile.

Immigrants to the United States accommodate to policies based on values that in large part reflect the autonomous cultural orientation of this society. Latino parents more accustomed to a collective view of the family (e.g., one where the elders command respect) may be unfamiliar with the US stance that highlights and privileges the rights of the child. From the perspective of child welfare, it is difficult to argue against socialization of practices that are common in some Latin American families, such as corporal punishment. Yet, for an immigrant parent, to have an acculturated child call an emergency hotline to report abuse is unconscionable from the perspective of Latino parental culture. Such actions, which are determined by cultural attitudes and beliefs, could have adverse effects on families in which parents are unfamiliar with their legal obligations in the United States. This is but one of many differences in cultural values and norms. Therefore, it is of the utmost importance that newcomers be educated regarding practices that violate US laws.

Changing Roles

The acculturation experience challenges families to reexamine their behaviors and may alter family roles and expectations in unforeseen ways. Wives often become employed while husbands face long periods of unemployment (Hondagneu-Sotelo 1994). In this new context, some families are challenged by the reversal of traditional gender roles and expectations (Hondagneu-Sotelo 1994). The family may also be challenged by other differences between their culture of origin and that of their host country.

Family Support

Although *familismo* (familism)—the support systems within Latino families that extend beyond immediate kin (Keefe et al. 1979)—is widely recognized as a resource for immigrant Latino youth (Gil-Rivas et al. 2003), the acculturation experience has the potential to change family dynamics and threaten family bonds. For example, *respeto* (respect) is frequently violated when the acculturating Latino youth, having internalized US cultural norms that emphasize individual rights and autonomy, assert their independence from the family. The strength of family has been observed to weaken with acculturation (Sabogal et al. 1987). Conflicts within families stemming from acculturation gaps between parents and their children have been shown to reduce family cohesion (Szapocznik and Kurtines 1993; Szapocznik et al. 1978). Youth can acculturate in substantially different ways, depending on macro-level forces in the regions in which they live, and these same factors may mediate or even determine how acculturation differences between them and their parents are resolved.

Segmented Assimilation

Differences in parental and child acculturation are at the heart of Portes and Rumbaut's (2001) segmented assimilation theory. Segmented assimilation theory recognizes that the United States is both a diverse and a stratified society. By virtue of their low levels of education and low-wage employment options, Latino immigrants and their children often occupy the poorer sectors of society (Portes and Rumbaut 2006). Thus, the children of Latino immigrants are described as experiencing downward assimilation—that is, entry to social sectors leading to downward mobility—because the pathway to higher social mobility is fraught with formidable obstacles, including discrimination and suboptimal inner-city schools that do little to prepare them for the challenges of the labor market (Portes and Rumbaut 2001). Overcoming such obstacles requires a concerted effort by both youth and their families. Toward this end, the pace of intergenerational differences in acculturation is an important factor in preservation of harmonious family relationships (Piedra and Engstrom 2009). Segmented assimilation theory describes three types of intergenerational acculturation patterns: dissonant, consonant, and selective.

Dissonant acculturation occurs when the youth rapidly learn English and adopt US mainstream ways at a much faster rate than their parents. In addition, knowledge of the original immigrant culture and language is lost, creating a gulf between the two generations that can undermine parental-child relationships (Hwang 2007). A role reversal occurs: instead of parents socializing their children, youth are the ones socializing their parents (Portes and Rumbaut 2006). *Consonant acculturation* occurs when there is congruence between the youth's rate of acculturation and that of their parents; that is, within a family, both parents and their offspring learn the new culture and language at the same pace. As parents and children adopt the new language, both simultaneously lose the home language. *Selective acculturation* occurs when youth and their parents are able to participate in both the native and the host cultures. This usually takes place when the acculturation process is embedded in a co-ethnic community with sufficient institutional diversity (e.g., Miami) to warrant retention of the native language and culture. In this context, parents and their offspring both go through a slower process of acculturation to the values and beliefs of the host society, but they are able to retain their native language and culture for much longer. This type of acculturation provides the greatest support for the social mobility of children, because parents and the wider co-ethnic community work jointly with the youth to overcome normative challenges that arise in the course of the acculturation process (Portes and Rumbaut 2001).

As the acculturation literature continues its rapid proliferation, one can hope that the effect of the numerous factors on acculturation outcomes will be better understood. The use of assessment scales upon intake can help providers to better administer agency staff and services, tailor outreach efforts, and develop interventions. Moreover, having a sense of the individual acculturation level of family members can help practitioners recognize the associated risks and protective factors at different points in the acculturation process (Lara et al. 2005).

Toward Greater Incorporation of Immigrants

Immigrants arriving in the United States from the late 1800s to the early 1900s from Southern and Eastern Europe had literacy levels comparable to those of today's Latino migrants and were also once considered inassimilable. Yet, over time, subsequent generations became incorporated into US life (Lieberson 1980). Unlike those earlier immigrants, today's immigrants face a labor market that presents a unique set of hurdles for economic advancement (Borjas 2001). Today's employment market is shaped like an hourglass, in which employment possibilities exist only for the most and the least skilled, and few or no possibilities exist for those in the middle (Sassen 1998); this allows Latinos with low skills and education little opportunity for advancement. The willingness of the large and growing number of Latino immigrants and their native-born children to incorporate fully into life in the United States underscores the need for structures that will facilitate that process. We know that acculturation is a long-term process that can span generations (Piedra and Engstrom 2009), and that facilitating this process requires access to the institutions of the host society (Portes and Rumbaut 2001). However, the extent to which the United States is willing to change to accommodate the needs of this new group remains an open question. The onus of adequate adjustment to and integration with the host society currently falls almost entirely on the individual immigrant. For example, the lack of comprehensive immigration reform, despite the presence of more than 11 million undocumented persons, impedes the incorporation of those persons and their children. The Development, Relief and Education of Alien Minors Act, also known as the DREAM Act, which was intended to help incorporate undocumented youth reared and educated in the United States and who know no other country, remains unresolved. Regardless of the determination and will of these undocumented youth, without structural changes at the federal level, their incorporation to US society will remain marginal at best.

Thus, it is imperative that the federal government focus on full incorporation of the immigrants within its borders, and take seriously its role in protecting them and regulating the admission of new immigrants and refugees (Jiménez 2007). The US government's current approach leaves much to the individual immigrants and the local communities in which they reside. Given this context, the plight of Latinos who hope to become fully incorporated merits attention.

The Role of the Federal Government

The US government is solely charged with setting and enforcing immigration policy. However, decisions made at the federal level can create local tensions when immigrants cluster in discrete areas of the country, creating a visible presence and by so doing testing the limits of tolerance of dominant societal groups (Shweder 2003). To improve the infrastructure, the federal government can grant subsidies to local communities with large immigrant populations to facilitate the incorporation of newcomers (Jiménez 2007). Such efforts could help reduce community tensions, especially in areas most threatened by the influx of newcomers, such as towns along the southern border and places where the cultural distance between immigrants and the local communities are the greatest.

Currently, there is no concerted federal effort to incorporate newcomers, linguistically or otherwise, into US society (Engstrom and Piedra 2006; Jiménez 2007; Piedra 2006). At a national level, some have argued that a commission to oversee the incorporation of immigrant families would help to formalize newcomers'acclimation (Fix et al. 2001). Others argue for more active approaches, such as immediate eligibility for health benefits, which have heretofore been reserved to refugees (Engstrom 2006; Jiménez 2007). Jiménez (2007, p. 1) has argued persuasively that "rather than dictate policy, the federal government should partner with state and local governments, NGOs, and the private sector in carrying out the business of integration." Such a partnership would go a long way toward reducing local community tensions that stem from sharing public space and institutional resources, such as when public school attendance by children of undocumented immigrants is perceived to occur at the expense of taxpayers.

Alternatively, federal funds—contributions from the taxes that immigrants are already paying—could be channeled into communities with high numbers of newcomers to assist in their settlement. These funds could be used to hire translators and teachers, and also to build or repair housing stock, create new businesses, and improve the existing structures of local communities. The public use of funds for the resettlement of Cuban refugees in the 1960s exemplifies this approach. These funds reduced public fears about what effect a sudden population influx would have on the local economy and contributed to the successful incorporation of that population. In the process, the city of Miami was transformed and today is recognized as a business gateway into Latin America. Resettlement plans for places such as Phoenix and border towns would go a long way toward alleviating local tensions brought on by sudden population changes (Jiménez 2007). The strength of such an approach would be in its national cohesion. By avoiding the patchwork efforts by states and local municipalities to resolve problems created by federal immigration policy, a carefully planned course of action by the federal government could mitigate local backlash.

At a minimum, the federal government can rethink its policies on the health benefits allowed to newcomers. Considering that Latino newcomers are healthier in the initial years of their arrival (Alegría et al. 2008; Escarce et al. 2006; Hernandez and Charney 1998; Nguyen 2006), it is ironic to think that the government coffers are much protected by barring these persons' eligibility for health benefits under PRWORA. Continuing to exclude recent immigrants from routine medical care creates an overuse of emergency medical services and, perhaps, a less healthy population in the long run—and this runs counter to national and local community interests.

Attention to immigrants who are more acculturated is equally important. Planned government efforts, including attention to corporate governance, can help Latinos who, by virtue of their higher education, meet the criteria for leadership but are not necessarily embraced by the institutions of majority society. Latinos have a long way to go to attain leadership positions in the private/corporate sector. According to a survey of 219 participating institutions by the only Democratic Latino senator, New Jersey's Robert Menendez (2010), Latinos represented only 3.4% of directors on corporate boards, and only 2.5% were found among the highest levels of management. In a country where so much of what occurs between minority and majority groups in society has to do with the voice given to particular social issues, it seems imperative that leadership be fostered, so that Latinos become full participants in the society to which they have dedicated their lives.

Building Stronger Infrastructures for Latino Mental Health at the Local Level

This chapter showed that acculturation level affects mental health, and that the precise relationship is unclear. Still, tailoring mental health services to accommodate each person's progress in the process of acculturation is warranted. The broad spectrum of acculturation levels along multiple dimensions (e.g., language, skills, education, immigration status), along with regional differences in the demand for services, complicate and hamper the ability of service providers to meet those needs. The problems are worse in areas where there are greater mismatches between providers and people in need.

One way to think about meeting the needs of Latinos in a given region is to understand the number of clients in need, according to their level of acculturation, compared to the ability of suppliers to meet those needs. Of course, estimating the number of people who need services could be particularly arduous in the mental health field, considering the stigma that such services carry and the lack of outreach characteristic of many communities. Still, in an ideal economic supply-and-demand graph, the optimal point occurs where suppliers of services are able to meet the demand for those services (Lewis and Widerquist 2001). In regions of the country with a high percentage of Latinos at low levels of acculturation, and also a high percentage of more acculturated compatriots who can meet their service needs through formal and informal helping systems (e.g., Miami), supply and demand do not suffer much of a mismatch. In other regions, where the demand for services exceeds supply or vice versa, more creative solutions must be found. For a start, programs could match informal helping networks with people in need. For instance, cultural brokers or Spanish-language speakers can be requested to volunteer to serve people in need in exchange for intangible rewards such as those associated with volunteerism (personal satisfaction and increased feelings of self-worth).

Regions Where Supply Meets Demand

High-density areas are more likely to have a sufficient number of available service providers to tailor services in culturally and linguistically appropriate ways. In these regions, useful infrastructure building strategies include providing language-appropriate outreach; offering ongoing training on issues of acculturation, language, and cultural competence; and creating cross-institutional collaborations to achieve higher levels of specialization. For example, in places such as Miami, parts of New York, New Jersey, Texas, and Chicago, agencies have the luxury of specializing in particular types of services. Working collaboratively, agencies can direct clients to the places most appropriate for their particular problem.

Specialized services can include focused programs that vary according to level of acculturation. Newcomers can be served by agencies whose sole responsibility is to acclimate them, much as the settlement houses of the past century did (Addams 1910). Newcomers from Latin America typically face short-term linguistic and economic struggles and lack familiarity with basis customs, norms, and laws of the United States. In addition to taking care of basic necessities—finding employment, obtaining housing and food, learning English, and understanding a new social world—immigrant families may need help reconciling differences across cultures and coping with their effects on emotional states.

Family tensions that arise during adaptation to a new society sometimes require intervention. In such families, workers may help bridge acculturation gaps between parents and offspring, using approaches as involved as family therapy initiatives or as simple as parent/youth outreach programs that supply appropriate literature. In Miami, José Szapocznik et al. (1986) have worked on bridging the acculturation gap, and there is evidence that the interventions treating Latino teens and their parents have been successful. Among the tactics of their treatment, called Bicultural Effectiveness Training (BET), parents are helped to increase their acculturation level while adolescents are taught the benefits of cultural retention.

Regions Where Demand Exceeds Supply

The demand for services and the ability to meet service needs can conflict for any number of reasons. In regions where there is a sudden influx of immigrants, there will be an urgent need for providers—and there are no easy solutions. Demand for services may also exceed supply in regions with a low density of Latino immigrants. In such areas, the few providers can be overwhelmed with people in need. The lack of federal funds further impairs communities' ability to bridge any service gaps that arise.

When the supply of services is constrained and exceeded by demand, the health of vulnerable groups is compromised. In places where immigrants are spread out over vast geographic distances and an established co-ethnic community is absent, even informal supports may be nonexistent. Furthermore, these communities are often unfamiliar with the problems commonly faced by immigrants and have little appreciation of the challenges that acculturation and language difficulties pose. The lack of a bilingual workforce further compounds the problem.

The problem of securing interpreters remains an ongoing challenge. In these areas, service providers need to be highly creative if their efforts are to be fruitful. For instance, it is now common for agencies to use translation services by telephone to assist their customers. Thoughtful use and training of ad hoc interpreters would be critical to agencies caring for Latinos in low-density areas (Larrison et al. 2010).

Spaces in local schools and other public institutions could be used for larger-scale programming efforts, which can be publicized through local Spanish-language stations and by word of mouth. For families experiencing tensions from the acculturation experience, large-scale education nights at a local school or church could enhance bridging efforts to unify parents and offspring. Over time, the development of Latino leaders and cultural brokers from within the community may enrich programming and could prove to be as rewarding to those who volunteer as to those in need.

Matching more acculturated Latinos with volunteer opportunities to help less acculturated Latinos can serve two purposes. Information and help given to low-acculturated individuals can be crucial to their incorporation. At the same, such work can be an important source of empowerment for more highly acculturated Latinos who feel disenfranchised or alienated. This chapter already noted that more-acculturated Latinos tend to compare their experiences to those of host-society members than to those of persons in their country of origin. At the same time, they are less protected by the native cultural factors (e.g., familism, respect for elders) to which their less acculturated kin still cling. Furthermore, by virtue of their ability to blend into host society and penetrate its institutions, more-acculturated Latinos are vulnerable to discrimination. Thus, agencies that play a role in helping acculturated Latinos to meet the needs of vulnerable less-acculturated populations can serve two purposes: essentially meeting the needs of each by putting them in contact with one another.

Conclusion

This chapter gave an overview of the many facets of the acculturation process, and the implications of this process for mental health. Certainly, institutions that provide mental health services to immigrants are well served by understanding how acculturation affects mental health; thus, this chapter also advances an argument for greater federal involvement in the settlement and incorporation of immigrants. Even so, as this chapter has demonstrated, acculturation tends to raise more questions than answers. The relationship between acculturation and mental health has been studied for some time and across a number of fields, but the effects and directions of influences remain unclear (Lara et al. 2005). We do not know the extent to which broad societal factors will hinder a person's ability to assimilate into the US mainstream. Likewise, for more-acculturated and educated Latinos, lack of representation in the higher levels of public and private institutions is an ongoing problem. Though all of these issues merit further investigation, this chapter has emphasized how, given these contextual factors, the processes of acculturation and subsequent assimilation—with all of their complexity and uncertainty—affect family relations and mental health services.

The provision of mental health services for Latinos rests on a keen appreciation for how the process of acculturation affects both the individual and the family. Such an understanding lays the groundwork for culturally appropriate assessments and services. However, greater governmental involvement is required to provide the policies and resources needed to assist communities in meeting the needs of Latinos. Through national policies and better-informed plans, the federal government can help local communities reduce social tensions spurred by the influx of people with dissimilar cultures and languages.

References

Addams, J. (1910). *Twenty years at Hull House*. New York, NY: Macmillan.

Ainslie, R. C. (1998). Cultural mourning, immigrants and engagement: Vignettes from the Mexican experience. In M. M. Suárez-Orozco (Ed.), *Crossings: Mexican immigration in interdisciplinary perspectives* (pp. 283–305). Cambridge, MA: Harvard University Press.

Alba, R. D., & Chamlin M. B. (1983). A preliminary examination of ethnic identification among Whites. *American Sociological Review, 48,* 240–242.

Alegría, M., Canino, G., Shrout, P. E., Woo, M., Duan, N., Vila, D., et al. (2008). Prevalence of mental illness in immigrant and non-immigrant U.S. Latino groups. *American Journal of Psychiatry, 165*(3), 359–369.

Araújo Dawson, B. (2009). Discrimination, stress, and acculturation among Dominican immigrant women. *Hispanic Journal of Behavioral Sciences, 31*(1), 96–111.

Araújo Dawson, B., & Panchanadeswaran, S. (2010). Discrimination and acculturative stress among first-generation Dominicans. *Hispanic Journal of Behavioral Sciences, 32*(2), 216.

Aron, A., Corne, S., Fursland, A., & Zelwer, B. (1991). The gender-specific terror of El Salvador and Guatemala: Post-traumatic stress disorder in Central American refugee women. *Women's Studies International Forum, 14*(1-2), 37-47.

Berry, J. W., Poortinga, Y. P., Segall, M. H., & Dasen, P. R. (1992). *Cross-cultural psychology: Research and applications*. New York, NY: Cambridge University Press.

Blau, P. M. (1994). *Structural contexts of opportunities*. Chicago, IL: The University of Chicago Press.

Borjas, G. J. (2001). *Heaven's door: Immigration policy and the American economy*. Princeton, NJ: Princeton University Press.

Bronfenbrenner, U. (1986). Ecology of the family as a context for human development: Research perspectives. *Developmental Psychology, 22*(6), 723–742.

Cabassa, L. J. (2003). Measuring acculturation: Where we are and where we need to go. *Hispanic Journal of Behavioral Sciences, 25*(2), 127–146.

Caldwell, A., Couture, A., & Nowotny, H. (2010). Closing the mental health gap: Eliminating disparities in treatment for Latinos. Retrieved June 1, 2010, from The Mattie Rhodes Center, https://www.mattierhodes.org/userfiles/file/samhsa_full_report.pdf

Caplan, S. (2007). Latinos, acculturation, and acculturative stress: A dimensional concept analysis. *Policy, Politics, & Nursing Practice, 8*(2), 93–106.

Cervantes, R., de Snyder, V., & Padilla, A. (1989). Posttraumatic stress in immigrants from Central America and Mexico. *Psychiatric Services, 40*(6), 615.

Chapman, M., & Perreira, K. (2005). The well-being of immigrant Latino youth: A framework to inform practice. *Families in Society: The Journal of Contemporary Social Services, 86*(1), 104–110.

Chiswick, B. R., & Miller, P. W. (2005). Do enclaves matter in immigrant adjustment? *City & Community, 4*(1), 5–35.

Chiswick, B. R., Miller, P. W., Barkan, E. R., Diner, H., & Kraut, A. M. (2008). Immigrant enclaves, ethnic goods, and the adjustment process. In E. R. Barkan, H. Diner & A. M. Kraut (Eds.), *From arrival to incorporation: Migrants to the U.S. in a global era.* (pp. 80–93). New York: New York University Press.

Cuéllar, I., Arnold, B., & Maldonado, R. (1995). Acculturation rating scale for Mexican Americans-II: A revision of the original ARSMA Scale. *Hispanic Journal of Behavioral Sciences, 17*(3), 275–304.

Cuéllar, I., Bastida, E., & Braccio, S. M. (2004). Residency in the United States, subjective well-being, and depression in an older Mexican-origin sample. *Journal of Aging & Health, 16*(4), 447–466.

Díaz Briquets, S. (1995). Relationship between U.S. foreign policies and U.S. immigration policies. In M. S. Teitelbaum (Ed.), *Threatened peoples, threatened borders: World migration and U.S. policy* (pp. 160–189). New York, NY: WW Norton.

Donà, G., & Berry, J. W. (1994). Acculturation attitudes and acculturative stress of Central American refugees. *International Journal of Psychology, 29*(1), 57–70.

Drachman, D., & Shen-Ryan, A. (1991). Immigrants and refugees. In A. Gitterman (Ed.), *Handbook of social work practice with vulnerable populations* (pp. 618–646). New York, NY: Columbia University Press.

Engstrom, D. W. (2006). Outsiders and exclusion: Immigrants in the United States. In D. W. Engstrom & L. M. Piedra (Eds.), *Our diverse society: Race and ethnicity—Implications for 21st century American society* (pp. 19–36). Washington, DC: NASW Press.

Engstrom, D. W., & Okamura, A. (2004). Working with survivors of torture: Approaches to helping. *Families in Society: The Journal of Contemporary Social Services, 85*(3), 301–309.

Engstrom, D. W., & Piedra, L. M. (2005). Central American survivors of political violence: An examination of contextual factors and practice issues. *Mental health care for new Hispanic immigrants: Innovative approaches in contemporary clinical practice, 85*, 301-310.

Engstrom, D. W., & Piedra, L. M. (Eds.). (2006). *Our diverse society: Race and ethnicity—Implications for 21st century American society.* Washington, DC: NASW Press.

Escarce, J. J., Morales, L. S., & Rumbaut, R. G. (2006). The health status and health behaviors of Hispanics. In M. Tienda & F. Mitchell (Eds.), *Hispanics and the future of America* (pp. 362–409). Washington, DC: National Academies Press.

Escobar, J. I., & Vega, W. A. (2000). Mental health and immigration's AAAs: Where are we and where do we go from here? *Journal of Nervous & Mental Disease, 188*(11), 736–740.

Fix, M. E. (1999). Trends in noncitizens' and citizens' use of public benefits following welfare reform: 1994–97. Retrieved from http://www.urban.org/url.cfm?ID=408086

Fix, M. E., Zimmerman, W., & Passel, J. S. (2001). The integration of immigrant families in the United States. *Immigration studies: The integration of immigrant families in the United States.* Retrieved from http://www.urban.org/url.cfm?ID=410227

Fry, R. (2010). Minorities and the recession-era college enrollment boom. Retrieved August 1, 2010. Retrieved from http://pewresearch.org/topics/demography/.

Fuligni, A. J. (1998). Authority, autonomy, and parent-adolescent conflict and cohesion: A study of adolescents from Mexican, Chinese, Filipino, and European backgrounds. *Developmental Psychology, 34*(4), 782–792. doi:10.1037/0012-1649.34.4.782

Gans, H. J. (1999). Toward a reconciliation of "assimilation" and "pluralism": The interplay of acculturation and ethnic retention. In C. Hirschman, P. Kasinitz, & J. DeWinde (Eds.), *The handbook of international migration: The American experience* (pp. 161–169). New York, NY: Russell Sage Foundation.

Gil-Rivas, V., Greenberger, E., Chen, C., & Montero y Lopez-Lena, M. (2003). Understanding depressed mood in the context of a family-oriented culture. *Adolescence, 38*(149), 93.

Gonzales, N. A., Knight, G. P., Birman, D., & Sirolli, A. A. (2004). Acculturation and enculturation among Latino youth. In K. I. Maton, C. J. Schellenbach, B. J. Leadbeater, & A. L. Solarz (Eds.), *Investing in children, youth, families, and communities: Strengths-based research and policy* (pp. 285–302). Washington, DC: American Psychological Association.

Gordon, M. M. (1964). *Assimilation in America: The role of race, religion, and national origins.* New York, NY: Oxford University Press.

Gzesh, S. (2006). Central Americans and asylum policy in the Reagan era. *Migration Information Source.* Retrieved from http://www.migrationinformation.org/

Hernandez, D. J., & Charney, E. (1998). *From generation to generation: The health and well-being of children in immigrant families.* Washington, DC: National Academies Press.

Hernandez, M. (2005). Central American families. In M. McGoldrick, J. Giordano, & N. Garcia-Preto (Eds.), *Ethnicity and family therapy* (pp. 178–191).: Guilford Press.

Hondagneu-Sotelo, P. (1994). *Gendered transitions: Mexican experiences of immigration.* Berkeley: University of California Press.

Hovey, J. (1999). Psychosocial predictors of acculturative stress in Central American immigrants. *Journal of Immigrant Health, 1*(4), 187–194.

Hunt, L. M., Schneider, S., & Comer, B. (2004). Should "acculturation" be a variable in health research? A critical review of research on U.S. Hispanics. *Social Science & Medicine, 59*(5), 973–986.

Huntington, S. P. (2004a). The Hispanic challenge. *Foreign Policy* (March/April), 30–45.

Huntington, S. P. (2004b). *Who are we? The challenges to America's national identity.* New York, NY: Simon & Schuster.

Hwang, W. (2007). Acculturative family distancing: Theory, research, and clinical practice. *Psychotherapy: Theory/Research/Practice/Training, 43*(4), 397–409.

Jensen, L., & Portes, A. (1992). The enclave and the entrants: Patterns of ethnic enterprise in Miami before and after Mariel. *American Sociological Review, 57*(3), 411–414.

Jiménez, T. (2007). From newcomers to Americans: An integration policy for a nation of immigrants. *Immigration Policy in Focus, 5*(11), Retrieved from www.immigrationpolicy.org

Jiménez, T. (2008). Mexican immigrant replenishment and the continuing significance of ethnicity and race. *American Journal of Sociology, 113*(6), 1527–1567.

Keefe, S. E., Padilla, A. M., & Carlos, M. L. (1979). The Mexican-American extended family as an emotional support system. *Human Organization, 38*(2), 144–152.

Kitayama, S. (2006). Does self-esteem matter equally across cultures? In M. H. Kernis (Ed.), *Self-esteem issues and answers: A sourcebook of current perspectives* (pp. 376–382). New York, NY: Psychology Press.

LaFromboise, T. (1998). Psychological impact of biculturalism: Evidence and theory. In P. B. Organista, K. M. Chun, & G. Marín (Eds.), *Readings in ethnic psychology* (pp. 123–155). New York, NY: Routledge.

Lambert, W. E., & Taylor, D. M. (1990). Language and culture in the lives of immigrants and refugees. In W. H. Holtzman & T. H. Bornemann (Eds.), *Mental health of immigrants and refugees* (pp. 103–128). Austin, TX: Hogg Foundation for Mental Health.

Lara, M., Gamboa, C., Kahramanian, M., Morales, L., & Bautista, D. (2004). Acculturation and Latino health in the United States: A review of the literature and its sociopolitical context. *Annual Review of Public Health, 26*, 367-397.

Lara, M., Gamboa, C., Kahramanian, M. I., Morales, L. S., & Bautista, D. E. H. (2005). Acculturation and Latino health in the United States: A review of the literature and its sociopolitical context. *Annual Review of Public Health, 26*, 367–397.

Larrison, C. R., Velez-Ortiz, D., Hernandez, P. M., Piedra, L. M., & Goldberg, A. (2010). Brokering language and culture: Can ad hoc interpreters fill the language service gap at community health centers? *Social Work in Public Health, 25*(3), 387–407.

Levitt, P. (2003). Transnational villagers. In J. Stone & D. Rutledge (Eds.), *Race and ethnicity: Comparative and theoretical approaches* (pp. 260–273). Malden, MA: Wiley-Blackwell.

Lewis, M. A., & Widerquist, K. (2001). *Economics for social workers: The application of economic theory to social policy and the human services.* New York: Columbia University Press.

Lieberson, S. (1980). *A piece of the pie.* Berkeley: University of California Press.

Mangold, D. L., Veraza, R., Kinkler, L., & Kinney, N. A. (2007). Neuroticism predicts acculturative stress in Mexican American college students. *Hispanic Journal of Behavioral Sciences, 29*(3), 366–382.

Markus, H. R., & Kitayama, S. (1991). Culture and self: Implications for cognition, emotion, and motivation. *Psychological Review, 98*, 224–253.

Massey, D. (1987). Understanding Mexican migration to the United States. *American Journal of Sociology, 92*(6), 1372–1403.

Menendez, S. R. (2010). *Corporate diversity report.* Retrieved from http://menendez.senate.gov/newsroom/press/release/?id=e8a1d85f-b9f9-4cb2-97dc-0c724f0a1ed2

Mitchell, W. (1962). The Cuban refugee program. *Social Security Bulletin, 25,* 3.

Murphy, H. (2009). Migration, culture and mental health. *Psychological Medicine, 7*(4), 677–684.

Nazario, S. (2007). *Enrique's journey.* New York, NY: Random House.

Nguyen, H. H. (2006). Acculturation in the United States. In D. L. Sam & J. W. Berry (Eds.), *The Cambridge handbook of acculturation psychology* (pp. 311–330). New York, NY: Cambridge University Press.

Ogbu, J. U. (1993). Differences in cultural frame of reference. *International Journal of Behavioral Development, 16*(3), 483–506.

Park, R. E. (1928). Human migrations and the marginal man. *American Journal of Sociology, 33*, 881–893.

Piedra, L. M. (Ed.). (2006). Revisiting the language question. In D. W. Engstrom & L. M. Piedra (Eds.), *Our diverse society: Race and ethnicity—Implications for 21st century American society* (pp. 67–87). Washington, DC: NASW Press.

Piedra, L. M., & Engstrom, D. W. (2009). Segmented assimilation theory and the Life Model: An integrated approach to understanding immigrants and their children. *Social Work, 54*(3), 270–277.

Pine, B. A., & Drachman, D. (2005). Effective child welfare practice with immigrant and refugee children and their families. *Child Welfare Journal, 84*(5), 537–562.

Portes, A., & Jensen, L. (1987). What is an ethnic enclave? The case for conceptual clarity. *American Sociological Review, 52*(6), 768–771.

Portes, A., & Mozo, R. (1985). The political adaptation process of Cubans and other ethnic minorities in the United States: A preliminary analysis. *International Migration Review, 19*(1), 35–63.

Portes, A., & Rumbaut, G. (2001). *Legacies: The story of the immigrant second generation.* New York, NY: Russell Sage Foundation.

Portes, A., & Rumbaut, R. G. (2006). *Immigrant America: a portrait* (3rd ed.). Berkeley: University of California Press.

Portes, A., & Stepick, A. (1994). *City on the edge: The transformation of Miami.* Berkeley: University of California Press.

Redfield, R., Linton, R., & Herskovits, M. J. (1936). Memorandum on the study of acculturation. *American Anthropologist, 38,* 149–152.

Rogler, L. H., Cortes, D. E., & Malgady, R. G. (1991). Acculturation and mental health status among Hispanics: Convergence and new directions for research. *American Psychologist, 46,* 585–597.

Ross, L. (1977). The intuitive psychologist and his shortcomings: Distortions in the attribution process. *Advances in Experimental Social Psychology, 10,* 173–220.

Rudmin, F. W. (2009). Constructs, measurements and models of acculturation and acculturative stress. *International Journal of Intercultural Relations, 33*(2), 106–123.

Rumbaut, R. G. (1997). Assimilation and its discontents: Between rhetoric and reality. *International Migration Review, 31,* 923–960.

Rumbaut, R. G. (1995). Vietnamese, Laotian, and Cambodian Americans. In P. G. Min (Ed.), *Asian Americans: Contemporary trends and issues* (pp. 232–270). Thousand Oaks, CA: Sage.

Sabogal, F., Marín, G., Otero-Sabogal, R., & Marín, B. V. (1987). Hispanic familism and acculturation: What changes and what doesn't? *Hispanic Journal of Behavioral Sciences, 9*(4), 397–412.

Sam, D. L., & Oppedal, B. (2002). Acculturation as a developmental pathway. *Online Readings in Psychology and Culture* (Unit 8, Chapter 6). Retrieved from http://orpc.iaccp.org/index. php?option=com_content&view=article&id=90%3Asam&catid=26%3Achapter&Itemid=4.

Sassen, S. (1998). *Globalization and its discontents.* New York, NY: New Press.

Shweder, R. A. (2003). The Moral Challenge in Cultural Migration. In N. Foner (Ed.), *American Arrivals: Anthropology Engages the New Immigration.* Santa Fe: School of American Research Press.

Singer, A. (2004). Welfare reform and immigrants: A policy review. In P. Kretsedemas (Ed.), *Immigrants, welfare reform, and the poverty of policy* (pp. 21–34). Westport, CT: Praeger.

Skerry, P. (2004). Citizenship begins at home: A new approach to the civic integration of immigrants. *Responsive Community, 14*(1), 26–37.

Smart, J., & Smart, D. (1995). Acculturative stress of Hispanics: Loss and challenge. *Journal of Counseling & Development, 73,* 390–390.

Smokowski, P. R., David-Ferdon, C., & Stroupe, N. (2009). Acculturation and violence in minority adolescents: A review of the empirical literature. *Journal of Primary Prevention, 30*(3), 215–263.

Sowell, T. (1981). *Ethnic America: A history.* New York, NY: Basic Books.

Stonequist, E. V. (1935). The problem of marginal man. *American Journal of Sociology, 7,* 1–12.

Suárez, Z. E., & Perez, R. M. (in press). Cuban-American families. In R. Wright , C. H. Mindel, R. W. Habenstein & T. V. Tran (Eds.), Ethnic families in America: Patterns and variations (5th ed.). New York: Elsevier.

Sullivan, T. (2000). A demographic portrait. In P. S. J. Cafferty & D. W. Engstrom (Eds.), *Hispanics in the United States: An agenda for the twenty-first century.* New Brunswick, NJ: Transaction Publishers.

Sullivan, T. A. (2006). Demography, the demand for social services, and the potential for civic conflict. In D. W. Engstrom & L. M. Piedra (Eds.), *Our diverse society: Race and ethnicity— Implications for 21st century American society* (pp. 9–18). Washington, DC: NASW Press.

Szapocznik, J., & Kurtines, W. M. (1993, April). Family psychology and cultural diversity: Opportunities for theory, research, and application. *American Psychologist, 48*(4), 400–407.

Szapocznik, J., Rio, A., Perez-Vidal, A., Kurtines, W., Hervis, O., & Santisteban, D. (1986). Bicultural Effectiveness Training (BET): An experimental test of an intervention modality for families experiencing intergenerational/intercultural conflict. *Hispanic Journal of Behavioral Sciences, 8*(4), 303–330.

Szapocznik, J., Scopetta, M. A., Aranalde, M. A., & Kurtines, W. (1978). Cuban value structure: Treatment implications. *Journal of Consulting & Clinical Psychology, 46*(5), 961–970.

Torres, M. d. l. A. (2006). Democracy and diversity: Expanding notions of citizenship. In D. W. Engstrom & L. M. Piedra (Eds.), *Our diverse society: Race and ethnicity—Implications for 21st century American society* (pp. 161–182). Washington, DC: NASW Press.

Waldinger, R. (1999). *Still the promised city?: African-Americans and new immigrants in postindustrial New York.* Cambridge, MA: Harvard University Press.

Ward, C. (1996). Acculturation. In D. Landis & R. Bhagat (Eds.), *Handbook of intercultural training* (2nd ed., pp. 124–147). Newbury Park, CA: Sage.

Ward, C., & Kennedy, A. (1993). Where's the "culture" in cross-cultural transition? Comparative studies of sojourner adjustment. *Journal of Cross-Cultural Psychology, 24*(2), 221–249.

Ward, C., & Kennedy, A. (1994). Acculturation strategies, psychological adjustment, and sociocultural competence during cross-cultural transitions. *International Journal of Intercultural Relations, 18*(3), 329–343.

Ward, C., Landis, D., & Bhagat, R. S. (1996). *Acculturation handbook of intercultural training* (2nd ed.) (pp. 124–147). Thousand Oaks, CA: Sage.

Warner, W. L., & Srole, L. (1945). *The social systems of American ethnic groups.* New Haven, CT: Yale University Press.

Weissbrodt, D. S., & Danielson, L. (2005). *Immigration law and procedure in a nutshell* (5th ed.). St. Paul, MN: Thomson/West.

Wilson, K., & Portes, A. (1980). Immigrant enclaves: An analysis of the labor market experiences of Cubans in Miami. *American Journal of Sociology, 86*(2), 295–319.

Zane, N., & Mak, W. (2003). Major approaches to the measurement of acculturation among ethnic minority populations: A content analysis and an alternative empirical strategy. In K. M. Chun, P. Balls Organista, & G. Marín (Eds.), *Acculturation: Advances in theory, measurement, and applied research* (pp. 39–60). Washington, DC: American Psychological Association.

Zhou, M., & Logan, J. R. (1989). Returns on human capital in ethnic enclaves: New York City's Chinatown. *American Sociological Review, 54*(5), 809–820.

Chapter 3
Building Response Capacity: The Need for Universally Available Language Services

Lissette M. Piedra, Flavia C. D. Andrade and Christopher R. Larrison

Abstract In this chapter, we discuss how the size and composition of the foreign-born Latino population and its dispersion throughout the United States create difficulties in the navigation of complex mental health and health care systems, yielding unfortunate consequences for individuals, their families, and communities. Given the challenges posed by the increasing number of people needing linguistically accessible services and the lack of a bilingual workforce, we use the idea of "building response capacity" as the central theme for this chapter. We argue that such a capacity must be multifaceted and grounded on demographic trends, sound social policy, and the institutional, cultural, and social context of health care delivery.

At the beginning of the twenty-first century, social tensions produced by immigration and growing language diversity are high. Perhaps at no other point in US history has the issue of language required such careful reflection and planning. There has been a large influx of new immigrants in the past four decades, and we have witnessed their unprecedented dispersal across the United States (Lichter and Johnson 2006; Durand et al. 2006; see also Chap. 1). Given the challenges posed by the increasing number of people needing linguistically accessible services and the lack of a bilingual workforce, solutions for building a response capacity must be multifaceted and grounded on demographic trends, sound social policy, and the institutional, cultural, and social context of health care delivery.

Any discussion about language diversity underscores two significant societal issues: (a) the right of all individuals to access mental health and health care, and (b) society's responsibility to guarantee that access. By this measure, Partida's indictment that "the absence of universally available language services is a national healthcare system failure (Partida 2007, p. 347)" simultaneously strikes at the core of the problem and offers a promising solution. She argues that instead of relying on the piecemeal efforts of individual institutions, providers, and health care plans, the solutions must be population-based (Partida 2007). She challenges us to imagine

L. M. Piedra (✉)
School of Social Work, University of Illinois at Urbana-Champaign, Champaign, IL, USA
e-mail: lmpiedra@illinois.edu

a system that invests in coordinated, population-based efforts to create universal access to language services in mental health and health care. Toward this end, we have borrowed her idea of "building response capacity" as the central theme for this chapter. Although we focus on Spanish speakers, many of the points discussed in this chapter apply to other linguistic minorities as well.

Three points frame the discussion throughout the chapter. First, the size and composition of the foreign-born Latino population and its dispersion throughout the United States are discussed. The problems posed by growing numbers of immigrants with limited English proficiency (LEP), who have difficulty accessing and navigating complex mental health and health care systems, yield unfortunate consequences not just for individuals but for their families and communities as well. The most stark manifestations of language tensions are found in those communities with new immigrant settlements whose small population size necessarily constrains the diversity of services offered (Cunningham et al. 2006; Elder et al. 2009; Sullivan 2006). Second, we draw attention to the sociopolitical context and the existing legal framework, both of which foster an ambivalent response to the heightened need for linguistically accessible services (Chen et al. 2007; Ku and Flores 2005; Piedra 2006, 2010). Finally, we explore staff- and agency-level solutions to creating language-accessible services by focusing on ways to improve the quality of interpretation and enhance its effect on the professional relationship between provider and client (Davidson 2000; Elderkin-Thompson et al. 2001; Flores 2005a; Flores et al. 2003).

Demographic Trends in the Latino Population: Language Implications for Services

Demographic trends have profound consequences for the kinds of mental health and health services, many communities will need (Caldwell et al. n.d.; Schneider et al. 2006; Sullivan 2006). Indeed, Latinos are experiencing dramatic demographic changes, and these will profoundly influence their service needs. In 2008, there were approximately 18 million Latino immigrant and 29 million native-born Latinos (Pew Hispanic Center 2010). Although fertility drives the current Latino population growth (Durand et al. 2006), high levels of immigration from Mexico and other parts of Latin America have contributed to rapid population change and, consequently, to an increased need for language-accessible services. As of 2005, nearly one-fourth (23%) of children live in immigrant families (Hernandez et al. 2008). As the baby boomer population approaches retirement, Latino immigrants and their native-born children will be poised to fill new jobs and support an aging population (Alba 2009; Sullivan 2006).

These population changes may prove to be a double-edged sword. On the one hand, the heightened immigration rates and the high birth rates of immigrants in the last decades relieve the United States of the inadequate population replacement plaguing other industrialized nations (Christie 2009). On the other hand, capacities of future labor forces rest on current social conditions. In this light, the outlook is cautionary: Latinos are younger, poorer, and less educated than the average population (Pew Hispanic Center 2010; see also Chap. 1). Because this group will one day make up nearly a quarter of the future labor force (Hernandez et al. 2008), investments in its health and well-being will become critical for strengthening the US economy in the coming decades. For many new immigrants, language proves to be a linchpin in the quest for upward social mobility and greater social inclusion—for entire families as well as for individuals (Borjas 2006).

Latinos with LEP and Their Children

Although concern rightfully centers on those directly affected by linguistically inaccessible mental health and health services, less attention is paid to those indirectly affected: namely, the children in immigrant families, who comprise the fastest growing segment of the child population (Hernandez 2004; Hernandez et al. 2008; Mather 2009). Because human beings live in families and are influenced by the context of institutions and communities in which they live, the well-being of each individual can affect family members; in some cases, these effects radiate across generations. For example, second-generation Latinos (i.e., the native-born of at least one immigrant parent) account for the majority of children in immigrant families (Fry and Passel 2009; Mather 2009). This suggests that for many Latino children—those projected to make up 23% of the US labor force growth from 2000 to 2020 (Mather 2009)—the tensions of language are part of everyday life and cut across multiple institutional sectors.

Data from 2008 show that most of the adult foreign-born population (72% or 11.9 million) have LEP (Pew Hispanic Center 2010). As with many demographic trends, the rates of LEP raise concerns for the children of immigrants. A quarter of preschool-age children are English-language learners (ELL), which is another way to say LEP, and more than half have at least one parent who is an ELL (Fortuny et al. 2010). Among children of Mexican and Central American origin, the rate of having at least one ELL parent jumps to 81% and 71%, respectively.

During a health crisis, the consequences of living in a household in which none of the adults speak English very well can be deadly, as illustrated by the case of Gricelda Zamora, a 13-year-old girl who died of a ruptured appendix after being misdiagnosed with gastritis (Scioscia 2000). Gricelda, who was bilingual, often served as an interpreter for her parents (Chen et al. 2007). When she was brought to the emergency room, Gricelda was too ill to communicate on her own behalf, and her parents, who spoke only Spanish, could not communicate with the hospital staff. Unable to provide the Zamoras with an interpreter, the family and the hospital staff relied on ad hoc interpreters and sent Gricelda home with instructions for her family to schedule a doctor's appointment within three days. The child died two days later. As highlighted by Gricelda's case, the potential dire consequences of linguistic isolation are heightened by the lack of English ability among adults in the household.

Growing Older Adult Population

At the other end of the life spectrum, service providers will find that language needs of older adults, which they already struggle to meet, will become a central and pressing issue. In the coming decades, the overall proportion of older adults (65 and over) is expected to increase from 6% in 2010 to 15% in 2050 (U.S. Census Bureau 2004). Similar to the general population, the growth rates among adult Latinos will be faster in comparison to the aging rate of the young population (U.S. Census Bureau 2004). However, unlike the general population, the aging Latino population will encounter particular challenges related to language. For many foreign-born older adults who have acquired proficiency in English, the cognitive decline that naturally accompanies the aging process often leads them to revert to the native language (McMurtray et al. 2009). The existence of such a phenomenon on a large scale creates difficulties for mental health and health providers—even for those with Spanish-language competencies—in delivering adequate care to these special populations (Vega et al. 2007).

The increase in this segment of the population will accentuate the social and economic disadvantages among the foreign-born and pose challenges to mental health and health care systems that are already encumbered with an increased demand for culturally and linguistically competent providers. Therefore, the growing number of older Latinos and the high number of immigrants and their children living in linguistic isolation underscore the urgency of providing linguistically accessible services. The increased need for services is particularly concerning because the demand for these services already often outstrips supply (Barrio et al. 2008; Clemans-Cope and Kenney 2007; Schur and Albers 1996). Service needs are particularly acute in communities with new immigrant populations, a topic we take up next.

New-Growth Communities

The geographic dispersion of the Latino population presents a significant challenge in the provision of linguistically accessible services. Even though most Latinos live in large cities within traditional immigration states, a relocation process to new destination areas is underway and growing fast (Fortuny et al. 2010; Fry 2008). Between 1996 and 2003, the total Latino population grew by about 10 million, or 35%, spreading out evenly across the nation (Cunningham et al. 2006). In "new-growth" communities (i.e., those with small but rapidly growing Latino populations), the proportion of Latinos almost doubled, with some areas experiencing even more pronounced growth (Suro and Singer 2002; see also Chap. 1).

Similar to other demographic trends, the effects of this geographic dispersion ripple through families and communities. The proportion of young children living in 22 new-growth states increased from 12% to 23% between 1990 and 2008 (Fortuny et al. 2010). Although the percentage of the Latino population in these areas remains relatively small, their growing number presents serious problems for communities lacking resources to meet their needs (Arroyo 2004). In the context of high numbers of immigrants and shifting settlement patterns, language issues that arise in the provision of mental health and health care are garnering increased local and national attention.

The Influence of Language Barriers on Access to Mental Health and Health Care

The current demographic trends are prompting us to move language proficiency to the forefront as critical to the quality of mental health and health care (Harmsen et al. 2008; Ponce et al. 2006). Legally mandating language services, though critical, has proven insufficient as a strategy to facilitate access (Ginde et al. 2009). Overwhelming evidence exists that language barriers persist and negatively influence access to services. For instance, non-English-speaking Latinos have significantly lower odds of receiving mental health services than their English-speaking counterparts (Sentell et al. 2007)—a particularly troubling finding even though immigrant Latinos have a lower need for mental health services than native-born Latinos (Alegría et al. 2007). For the smaller number of immigrant Latinos who need mental health services, LEP Latinos are significantly less likely to receive care.

Linguistic minorities are less likely than English speakers to receive adequate health information, undergo screening services, be referred to a specialist, or engage in preventive medical and mental health services (for a review on health disparities in the Latino population, see Vega et al. 2009). Traditionally, low socioeconomic status, low insurance coverage rates, and undocumented legal status have been associated with lower rates of health care access among Latinos; however, health disparities remain after these factors are taken into account (DuBard et al. 2006; Jerant et al. 2008; Kirk et al. 2005; Kramer et al. 2004; Reimann et al. 2004). Language barriers are likely to play a role in these disparities. Latinos, particularly those who are Spanish monolingual, report less satisfaction with their health care providers and with their access to health care than their English-speaking counterparts (Morales et al. 1999; Wallace and Villa 2003). Language barriers complicate their ability to understand medical terminology and can potentially undermine treatment adherence because they have difficulty accepting the validity of the diagnosis and the treatment plan and in complying with treatment plans (Davidson 2000; Wilson et al. 2005). Should LEP patients prefer a Spanish-speaking doctor, they are likely to have their treatment delayed (Insaf et al. 2010), further contributing to an unequal burden of disease, including disparities in mental health, dental health, and occupational health (Mui et al. 2007; Premji et al. 2008; Sentell et al. 2007). Therefore, those who do not speak English well have more unmet service needs and worse self-rated health (Borrell and Crawford 2006; Sentell et al. 2007).

Taken together, demographic trends and service disparities among linguistic minorities create the need for broader cultural changes to accommodate the language needs of emerging populations (Partida 2007). Although one can hardly contest the role language plays in erecting service barriers to mental health and health care, many in the United States, including health care professionals, are ambivalent about the cultural implications of responding to the needs of linguistic minorities (Flores 2005b). Arguably, service disparities arise within a larger historical, geographic, sociocultural, economic, and political context (Williams and Jackson 2005). Consequently, understanding the sociocultural backdrop that underlies language concerns can be useful to practitioners, administrators, and policymakers in developing strategies for building greater response capacity (Piedra 2006, 2010).

Sociopolitical Context of Language Services

The United States has a long history both of accepting immigrants into the country and of expecting them to learn English. This expectation is culturally American, rooted partly in myths about assimilation and partly in the economic necessity to function in the dominant language. Even so, the United States has always been a multilingual society (Sollors 1998). Foreign-language presses, in fact, played a vital role in immigrant communities throughout the nineteenth and early twentieth centuries. Hardly an outdated oddity, linguistic diversity remains a feature in our country's landscape: The 2000 census identified 380 single languages or language families spoken in the United States (Shin 2003).

Yet, despite the presence of multiple languages, English dominance prevails, with a corresponding national pride arising from this fact. Globalization, the Internet, and smart phones further reinforce English dominance (Saha and Fernandez 2007). Thus, many Spanish-speaking immigrants encounter a larger social context that reflects the mixed feelings of its citizens about the legitimacy of bilingual services. This ambivalence is reflected in our laws, in the fact that we spend too few resources to provide linguistically accessible services, and in mental health and health professionals' perceptions of bilingual services. Some may wonder privately, "Why don't they just learn English?" (Flores 2005b).

Indeed, such a question begs another: "How much accommodation is too much?" Linguistically accessible services are really about institutional access, and about the extent to which society must change to accommodate those needs (Partida 2007; Piedra 2006). After the Zamora tragedy, one emergency-department clinician bristled at the idea that it was the health community's responsibility to provide language-accessible services (O'Beirne 2000). In a letter to the editor, he raised the question of whether, in the presence of an interpreter program, "is it really the responsibility of the medical community to take it upon ourselves to be yet more 'consumer-friendly'?" Rather, he advised readers that "if you have trouble in the ER (Emergency Room) or any situation because you don't speak English, *learn English*, and do it soon. Until then, at least try to bring along a bilingual friend or family member."

Some providers believe that offering language access creates both a financial drain and an incentive that attracts more LEP patients. For example, the costs and burdens associated with language services are unevenly distributed across providers, unlike the costs of providing usual care (Ku and Flores 2005). Communities with high immigrant concentrations will have a greater need to provide language assistance than those with lower levels. Accordingly, special-interest groups such as the American Medical Association have raised concerns over the financial burden of providing interpretation services (Ku and Flores 2005).

As reflected in a growing chorus of anecdotal evidence, a strong national bias in favor of English means that we frequently underestimate the difficulties of moving between two languages in different service contexts (Engstrom et al. 2009; Piedra 2010; Saha and Fernandez 2007). Conversational language skills, for instance, are mistaken for fluency in professional terminology (Engstrom et al. 2009; Piedra 2010). Such mistakes reflect a poor understanding of the complexity of the interpreted interaction and lead providers to lose sight of the additional roles the interpreter plays (e.g., advocate, cultural broker, team member, co-diagnostician) that can either facilitate or interfere with the accuracy of the exchange (Hsieh 2006a, 2006b, 2007). Our underestimation of the public's language needs and of the complexity of language services is reflected in legislation that establishes no expectations that mental health and health providers should learn how to work with interpreters and, further, offers few opportunities for ongoing training for interpreters. Moreover, existing language laws mandate the right to language access, but do not provide funds for implementation or enforcement, impeding accountability (Butera et al. 2000). Even more troubling, the laws as they stand may create institutional disincentives to expand language services and fail to promote the coordination of language access.

Legal Framework for Language Services

Our current legal framework mandates language access for mental health and health care settings that receive federal funds such as Medicare. Specifically, the federal government stipulates, through Title VI of the Civil Rights Act of 1964, that no person should "on the grounds of race, color, or national origin, be excluded from participation in, be denied the benefits of, or be subject to discrimination under any program or activity receiving Federal financial assistance" (Civil Rights Act of 1964, Sect. 601). Although this legislation does not specifically mention language, because those with LEP tend to be foreign-born, the denial of services due to language barriers is seen as a violation of Title VI and the Civil Rights Act of 1964 (Snowden et al. 2007). The subsequent Executive Order (EO) 13166 and related policy guidelines reaffirm the spirit of Title VI and the Civil Rights Act of 1964 (Snowden et al. 2007).

EO 13166, "Improving Access to Services for Persons with Limited English Proficiency," extends beyond those programs that receive federal funding and directs all federal agencies to ensure that their programs provide equal access to LEP persons. Although EO 13166 has enjoyed bipartisan support, the accompanying Policy Guidance balances federal mandates for language-assisted services with the need of small business, local governments, and small nonprofit organizations to remain solvent (Chen et al. 2007). Most states have responded by enacting "threshold policies," which set a minimum number of speakers of a language that, when exceeded, triggers a variety of programmatic steps to accommodate the group's language-related needs (Snowden et al. 2007). Although these policies are important legal protections for linguistic minorities, they are increasingly being shown to be insufficient. For example, since 2001, Massachusetts state law has dictated that emergency department (ED) patients with LEP have the right to a professional interpreter. However, researchers found that one year later, among the 11% of ED patients who had significant language barriers, the use of professional medical interpreters remained low (Ginde et al. 2009). Part of the reason for this finding reflects the more extensive assessment used by researchers to determine significant language barriers compared to that of treating clinicians. Even so, the discrepancy in assessments and the persistence of unmet need underscore the limitations of legal mandates.

The lack of federal funds associated with EO 13166 creates a serious obstacle to its implementation. Although EO 13166 technically is not an unfunded mandate, no federal funds have been set aside for its implementation (Snowden et al. 2007). Therefore, based on this executive order, programs that receive federal funding (e.g., Medicare) must provide language assistance for clients who need it, but do not receive additional resources to help meet that obligation. They must find the means to comply, with the added constraint that private insurers usually do not pay or reimburse for interpretation services, written translations, or telephone language lines (Ku and Flores 2005). Moreover, neither EO 13166 nor the accompanying Policy Guidance provides any direction on how to develop a coordinated nationwide system to address language barriers. Thus, in the end, these services are provided half-heartedly, with language assistance varying by state, region, language, medical condition, and institution (Chen et al. 2007).

Barriers to the Provision of Linguistically Accessible Mental Health and Health Care

The problems posed by language barriers have drawn increased attention to the need for bilingual providers (Chapa and Acosta 2010). However, there is a growing recognition that developing a bilingual workforce large enough to meet the increasing need for language services will entail a long-term effort (Chapa and Acosta 2010). In light of the limited pool of bilingual providers, organizations usually respond to Title VI and EO 13166 by providing translated written materials and interpreters. Although both are necessary resources for LEP clients, they often prove insufficient to overcome language barriers independent of other efforts (Gregg and Saha 2007). Translated literature requires a level of literacy that may render the information inaccessible to immigrants with low levels of formal education (Cunningham et al. 2006).

In addition, the lack of funds and regulatory oversight has led to the use of "ad hoc" interpreters: individuals who are chosen due to convenience (e.g., janitor, family member, volunteer, and dual-role staff) but may have limited or no professional training as medical interpreters. Increasingly, scholars underscore the problems associated with untrained interpreters (Flores et al. 2003), such as tensions in the types of roles an interpreter should assume during the interpreted encounter, and ethical issues related to the interpreters' degree of discretionary power during the interpretation session (Hsieh 2007, 2008). To build universally responsive systems, it is important for providers to understand how the presence of an interpreter adds complexity to clinical encounters and how to avoid the pitfalls of unreflectively use of interpreters who are untrained, dual-function staff, or family members.

The Triad Relationship

In language-concordant services, both the service provider and the client use the dominant language as the common context of exchange. The presence of an interpreter transforms this two-way relationship into a triadic relationship, altering the dynamics of the interaction between the provider and the client (Sluzki 1978). In a triadic relationship, all parties involved in the interpretation (i.e., the client, the service provider, and the interpreter) must cooperate to create a common context of exchange and minimize translation error. For example, one study, which found communication errors in 50% of the encounters interpreted by bilingual nurses, also found that these errors were not random; they reflected interaction patterns among the health care provider, the dual-role staff member, and the patient (Elderkin-Thompson et al. 2001). Miscommunication occurred when interpretations did not match what the patient had actually said. Instead, the interpretations reflected the nurse-interpreter's clinical expectations. In some cases, the nurse-interpreters slanted their interpretations unfavorably against the patient, undermining the patient's credibility. Physicians contributed to inaccuracies in interpretation by not verifying information when presented with contradictory data. Patients compounded the problem by using cultural metaphors to explain or describe symptoms.

Successful interpretations also showed discernible communication patterns (Elderkin-Thompson et al. 2001). In these interpretations, nurse-interpreters translated the data as completely as possible so that the physician could extract relevant clinical information. The physician used simple sentences and presented them slowly and systematically. Patients were encouraged by the doctor to provide additional information. Physicians verified the accuracy of the interpretation by summarizing their perception of the problem, requesting an interpretation of that summary back to the patient, and checking for the patient's assent. In addition, the nurse-interpreters and physicians used nonverbal communication cues such as eye contact, smiling, and nodding to establish rapport with the patient. In other words, *all three actors* contributed to the accuracy of interpretations.

Arguably, triadic cooperation requires a recognition that interpreter-mediated communications are dynamic situations in which each person is more than a conduit/receptor of language (Hsieh 2006a, b). It also requires a recognition that the reduction of language barriers requires a coordinated effort among all three parties. Thus, a successful partnership necessitates that the health care professional and interpreter agree on the roles the interpreter can assume, the style of interpretation, the communicative goals for each interpreted encounter, and the strategies for meeting those goals (Beeber et al. 2009; Davidson 2000; Hsieh 2006a, 2006b, 2007, 2008). When handled sensitively, the process can strengthen the patient's trust in the care he or she is receiving, an important factor in treatment adherence (Kimbrough 2007).

The Importance of Assessing Language Skills

Organizations commonly use dual-role staff—bilingual persons who function both as a health care provider (though typically not as a physician) and as an interpreter (Elderkin-Thompson et al. 2001; Engstrom & Min 2004; Engstrom et al. 2009; Moreno et al. 2007). Much like family members, such workers lack training in interpretation protocols, may not be fluent in either English or the second language, or may be unfamiliar with technical terminology in one of the languages (Engstrom et al. 2009; Moreno et al. 2007). In the absence of professionally trained interpreters, assessing the language skills of dual-role staff is critical. These assessment practices transmit an important message to the broader members of the organization that language skills vary and that the clinical encounter requires a high level of language ability. Importantly, language assessments discourage the inappropriate use of dual-staff by monolingual staff.

In one study, researchers assessed the language skills of staff who were also working as medical interpreters. They found that one in five (20%) had insufficient bilingual skills to serve as an interpreter in a medical encounter (Moreno et al. 2007). The researchers measured comprehension, completeness, and vocabulary in both English and the second language, and then scored the assessment for three possible outcomes: not passing, passing at the basic interpreter level, and passing at the medical interpreter level. Staff who did not pass possessed a limited ability to read, write, and speak *either* English or the second language. Those who passed at the basic level could manage conversational exchanges such as scheduling an appointment or conveying general information, but lacked sufficient fluency in both languages to interpret for a clinical encounter. Staff whose language skills were at the medical interpreter level demonstrated enough language skills to assist in clinical encounters. Interestingly, participants in this large organization appreciated having their skill level tested. These language assessments eliminate the pressure placed on those who have limited language skills to serve as interpreters when there are few other alternatives (Engstrom et al. 2009; Moreno et al. 2007).

Consequences of the Unreflective Use of Interpreters

Although the assessment of language skills matters, the fact that LEP patients may rely on the interpreter to serve as a cultural broker or as an advocate increases the potential for miscommunication, especially if the interpreter feels compelled to assume roles outside of his or her expertise (Beeber et al. 2009; Hsieh 2006a, 2006b, 2007, 2008). When interpreters feel pressure—either from the patient, the provider, or both—to go beyond their expertise, they may act as co-diagnosticians or may omit information in an effort to save time (Hsieh 2007). Providers who are unaware of this possibility might unreflectively use interpreters and naively assume that the encounters are interpreted accurately. In doing so, providers undermine the value of their expertise and lower the quality of service. In such cases, the interpreter can leverage power by serving as the center of negotiation and exchange between the client and the professional (Davidson 2000; Kaufert et al. 1985). For example, one study found that interpreters, responding to time constraints, would manage the interpreted encounter by engaging in parallel dialogue with the patient and the doctor, summarizing content, *and* deciding which information and questions would be directly interpreted (Davidson 2000). When the researcher compared the number of patient questions answered by the physician in language-concordant encounters to those answered in interpreted encounters, he found that more than half of the questions in the interpreted encounters went unanswered because the interpreter had not forwarded the patient's questions to the doctor (Davidson 2000).

When mental health and health providers allow interpreters to act as the center of language exchange instead of as facilitators, there are serious consequences. Findings reveal that when interpreters have the power to decide what to translate and how to translate it, they tend to significantly reduce and revise speech, compromising the provider–client relationship (Aranguri et al. 2006; Beeber et al. 2009; Davidson 2000). Some of the content and meaning lost in interpreted encounters included conversational niceties that generate "small talk" and facilitate rapport between patient and provider (Aranguri et al. 2006). Such alterations negatively affect the emotional engagement of these two parties, and hinder the provider's ability to collect relevant social history and clinical data (Aranguri et al. 2006). Studies by Davidson et al. illustrate that despite laws mandating the right to language access, providers frequently misunderstand their responsibility (Chen et al. 2007) and fail to recognize the importance of learning to work with interpreters (Hsieh 2006b).

Building Response Capacity for Language Accessibility

The serious shortage of bilingual providers and professional medical interpreters continually threatens the quality of care for Latinos (Chapa and Acosta 2010; Vega and Lopez 2001). The limited opportunities to hire bilingual providers and professionally trained interpreters create incentives for health and social service administrators to use family members, friends, and paraprofessional staff as ad hoc interpreters (Casey et al. 2004). In turn, unreflectively using interpreters, underestimating the challenges in interpreted clinical encounters, dedicating insufficient resources to this task, and poor administrative planning undermine language access to high-quality services. Although these obstacles pose serious problems, they are surmountable. Consistent with Partida (2007), we argue for building response capacity by promoting greater communicative competence within mental health and health agencies, across health care systems, and for all health care professionals.

Communicative Competence

To achieve accurate communication exchanges between providers and patients, it is important to distinguish between communicative and linguistic competence. Increasingly, researchers recognize that straightforward language interpretation during a clinical encounter is necessary but not always sufficient to overcome barriers to care (Gregg and Saha 2007). Communicative competence includes the ability to recognize how the context shapes the meanings of words (Gregg and Saha 2007; Imberti 2007). Specifically, it includes everything that is commonly referred to as *cultural competence*, that is, having the knowledge, awareness, and skills to make services culturally relevant and effective (Marsiglia and Kulis 2009). Gregg and Saha (2007, p. 369) drew on linguist Gumperz's definition of communicative competence:

> Whereas linguistic competence covers the speaker's ability to produce grammatically correct sentences, communicative competence describes his [or her] ability to select, from the totality of grammatically correct expressions available to him [or her], forms which appropriately reflect the social norms governing behavior in specific encounters (Gumperz 1972).

This subtle distinction between linguistic competence and communicative competence is critical in managing language issues in a clinical encounter. For example, Hsieh (2008) noted that interpreters varied their roles and interpreting style to achieve a particular communication goal between provider and patient (e.g., fostering the provider–patient relationship). She noted that even when interpreters assumed a conduit role (translating word for word) to create the illusion of a dyadic provider–patient exchange, they would deviate from that strict conduit role and assume the role of facilitator to achieve the more important goal of fostering a two-way communication pattern between the providers and the patient. For example, they would maintain a first-person singular interpreting style (i.e., speaking as if he or she were the original speaker), even when the provider used second-person speech (Hsieh 2008). Hsieh's transcript excerpt illustrates a provider asking, "Is she taking any medication?" being translated as "Are you taking any medication?" (p. 1372). Because language, as a dynamic communication medium, includes much more than a system of words and grammatical rules, its utility rests more in the meaning conveyed than in the words used (Gregg and Saha 2007). Communicative competence requires attention to language *and* to contextual factors that shapes its meaning, including social status and group identity. Thus, although the aforementioned interpretation is linguistically inaccurate, the meaning conveyed (the doctor asking a direct question) captures the communication intent.

As the previous example illustrates, achieving communicative competence in interpreted encounters requires a coordinated effort among the members in the triadic relationship. The physician who understands how to work effectively with interpreters would not frame questions to a patient in the second person (asking the question of the interpreter rather than of the patient). By speaking to the interpreter instead of to the patient, the physician created a scenario in which the interpreter had to choose between the role of language conduit and relationship facilitator. In certain circumstances, referring to a patient in the second person could lead the interpreter to take on the role of co-diagnostician. Arguably, the nature of interpretation will create situations in which interpreters must assume roles other than that of a language conduit. However, the lack of awareness among providers of ways to communicate competently within an interpreted encounter creates an additional and unnecessary layer of complexity for interpreters and patients. Given the role of language in limiting access to services, in the next section we focus on organizational practices that enhance communicative competence in interpreted encounters.

Organizational Support for Communicative Competence

Mental health and health agencies can help create an organizational context for communication competence by institutionalizing rules that focus on enhancing interactions between medical professionals and clients. Because formal rules exert direct influence on beliefs and behaviors, these rules influence how service providers and clients relate (Glisson et al. 2006; Muldrow et al. 2002). The establishment of formal rules that apply to all patient communications also helps to create an organizational culture that fosters communication competency. Although LEP clients have specific language needs, many other clients with low levels of education and/or literacy need help with provider–patient communications. Thus, organizations that encourage communication competence are facilitating a solution-focused approach to communication rather than merely the identification of communication barriers specific to LEP clients.

The Commonwealth Fund and Kaiser Permanente have identified five key organizational practices that help improve health care agencies' communicative competence with clients (Barrett et al. 2008). First, agency administrators and staff must recognize that a team effort begins at the front desk, where services are coordinated. Second, mental health and health agencies should use standardized communication tools. Most clinicians are unfamiliar with existing communication strategies, such as Teach Back, Ask Me 3, or Motivational Interviewing, that have been found effective in enhancing communication (for a discussion of these strategies, see Appendix D in Barrett et al. 2008). Third, at every point possible, staff should use plain language, face-to-face communications, pictorials, and educational materials. For example, the *Hablamos Juntos* Project—an organization sponsored by the Robert Wood Johnson Foundation to improve communication between health care providers and their patients with LEP—encourages the use of universal health care symbols as part of an overall system that aids diverse populations in navigating a health care system with ease and comfort (Berger n.d.). Such symbols are useful for linguistically diverse populations and for English speakers with low literacy skills. Fourth, providers and interpreters should collaborate with clients to achieve communication goals; fifth, administrators should create an organizational environment in which high levels of health literacy in clients are not assumed (Barrett et al. 2008).

A Coordinated System of Interpretation

The implementation of the aforementioned organizational practices would enhance the quality of care for the general patient population, not only those with LEP. To be optimally effective with the LEP population, organizational policies must go beyond by making the best use of limited resources and having targeted mandates. Given the problems associated with using interpreters, an argument could be made that adherence to Title VI and EO 13166 *includes* the design of communications protocols—which will vary by specialization—and the creation of training programs for all mental health and health professionals who work with LEP clients on *how to work with interpreters* (Hsieh 2006b). Such an approach would be part of a coordinated system of interpretation. In a coordinated system of interpretation, organizations would provide language skills assessments for all employees used as interpreters, and would have guidelines for matching those skills with appropriate tasks. Moreover, all service providers would have access to protocols for those working with interpreters, which would include guidelines for ensuring accuracy during an interpreted clinical encounter. In the same way that organizations require ethics and safety trainings, mental health and health staff could be trained on how to work with interpreters and how to use alternative communication or interpretation methods in the absence of trained interpreters. This latter point is particularly important because service providers often underestimate the value of remote forms of interpretation services such as telephone, video (Cunningham et al. 2008), and remote simultaneous medical interpreting, a strategy used by the United Nations (Gany et al. 2007a, 2007b).

In addition to leading to better treatment outcomes and satisfaction with services, a coordinated system of interpreters could lower the overall cost of health care by increasing the effectiveness of services provided. Therefore, under a coordinated system of interpretation, communication competence would go beyond hiring an adequate number of interpreters and providing translated materials. The overarching goal would be the efficient use of existing resources by all staff members throughout the organization, such that high level of communicative competence is achieved in clinical encounters with all patients. Thus, major investments for a coordinated system of interpretation would be offset by improvements in the health and well-being of current patients (Jacobs et al. 2007). In the long term, this would benefit society at large by optimizing health and well-being in the population, and ensuring a productive labor force.

Organizational Climate That Encourages a Proactive Use of Interpreters

Whereas operational policies and procedures formally regulate activities within an organization, the organizational climate influences behavior through a shared set of expectations, unwritten rules, and social mores (Frederickson 1966; Glisson 2000). When administrators pay attention to the organizational climate, they become more aware of discretionary practices that interpreters may employ to accommodate (a) the organization's needs to save time, (b) the patient's needs for advocacy, and (c) their own need to save face when uncertain about an interpretation (Hsieh 2008). In the latter case, a health care setting with a coordinated approach to interpretation might develop an organizational climate in which a provider anticipates content that might be difficult to interpret. In such a context, the provider would cue the interpreter accordingly, signaling the appropriateness of seeking clarification before conveying the information (Hsieh 2008).

The cultivation of such an organizational climate is multifaceted. The literature suggests that the training, perceived role, and length of employment of interpreters may influence their relationship with the organizations they work for and the clients they serve (Flores 2005a; Karliner et al. 2007). Supervision of interpreters and providers is another conduit through which organizations can foster formal expectations and informal attitudes that support compliance with established protocols (Beeber et al. 2009). In addition, the use of positive feedback to reinforce attitudes should not be underestimated. One study found that when health providers were shown evidence of patients' satisfaction with interpretive services, their attitude toward those services changed and there was an increase in use (Cunningham et al. 2008). Because it is impossible to establish formal rules to cover all the possible scenarios that might emerge, the organization's climate plays an essential role in creating a context in which professional staff, interpreters, and clients *collaborate* with one another to maximize communicative competence.

Planning for the Future

An immediate strategy toward building response capacity would be to train current health and mental health care professionals on how to work with interpreters, and to require interpreters to undergo a universal certification program that would include specific standards for interpretation (Vega and Lopez 2001). Several training programs already in existence could serve as models and foundations for this expansion of efforts. Perhaps the most ambitious plan for building response capacity is the development of a coordinated system of interpreters across mental health and health organizations in a given geographic region (Partida 2007). Such an approach would require the pooling of resources from multiple organizations and the development of a system for sharing those resources efficiently and equitably.

Technology, such as use of telephone and video conferencing, and the coordinated translation of materials and documents would play a central role in the provision of interpretation services. Patients in new-growth communities would benefit immediately from such an approach.

Another way to improve the response capacity for language-assisted services in coming decades is to increase the educational investment in Latinos and facilitate the retention of the second language, Spanish, commonly learned at home. Currently, two out of five adult Latinos have not completed high school, and about only one in ten has completed college (Pew Hispanic Center 2010; see also Chap. 1). The loss of this population in higher education affects multiple service sectors, which face dramatic bilingual labor shortages. Educational investments in the Latino population will facilitate language-assisted services in the long run. For this population, many of whom are children of immigrants, embracing English does not necessarily mean abandoning Spanish (Pew Hispanic Center 2009). About two-thirds (64%) of Latinos aged 16 to 25 are either bilingual (41%) or Spanish dominant (23%) (Pew Hispanic Center 2009). Among the children of immigrants, 79% report that they are proficient in speaking Spanish (Pew Hispanic Center 2009). Even so, the retention of a second language learned in childhood—a much easier enterprise that learning a new foreign language as an adult—must be met with adequate educational supports. As this chapter has illustrated, there is a world of difference between possessing conversational skills and having a professional command of language.

Conclusion

Despite the difficulties that language barriers pose, these problems are not insurmountable. The resolution of language barriers requires thoughtful service planning that includes the use of language assessments for bilingual workers, a team approach focused on enhancing communication competence in the triadic relationship, and increased attention to how language affects service access. Agency-level solutions to language barriers require instituting formal rules and regulations (e.g., creating an organizational culture) that will lead to enhanced communication competence and attention to the norms, practices, and beliefs of staff (e.g., the organizational climate) that raise or reduce language barriers.

However, underlying this discussion of language and the need for building response capacity within institutions, we must acknowledge that the nation is on the precipice of a sweeping cultural change, where language—specifically, Spanish—is at the center of the change. The United States will never become bilingual—English dominance will prevail—but the way health and social services plan and deliver linguistically and culturally accessible services must change to meet the needs of this population. There is an urgent need for service providers from all sectors to know how to work with interpreters. Mental health and health care organizations must develop protocols for using interpreters.

Moreover, given the dearth of adequately trained interpreters and bilingual staff, especially in new-growth areas, there remains a pressing need for regional coordination of language services. State and federal government have a role in increasing incentives for such service coordination. The emerging cultural and linguistic reality will also call into question the role of educational institutions, as the demand for Spanish proficiency continues to outstrip available resources. As a nation, much of our future prosperity is linked with the well-being of the Latino population; hence, the time and resources invested in building response capacity is well spent.

References

Alba, R. D. (2009). *Blurring the color line: The new chance for a more integrated America.* Boston, MA: Harvard University Press.

Alegría, M., Mulvaney-Day, N., Woo, M., Torres, M., Gao, S., & Oddo, V. (2007). Correlates of past-year mental health service use among Latinos: Results from the national Latino and Asian American study. *American Journal of Public Health, 97*(1), 76–83.

Aranguri, C., Davidson, B., & Ramirez, R. (2006). Patterns of communication through interpreters: A detailed sociolinguistic analysis. *Journal of General Internal Medicine, 21,* 623–629.

Arroyo, L. E. (2004). *The health of Latino communities in the South: Challenges and opportunities.* Retrieved from http://www.nclr.org/content/publications/download/26898

Barrett, S. E., Puryear, J. S., & Westpheling, K. (2008). *Health literacy practices in primary care settings: Examples from the field.* Retrieved from http://www.commonwealthfund.org

Barrio, C., Palinkas, L. A., Yamada, A. M., Fuentes, D., Criado, V., Garcia, P., & Jeste, D. V. (2008). Unmet needs for mental health services for Latino older adults: Perspectives from consumers, family members, advocates, and service providers. *Community Mental Health Journal, 44*(1), 57–74. doi:10.1007/s10597-007-9112-9

Beeber, L. S., Lewis, V. S., Cooper, C., Maxwell, L., & Sandelowski, M. (2009). Meeting the "now" need: PMH-APRN–interpreter teams provide in-home mental health intervention for depressed Latina mothers with limited English proficiency. *Journal of the American Psychiatric Nurses Association, 15*(4), 249–259. doi:10.1177/1078390309344742

Berger, C. (n.d.). *Universal symbols in health care workbook: Executive summary*—Best practices for sign systems. Retrieved from http://www.hablamosjuntos.org/signage/PDF/Best%20Practices-FINALDec05.pdf

Borjas, G. (2006). Making it in America: Social mobility in the immigrant population. *The Future of Children, 16*(2), 55–71. doi:10.1353/foc.2006.0013

Borrell, L. N., & Crawford, N. D. (2006). Race, ethnicity, and self-rated health status in the behavioral risk factor surveillance system survey. *Hispanic Journal of Behavioral Sciences, 28*(3), 387–403.

Butera, G., McMullen, L., & Phillips, R. (2000). Energy express: Connecting communities and intervention on behalf of schoolchildren in West Virginia. *Journal of Research in Rural Education, 16*(1), 30–39.

Caldwell, A., Couture, A., & Nowotny, H. (n.d.). Closing the mental health gap: Eliminating disparities in treatment for Latinos. Retrieved June 1, 2010, from Mattie Rhodes Center http://www.mattierhodes.org/UserFiles/File/SAMHSA_full_report.pdf

Casey, M. M., Blewett, L. A., & Call, K. T. (2004). Providing health care to Latino immigrants: Community-based efforts in the rural Midwest. *American Journal of Public Health, 94,* 1709–1710.

Chapa, T., & Acosta, H. (2010). *Movilizandonos por nuestro futuro:* Strategic development of a mental health workforce for Latinos—Consensus statements and recommendations.

Retrieved from http://minorityhealth.hhs.gov/Assets/pdf/Checked/1/MOVILIZANDONOS_POR_NUESTRO_FUTURO_CONSENSUS_REPORT2010.pdf

Chen, A. H., Youdelman, M. K., & Brooks, J. (2007). The legal framework for language access in healthcare settings: Title VI and beyond. *Journal of General Internal Medicine, 22*(Suppl. 2), 362–367.

Christie, L. (2009). *Hispanic population boom fuels rising U.S. diversity.* Retrieved from http://www.cnn.com/2009/US/05/14/money.census.diversity/index.html

Clemans-Cope, L., & Kenney, G. (2007). Low income parents' reports of communication problems with health care providers: Effects of language and insurance. *Public Health Reports, 122*(2), 206–216.

Cunningham, H., Cushman, L. F., Akuete-Penn, C., & Meyer, D. D. (2008). Satisfaction with telephonic interpreters in pediatric care. *Journal of the National Medical Association, 100*(4), 429–434.

Cunningham, P., Banker, M., Artiga, S., & Tolbert, J. (2006). *Health coverage and access to care for Hispanics in "new growth communities" and "major Hispanic centers."* Washington, DC: The Henry J. Kaiser Family Foundation.

Davidson, B. (2000). The interpreter as institutional gatekeeper: The socio-linguistic role of interpreters in Spanish-English medical discourse. *Journal of Sociolinguistics, 2000*(4/3), 379–405.

DuBard, C. A., Garrett, J., & Gizlice, Z. (2006). Effect of language on heart attack and stroke awareness among U.S. Hispanics. *American Journal of Preventive Medicine, 30*(3), 189–196.

Durand, J., Telles, E., & Flashman, J. (2006). The demographic foundations of the Latino population. In M. Tienda & F. Mitchell (Eds.), *Hispanics and the future of America* (1st ed., pp. 66–99). Washington, DC: National Academies Press.

Elder, J. P., Ayala, G. X., Parra-Medina, D., & Talavera, G. A. (2009). Health communication in the Latino community: Issues and approaches. *Annual Review of Public Health, 30,* 227–251. doi:10.1146/annurev.publhealth.031308.100300

Elderkin-Thompson, V., Silver, R. C., & Waitzkin, H. (2001). When nurses double as interpreters: A study of Spanish-speaking patients in a U.S. primary care setting. *Social Science & Medicine (1982), 52*(9), 1343–1358.

Engstrom, D. W., & Min, J. W. (2004). Perspectives of bilingual social workers: "You just have to do a lot more for them." *Journal of Ethnic & Cultural Diversity in Social Work, 13*(1), 59–82.

Engstrom, D. W., Piedra, L. M., & Min, J. W. (2009). Bilingual social workers: Language and service complexities. *Administration in Social Work, 33*(2), 167–185.

Flores, G. (2005a). The impact of medical interpreter services on the quality of health care: A systematic review. *Medical Care Research & Review, 62*(3), 255–299.

Flores, G. (2005b). She walked from El Salvador. *Health Affairs, 24*(2), 506–510.

Flores, G., Laws, M. B., Mayo, S. J., Zuckerman, B., Abreu, M., & Medina, L. (2003). Errors in medical interpretation and their potential clinical consequences in pediatric encounters. *Pediatrics, 111*(1), 6–14. doi:10.1542/peds.111.1.6

Fortuny, K., Hernandez, D. J., & Chaudry, A. (2010). *Young children of immigrants: The leading edge of America's future.* Retrieved from http://www.urban.org/UploadedPDF/412203-young-children.pdf

Frederickson, N. (1966). Some effects of organizational climates on administrative performance. In N. Frederickson, *Research memorandum RM-66-21.* Washington, DC: Educational Testing Services.

Fry, R. (2008). *Latino settlement in the new century.* Retrieved June 1, 2010, from Pew Hispanic Center http://pewhispanic.org/files/reports/96.pdf

Fry, R., & Passel, J. S. (2009). *Latino children: A majority are U.S.-born offspring of immigrants.* Retrieved from http://pewhispanic.org/files/reports/110.pdf

Gany, F., Kapelusznik, L., Prakash, K., Gonzalez, J., Orta, L. Y., & Tseng, C.-H. (2007a). The impact of medical interpretation method on time and errors. *Journal of General Internal Medicine, 22*(Suppl. 2), 319–323.

Gany, F., Leng, J., Shapiro, E., Abramson, D., Motola, I., & Shield, D. C. (2007b). Patient satisfaction with different interpreting methods: A randomized controlled trial. *Journal of General Internal Medicine, 22*(Suppl. 2), 312–318.

Ginde, A. A., Clark, S., & Camargo, C. A. (2009). Language barriers among patients in Boston emergency departments: Use of medical interpreters after passage of interpreter legislation. *Journal of Immigrant & Minority Health, 11,* 527–530.

Glisson, C. (2000). Organizational climate and culture. In R. J. Pattie (Ed.), *The handbook of social welfare management* (pp. 195–218). Thousand Oaks, CA: Sage.

Glisson, C., Dukes, D., & Green, P. (2006). The effects of the ARC organizational intervention on caseworker turnover, climate, and culture in children's service systems. *Child Abuse & Neglect, 30*(8), 855–880.

Gregg, J., & Saha, S. (2007). Communicative competence: A framework for understanding language barriers in health care. *Journal of General Internal Medicine, 22*(Suppl. 2), 368–370.

Gumperz, J. (1972). Sociolinguistics and communication in small groups. In J. B. Pride & J. Holmes (Eds.), *Sociolinguistics* (pp. 203–224). Harmondsworth, UK: Penguin Books.

Harmsen, J. A. M., Bernsen, R. M. D., Bruijnzeels, M. A., & Meeuwesen, L. (2008). Patients' evaluation of quality of care in general practice: What are the cultural and linguistic barriers? *Patient Education & Counseling, 72*(1), 155–162.

Hernandez, D. J. (2004). Demographic change and the life circumstances of immigrant families. *The Future of Children, 14*(2), 17–47. Retrieved from http://futureofchildren.org/futureofchildren/publications/docs/14_02_03.pdf

Hernandez, D. J., Denton, N. A., & Macartney, S. E. (2008). Children in immigrant families: Looking to America's future. *Society for Research in Child Development, 22*(3), 3-22.

Hsieh, E. (2006a). Conflicts in how interpreters manage their roles in provider-patient interactions. *Social Science Medicine, 62*(3), 721.

Hsieh, E. (2006b). Understanding medical interpreters: Reconceptualizing bilingual health communication. *Health Communication, 20*(2), 177–186. doi:10.1207/s15327027hc2002_9

Hsieh, E. (2007). Interpreters as co-diagnosticians: Overlapping roles and services between providers and interpreters. *Social Science & Medicine, 64,* 924–937. doi:10.1016/j.socscimed.2006.10.015

Hsieh, E. (2008). "I am not a robot!" Interpreters' views of their roles in health care settings. *Qualitative Health Research, 18*(10), 1367–1383. doi:10.1177/1049732308323840

Imberti, P. (2007). Who resides behind the words? Exploring and understanding the language experience of the non-English-speaking immigrant. *Families in Society, 88*(1), 67–73.

Insaf, T. Z., Jurkowski, J. M., & Alomar, L. (2010). Sociocultural factors influencing delay in seeking routine health care among Latinas: A community-based participatory research study. *Ethnicity & Disease, 20*(2), 148–154.

Jacobs, E. A., Sadowski, L. S., & Rathouz, P. J. (2007). The impact of an enhanced interpreter service intervention on hospital costs and patient satisfaction. *Journal of General Internal Medicine, 22*(Suppl. 2), 306–311.

Jerant, A. F., Fenton, J. J., & Franks, P. (2008). Determinants of racial/ethnic colorectal cancer screening disparities. *Archives of Internal Medicine, 168*(12), 1317–1324.

Karliner, L. S., Jacobs, E. A., Chen, A. H., & Mutha, S. (2007). Do professional interpreters improve clinical care for patients with limited English proficiency? *Health Services Research, 42*(2), 727–754.

Kaufert, J. M., O'Neil, J. D., & Koolage, W. W. (1985). Culture brokerage and advocacy in urban hospitals: The impact of native language interpreters. *Sante Culture Health, 8*(2), 3–9.

Kimbrough, J. B. (2007). Health literacy as a contributor to immigrant health disparities. *Journal of Health Disparities Research & Practice, 1*(2), 93–106.

Kirk, J. K., Bell, R. A., Bertoni, A. G., Arcury, T. A., Quandt, S. A., Goff, D. C., Jr., et al. (2005). Ethnic disparities: Control of glycemia, blood pressure, and LDL cholesterol among US adults with type 2 diabetes. *Annals of Pharmacotherapy, 39*(9), 1489–1501.

Kramer, H., Han, C., Post, W., Goff, D., Diez-Roux, A., Cooper, R., et al. (2004). Racial/ethnic differences in hypertension and hypertension treatment and control in the multi-ethnic study of atherosclerosis (MESA). *American Journal of Hypertension, 17*(10), 963–970.

Ku, L., & Flores, G. (2005). Pay now or pay later: Providing interpreter services in health care. *Health Affairs, 24*(2), 435–444.

Lichter, D. T., & Johnson, K. M. (2006). Emerging rural settlement patterns and the geographic redistribution of America's new immigrants. *Rural Sociology, 71*(1), 109–131.

Marsiglia, F. F., & Kulis, S. (2009). *Diversity, oppression, and change*. Chicago, IL: Lyceum Books.

Mather, M. (2009). *Children in immigrant families chart new path*. Retrieved from http://prb.org/pdf09/immigrantchildren.pdf

McMurtray, A., Saito, E., & Nakamoto, B. (2009). Language preference and development of dementia among bilingual individuals. *Hawai'i Medical Journal, 68*(9), 223–226.

Morales, L. S., Cunningham, W. E., Brown, J. A., Liu, H., & Hays, R. D. (1999). Are Latinos less satisfied with communication by health care providers? *Journal of General Internal Medicine, 14*(7), 409–417.

Moreno, M. R., Otero-Sabogal, R., & Newman, J. (2007). Assessing dual-role staff-interpreter linguistic competency in an integrated health system. *Journal of General Internal Medicine, 22*(Suppl. 2), 331–335.

Mui, A. C., Kang, S. Y., Kang, D., & Domanski, M. D. (2007). English language proficiency and health-related quality of life among Chinese and Korean immigrant elders. *Health & Social Work, 32*(2), 119–127.

Muldrow, T. W., Buckley, T., & Schay, B. W. (2002). Creating high-performance organizations in the public sector. *Human Resource Management, 41*(3), 341–354.

O'Beirne, E. (2000). Letters 07-13-2000. *Phoenix New Times.* Retrieved from http://www.phoenixnewtimes.com/2000-07-13/news/letters-07-13-2000/

Partida, Y. (2007). Addressing language barriers: Building response capacity for a changing nation. *Journal of General Internal Medicine, 22*(Suppl. 2), 347–349.

Pew Hispanic Center. (2009). Between two worlds: *How young Latinos come of age in America.* Retrieved from http://pewhispanic.org/files/reports/117.pdf

Pew Hispanic Center. (2010). *Statistical portrait of Hispanics in the United States, 2008.* Retrieved from http://pewhispanic.org/factsheets/factsheet.php?FactsheetID=58

Piedra, L. M. (2006). Revisiting the language question. In D. W. Engstrom & L. M. Piedra (Eds.), *Our diverse society: Race and ethnicity—Implications for 21st century American society* (pp. 67–87). Washington, DC: NASW Press.

Piedra, L. M. (2010). Latinos and Spanish: The awkwardness of language in social work practice. In R. Furman & N. Negi (Eds.), *Social work practice with Latinos* (pp. 262–281). Chicago, IL: Lyceum Books.

Ponce, N. A., Hays, R. D., & Cunningham, W. E. (2006). Linguistic disparities in health care access and health status among older adults. *Journal of General Internal Medicine, 21*(7), 786–791.

Premji, S., Messing, K., & Lippel, K. (2008). Broken English, broken bones? Mechanisms linking language proficiency and occupational health in a Montréal garment factory. *International Journal of Health Services: Planning, Administration, Evaluation, 38*(1), 1–19.

Reimann, J. O. F., Talavera, G. A., Salmon, M., Nuñez, J. A., & Velasquez, R. J. (2004). Cultural competence among physicians treating Mexican Americans who have diabetes: A structural model. Social Science & Medicine, 59(11), 2195-2205.

Saha, S., & Fernandez, A. (2007). Language barriers in health care. *Journal of General Internal Medicine, 22*(Suppl. 2), 281–282.

Schneider, B., Martinez, S., & Owens, A. (2006). Barriers to educational opportunities for Hispanics in the United States. In M. Tienda & F. Mitchell (Eds.), *Hispanics and the future of America* (pp. 179–221). Washington, DC: National Academies Press.

Schur, C. L., & Albers, L. A. (1996). Language, sociodemographics, and health care use of Hispanic adults. *Journal of Health Care for the Poor & Underserved, 7*(2), 140–158.

Scioscia, A. (2000). Critical connection. *Phoenix New Times.* Retrieved from http://www.phoenixnewtimes.com/2000-06-29/news/critical-connection/

Sentell, T., Shumway, M., & Snowden, L. (2007). Access to mental health treatment by English language proficiency and race/ethnicity. *Journal of General Internal Medicine: Official Journal of the Society for Research & Education in Primary Care Internal Medicine, 22* (Suppl. 2), 289–293.

Shin, H. B. (2003, April 5). Language use and the English-speaking ability: 2000 (Census 2000 Brief, 2006 (April 5)). doi:http://www.census.gov/prod/2003pubs/c2kbr-29.pdf. Retrieved from http://www.census.gov/prod/2003pubs/c2kbr-29.pdf

Sluzki, C. E. (1978). The patient-provider-translator triad: A note for providers. Family Systems Medicine *(currently Family Systems & Health), 2*(4), 379–400.

Snowden, L., Masland, M., & Guerrero, R. (2007). Federal civil rights policy and mental health treatment access for persons with limited English proficiency. *American Psychologist, 62*(2), 109–117.

Sollors, W. (Ed.). (1998). *Multilingual America: Transnationalism, ethnicity, and the languages of American literature.* New York: New York University Press.

Sullivan, T. A. (2006). Demography, the demand for social services, and the potential for civic conflict. In D. W. Engstrom & L. M. Piedra (Eds.), *Our diverse society: Race and ethnicity— Implications for 21st century American society* (pp. 9–18). Washington, DC: NASW Press.

Suro, R., & Singer, A. (2002). *Latino growth in metropolitan America: Changing patterns, new locations* (pp. 1–18). Washington, DC: The Brooking Institution, Center on Urban & Metropolitan Policy, and The Pew Hispanic Center.

U.S. Census Bureau. (2004). *U.S. interim projections by age, sex, race, and Hispanic origin.* Retrieved from http://www.census.gov/population/www/projections/usinterimproj/

Vega, W. A., & Lopez, S. R. (2001). Priority issues in Latino mental health services research. *Mental Health Services Research, 3*(4), 189–200.

Vega, W. A., Karno, M., Alegria, M., Alvidrez, J., Bernal, G., Escamilla, M., & Loue, S. (2007). Research issues for improving treatment of U.S. Hispanics with persistent mental disorders. *Psychiatric Services, 58*(3), 385–394. doi:10.1176/appi.ps.58.3.385

Vega, W. A., Rodriguez, M. A., & Gruskin, E. (2009). Health disparities in the Latino population. *Epidemiologic Reviews, 31*(1), 99–112. doi:10.1093/epirev/mxp008

Wallace, S. P., & Villa, V. M. (2003). Equitable health systems: Cultural and structural issues for Latino elders. *American Journal of Law & Medicine, 29*(2–3), 247–267.

Williams, D. R., & Jackson, P. B. (2005). Social sources of racial disparities in health. *Health Affairs, 24*(2), 325–334.

Wilson, E., Chen, A. H., Grumbach, K., Wang, F., & Fernandez, A. (2005). Effects of limited English proficiency and physician language on health care comprehension. *Journal of General Internal Medicine, 20*(9), 800–806.

Part II
Building Infrastructures Across Service Sectors

Chapter 4
Increasing Service Parity Through Organizational Cultural Competence

I. David Acevedo-Polakovich, Elizabeth A. Crider,
Veronica A. Kassab and James I. Gerhart

Abstract US Latinos' limited access to existing services leads to lower service use which, in turn, leads to increased impairment as a result of behavioral health conditions. Although discussions of cultural-responsiveness efforts to address this limited access most often focus on specific practices or on the characteristics of service providers, the long-term success of efforts to incorporate culturally responsive interventionists and practices into service settings depends on broader organizational changes. This chapter introduces Hernandez et al.'s (2009) organizational cultural-competence framework, and expands upon this framework by introducing evaluation and assessment approaches that might be used to guide its implementation and by providing examples from the recent literature that illustrate its application in various Latino communities. By doing so, this chapter provides a road map for efforts to bring about organizational cultural competence.

Although the prevalence of behavioral health conditions is fairly consistent across ethnic groups in the United States, Latinos and other US ethnic minority groups are less likely than European Americans to have accessible mental health services available to them (Alegría et al. 2002). The lower availability and accessibility of mental health services lead to less use, which in turn seems to increase the risk that behavioral health conditions will lead to significant functional impairment (Isaacs et al. 2008). For this reason, efforts that seek to eliminate the increased impairment burden imposed by behavioral health conditions on US Latinos and other ethnic minority group members are more likely to be successful when targeted at addressing the availability, accessibility, and utilization barriers faced by members of these groups (Hernandez et al. 2009).

This chapter presents a model that seeks to guide efforts at addressing ethnic disparities in the availability, accessibility, and utilization of mental health services.

I. D. Acevedo-Polakovich (✉)
Central Michigan University, MI, USA
e-mail: david.acevedo@cmich.edu

The model was developed to summarize and organize the findings of a comprehensive review of the literature on culturally competent children's mental health services published between 1994 and 2004 (Hernandez et al. 2006). According to the model, disparities regarding service availability, accessibility, and utilization arise from a fundamental incompatibility between the conceptualization of behavioral health and behavioral health interventions typically reflected in service settings and the conceptualization of behavioral health and behavioral health interventions within ethnic minority communities. Hence, to address service disparities organizations must increase their compatibility with local conceptualizations of behavioral health and behavioral health interventions.

This model uses the term *organizational cultural competence* to capture the compatibility between service environments and local conceptualizations of behavioral health and behavioral health interventions (Hernandez et al. 2006, 2009). Organizational cultural competence is a characteristic of behavioral health service organizations that includes, but extends beyond, other dimensions of cultural competence such as individual cultural competence (e.g., Sue et al. 1982) and specific culturally competent practices (e.g., Bernal et al. 1995). Without organizational change, efforts to develop a culturally competent workforce and implement culturally competent practices are less likely to be successful (Alegría et al. 2007; Skyttner 2005).

The focus on an organization's compatibility with the needs and conditions of local populations offers at least two important advantages (Hernandez et al. 2009). First, it avoids a frequent criticism of approaches that focus on cultural generalizations: The fact that they do not capture the meaningful variance associated with the diversity that can exist within ethnicity-based groups. In avoiding this problem, the focus on compatibility facilitates culturally competent services in contexts often overlooked by generalized approaches, such as small ethnic communities and subcultures within larger ethnic groups. Second, cultural competence is highlighted as an inherent aspect of all behavioral health organizations, not only of those serving ethnic minority groups. In this sense, the traditional approach to behavioral health services, which has successfully served the relatively affluent proportion of the US population, is a culturally competent one, but only with regard to this particular constituency (U.S. Department of Health and Human Services [USDHHS] 2001). An understanding of the local community context can reveal the degree to which the concepts, practices, and policies that dominate traditional approaches to behavioral health services are appropriate and relevant.

Hoping to facilitate efforts at understanding and addressing the behavioral health service disparities faced by US Latinos and other ethnic groups, this chapter describes Hernandez et al.'s (2006, 2009) organizational cultural competence model, and expands on their work by introducing assessment approaches that might be used to guide efforts at developing culturally competent behavioral health organizations. Although each of the model's components is described in a separate section of this chapter, they do in fact overlap. In practice, organizational cultural competence is achieved (along with the reduction or elimination of service disparities) when there is congruence across components. A final section

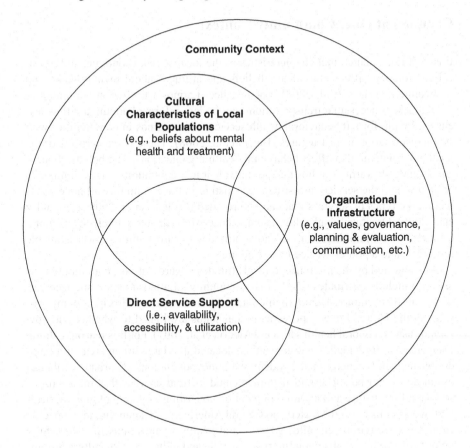

Fig. 4.1 A culturally competent organization

of this chapter draws overall conclusions and makes recommendations for future research and practice in organizational cultural competence. Examples from the recent literature are used to illustrate the application of the model in various Latino communities.

Figure 4.1, adapted from Hernandez et al. (2006), gives a visual representation of the model. The components of the model are: (a) community context, (b) cultural characteristics of local populations, (c) organizational infrastructure, and (d) direct service support. The figure illustrates a model organization whose infrastructure and direct service support are fully integrated with the characteristics of the local community, and are responsive to the characteristics of local populations. By comparison, a figure could be envisioned where the circular areas representing infrastructure and service support are located outside of the community context and do not overlap with cultural characteristics. Such a figure would represent an organization low in cultural competence.

Component One: Community Context

It is well documented that characteristics of the local social, economic, and physical environment affect individuals' beliefs and attitudes about mental health and its treatment (Isaacs et al. 2008). For instance, Latinos who live in communities with a lack of accessible transportation may be less informed about, and thus less engaged with, formal behavioral health services than Latinos in communities with rich transportation infrastructures (Barrio et al. 2008). These characteristics of the local environment also affect behavioral health organizations. The beliefs about— and attitudes toward—Latinos that are prevalent in a community, the community's affluence, and the service infrastructures existing in the community all have an effect on the types of services that can be provided (Callejas et al. 2009; Hernandez et al. 2006). Organizational cultural competence efforts are more likely to encounter obstacles in communities with negative attitudes toward Latinos, fewer available resources, and a poorer service infrastructure.

As suggested by the reference to local attitudes toward Latinos, community context also includes attributes related to a community's Latinos that are not necessarily tied to their culture. Demographic factors such as country of origin, number of years in the United States, and generational status are linked to whether and how Latinos use behavioral health services (Alegría et al. 2007). For this reason, cultural competence efforts made by organizations located in a large urban area with long-established multigenerational residential Latino populations of urban Caribbean origin might not be successful if implemented in rural areas with a more limited service infrastructure and a Latino population consisting of young migrant agricultural workers from rural Mexico and Central America. Understanding their specific community's environment allows behavioral health organizations to successfully tailor their services to the community as a whole and to the specific cultural groups represented within that community (Añez et al. 2005). Approaches to the assessment of community context are presented in the following section.

Component Two: Cultural Characteristics of Local Populations

Culture exerts a strong influence over individuals' understanding of mental health and its treatment (Isaacs et al. 2008). However, over time local conditions can interact with broader cultural forces to create highly localized manifestations of culture. For example, in one Mexican American community, Newton (1978) documented a belief system regarding mental illness that incorporated a key distinction between emotional and mental problems, the first being seen as relatively less impairing than the latter. Although emotional problems closely overlapped with the issues usually treated by mental health providers, that community's belief system also suggested that formal providers only treated the mental problems. This mismatch between the types of problems that formal providers do in fact treat and the types of problems they were believed to treat reduced the use of formal care, even when it was needed. The conceptualization of mental health and its treatment documented by Newton (1978) reflects both general cultural views common to many Mexican-origin populations and idiosyncrasies that are specific to the local community (Guarnaccia et al. 2003), underscoring the importance of developing services that are responsive to local cultural nuances and not broad generalizations of Latino cultural views (Weisman et al. 2005).

The remainder of this section introduces four assessment approaches that can guide efforts at understanding aspects of the local context and culture that are directly relevant to service needs: action-oriented community diagnosis, rapid assessment, rapid ethnographic assessment, and community readiness assessments. Regardless of the specific approach utilized, these approaches should be implemented with the aim of understanding the cultural and social context surrounding mental health and its treatment (Posavac and Carey 2007).

It is important to note that the assessments discussed in this section provide information on only two of four issues useful in the design and oversight of organizational cultural competence efforts. Subsequent sections of this chapter discuss assessment focused on the other two types of information used in these efforts (i.e., a behavioral health organization's level of cultural competence and its readiness to engage in cultural competence efforts). It should be noted that although these different types of information are discussed separately, they can all be gathered during one overall assessment focused on four objectives:

1. Describing the characteristics of local context and culture as related to mental health services.
2. Describing a target community's readiness for change as regards mental health services.
3. Describing a mental health service organization's current level of cultural competence across its various functions and domains.
4. Describing a mental health service organization's readiness to engage in cultural competence efforts.

Action-Oriented Community Diagnosis

Action-oriented community diagnosis (AOCD) is a community assessment technique, based on case study research designs, that focuses on examining the contextual factors affecting a given area of interest within communities (e.g., the cultural competence of behavioral health services) (Quinn 1999; Steckler et al. 1993). It typically involves several stages (Eng and Blanchard 1991):

1. Identifying the target population
2. Reviewing secondary data sources
3. Interviewing service providers
4. Interviewing community members

5. Analyzing data
6. Presenting findings to the community and incorporating community feedback.

Although the analysis of data in AOCD most often occurs in an iterative fashion based on qualitative grounded-theory approaches, quantitative data are also frequently used throughout course of the assessment (Eng et al. 2005). AOCD is typically conducted by small teams of evaluators under the supervision of two coordinators. Often, one coordinator is an expert in the local community, whereas the other is an expert in service planning. Because meaningful community involvement is at the core of successful organizational cultural competence efforts (Hernandez et al. 2006, 2009), an advantage of AOCD is that it is as much a process of relationship building and community engagement as it is an assessment and service development process (Eng and Blanchard 1991). Additionally, its results are highly reflective of the local context and directly relevant to service development.

Maciak et al.'s (1999) creation of a partnership to develop and implement services to ameliorate intimate partner violence against Latina women in southwest Detroit illustrates the benefits of AOCD. After reviewing secondary data sources to generate hypotheses about local conditions, focus groups were conducted with local stakeholders (community members, service providers, and clergy) to better understand local conditions and identify possible intervention strategies. To promote community involvement, trained community members co-facilitated some of these focus groups.

The AOCD assessment yielded several important findings. For instance, whereas Latinas in this community were not inclined to report intimate partner violence to authorities, they were comfortable seeking help from family or clergy. This suggested that family and clergy members could provide important points of access to this population. A related finding was that mother and toddler groups held weekly at local churches could be used to engage Latinas who are victims of intimate partner violence. Other findings uncovered a need for cultural competence training among non-Latino personnel working with Latinas.

The findings of the AOCD assessment guided the development of a coordinated set of strategies to ameliorate intimate partner violence and the formation of a stakeholder partnership that would guide its implementation. This set of strategies included providing cultural competence training where needed, building the capacity of church-based mother and toddler groups to adequately identify and address intimate partner violence, and the creation of culturally responsive social marketing materials that raised awareness about intimate partner violence, its effects, and the services available in the community.

Rapid Assessment

Rapid assessment utilizes techniques from ethnography, action research, and participatory action research to quickly and cost-effectively integrate available evidence on a pragmatic area of importance (such as organizational cultural competence) (McNall and Foster-Fischman 2007). As a first step in rapid assessment, a small team of evaluators identifies informants who may have access to key information about the assessment's focus area. Data are then collected from these informants and the information they provide is integrated with any available secondary data in order to describe community conditions and make recommendations for change (McNall and Foster-Fischman 2007). Depending on the nature and scope of the issue being addressed and on the size and accessibility of the community in which it occurs, a rapid assessment process may last from a few weeks to a few months (McNall and Foster-Fischman 2007).

New data in rapid assessment are typically collected through a combination of surveys, focus groups, transect walks, and behavior mapping, to complement information identified through review and interviews with key informants (McNall and Foster-Fischman 2007). Because focus groups, interviews, and surveys are usually familiar in service settings, we briefly introduce some of the additional data-gathering tools used in rapid assessment. *Behavior mapping* involves documenting behavioral observations on the type of people, their activities, and time spent at a particular site in the community (Taplin et al. 2002). Mapping can also involve documenting the geographic areas and populations that are affected by a problem or the location of the various resources that can aid in resolution of a problem (McNall and Foster-Fischman 2007). *Transect walks* are used to provide field-based information that might be overlooked by other approaches (Taplin et al. 2002). They involve visiting an area of particular relevance to the problem being evaluated in the company of key informant (Taplin et al. 2002). For instance, a neighborhood or service setting might be visited in the company of a key stakeholder with expertise in the area, or in the company of an individual who is looking for services. These visits allow evaluators to document practical information about the actual conditions surrounding the objectives of the assessment.

Valdez et al. (2009) employed rapid assessment to examine adaptation and well-being among the large number of Latino day laborers who moved into the New Orleans area to take advantage of employment opportunities created by the rebuilding efforts following Hurricane Katrina. Because there was little preexisting information on this newly established group, the assessment involved conducting open-ended interviews with 52 Latino men. Results revealed that almost half of these men used crack cocaine, a surprising finding given that the use of this drug is not usually encountered among Latino day-laborer populations elsewhere in the country. Analysis of the qualitative data suggested that the high use was associated with high accessibility of crack and drug paraphernalia, social isolation, vulnerability to victimization by employers, and the lack of an established Latino community in the area. These findings documented a need for additional HIV and addiction screening services, and for interventions addressing the accessibility to drugs, the social isolation, and the vulnerability associated with this pattern of drug use.

Rapid Ethnographic Assessment

Rapid ethnographic assessment employs ethnography to understand health issues among target populations (McNall and Foster-Fischman 2007). For example, in response to previous research documenting a rapid decline in breastfeeding among residents in the outskirts of Mexico City, Guerrero et al. (1999) conducted a rapid ethnographic assessment to guide the development and implementation of an intervention to promote breastfeeding. During the assessment process, the researchers gathered data from 150 mothers through interviews and questionnaires. Data analyses revealed that physician advice was the most important factor in their decisions about breastfeeding. Other factors that contributed to their decisions included certain cultural syndromes, such as *susto* (associated with fright) or *coraje* (associated with anger). Service solutions developed in response to this information included training seminars with community physicians, to address their influence on mothers; and a program to train peer counselors to promote breastfeeding in a manner that appropriately addressed local beliefs and conditions.

Community Readiness Assessments

Community readiness assessments are specifically geared to provide information regarding a community's preparation to address a defined set of issues, including provision of culturally responsive mental health services (Oetting et al. 2001). Because a community's readiness level has direct implications for the types of interventions needed to advance cultural competence efforts, readiness assessments complement and expand the information gathered in assessments of the local context and culture. Like the other assessment processes described in this chapter, readiness assessments usually involve the collection of data using semistructured interviews with key stakeholders (e.g., local leaders, community representatives) and the review of available information (e.g., local service or needs reports). In the case of organizational cultural competence efforts, interviewees might include individuals who use services, care providers, individuals who needed services but did not use them, and administrators of behavioral health organizations.

According to one prevalent model, community readiness assessment should focus on determining a community's current status in six specific areas (Edwards et al. 2000): (1) existing efforts (programs, activities, policies, etc.), (2) knowledge of existing efforts by community members, (3) leadership (includes appointed leaders and influential community members), (4) community climate (prevailing attitudes about the issue in the community), (5) knowledge about the issue, and (6) resources related to the issue. The data collected on each of these areas is then used to establish a community's readiness to engage with an issue, which in turn points to specific types of interventions that might prove most beneficial.

Edwards et al. (2000) have identified nine stages of community readiness. These are presented in Table 4.1, along with a description of the suggested goals of organizational interventions to increase the use of mental health services. A more com-

Table 4.1 Stages of community readiness and intervention goals

Stage	Intervention Goal
No Awareness	Increase general awareness about mental health services.
Denial/Resistance	Increase awareness of the relevance of mental health services in the community.
Vague Awareness	Increase awareness that community efforts can improve mental health service availability, accessibility, and use.
Pre-planning	Increase awareness about potential improvements to mental health services.
Preparation	Gather information to guide the development of new services and the improvement of existing services.
Initiation	Disseminate information about available services.
Stabilization	Ensure the sustainability of current services.
Confirmation/Expansion	Improve and enhance available services.
Community Ownership	Maintain momentum and continue growth.

prehensive discussion of these stages is beyond the scope of this chapter, but can be found in Plested et al. (2006).

Hull et al. (2008) employed a community readiness assessment to examine issues surrounding health service access among Latinos in Nashville, Tennessee, an area that had experienced a 763% growth in its Latino population since 1990. Because of this rapid growth, concerns arose that the existing services infrastructure did not adequately meet the needs of Latinos. Hull et al. administered a version of Plested et al.'s (2006) Community Readiness Assessment, after adapting it to reflect the specific needs of their assessment. The adapted questionnaire was administered to two groups of key informants: Latino community members and representatives of health service organizations. Their results suggested that the average level of readiness among health service organizations corresponded to the preparation stage, whereas the average level of readiness among community members corresponded to the pre-planning stage. Based on these findings, Hull et al. developed a set of recommendations designed to raise readiness among community members and organizations before pursuing further change. Sample recommendations include community and service provider workshops designed to raise awareness about health issues that are important to local Latinos, and community forums to discuss the readiness assessment findings. More recently, Piedra and Buki (2010) published an article describing an adaptation of the Community Readiness Assessment specifically for measuring a community's readiness to address mental health issues of immigrant Latinos. (The article includes both English and Spanish versions of the measure.)

Component Three: Organizational Infrastructure

As presented in Fig. 4.1, which provides a visual representation of the main components of organizational cultural competence, there are two important organizational domains that must be responsive to the local culture and context: organizational infrastructure and direct service support. The key distinction between the organizational functions included in each of these domains is their relation to service. The eight functions included in organizational infrastructure are necessary for an organization's successful functioning, but are not directly related to services. This section of the chapter introduces each of these eight functions: planning and evaluation, organizational values, communication, community participation, governance, human resources, service array, and technical support.

Planning and Evaluation

Within the domain of organizational infrastructure, *planning and evaluation* refer to an organization's collection and use of data for the purposes of directing cultural competence efforts. Evaluation includes the community assessments discussed previously in this chapter, along with the organizational assessments discussed in this section. As mentioned earlier, because the data collection methods used in all of these assessments are overlapping and complementary, it may be most efficient to conduct one overall assessment with multiple objectives.

Organizational Cultural Competence Assessment

This type of organizational assessment focuses on understanding the degree to which each of the essential functions of a mental health service organization is culturally competent (i.e., reflective of, and responsive to, local conditions). In a review of the relevant literature, Harper et al. (2006) identified 35 approaches to the assessment of organizational cultural competence and examined the ability of each approach to account for the organizational infrastructure domains included in Hernandez et al.'s (2006, 2009) model. Harper et al. conducted a more in-depth examination of 17 of these assessment approaches, each of which met their criteria for further examination (i.e., a focus on cultural competence in mental health, going beyond a planning/screening checklist, going beyond consumer ratings).

Harper et al. (2006) concluded that most of the available assessment approaches focused on ensuring alignment with a theoretical model or policy regarding cultural competence and were not informed by validity or reliability research. For example, the Office of Minority Health's Cultural and Linguistic Standards (CLAS) Assessment Tool (Office of Minority Health, n.d.) was the only approach that rendered information relevant to all of the organizational infrastructure domains; however, Harper et al. were not able to identify any validity or reliability research to support the use of this measure. Similarly, of the seven additional assessment approaches that included information about all but one of the organizational infrastructure domains, only the Ohio Department of Mental Health's (2003) Consolidated Culturalogical Assessment Tool Kit (CCATK) was developed through a process that included validity and reliability testing.

Harper et al.'s (2006) findings suggest that although organizations undertaking cultural competence assessment efforts have at their disposal a variety of approaches, there is great variability in whether the approaches account for all functions involved in organizational cultural competence, and there is little data to aid organizations in selecting among approaches. Given this state of affairs, organizations might increase the comprehensiveness and reliability of their results by deploying a multiple-method assessment approach that includes more than one of the existing approaches (e.g., both the CLAS Assessment Tool and the CCATK). It is important to note that approximately half of the assessment approaches reviewed by Harper et al. were explicitly tied to guidelines for planning organizational cultural competence efforts, a feature that might be attractive to administrators and planners. This is the case for both the CLAS Assessment Tool and the CCATK.

Organizational Readiness Assessment

Paralleling community readiness, *organizational readiness* refers to the various factors influencing an organization's preparation to address a defined set of issues, including cultural competence efforts (Weiner et al. 2008). As with community readiness, the primary principle underlying organizational readiness is that efforts to implement change in an organization will be compromised if they are pursued in an organization that is not ready to support this change (Lehman et al. 2002). For this reason, it is recommended that organizational planning and evaluation focused on cultural competence include a consideration of organizational readiness.

As is the case with organizational cultural competence assessment, there is a variety of instruments available that have been designed to assess organizational readiness. However, a recent review of 43 instruments uncovered limited evidence of reliability or validity for most publicly available measures (Weiner et al. 2008). The Texas Christian University (TCU) Organizational Readiness for Change Assessment (ORC; Lehman et al. 2002) is one promising exception. Developed from established measures of organizational characteristics known to predict program change, it provides an assessment of four major organizational domains: motivation, resources, staff attributes, and climate. Two versions of the ORC have been developed, one designed for interventionists and another for program administrators. Both of these versions, along with scoring norms and detailed technical information, are available free of charge through the Institute for Behavioral Research at TCU (www.ibr.tcu.edu).

Organizational Values

An organization's approach to services is usually guided by larger values that are often explicitly recognized. For instance, the system-of-care approach embraced by some behavioral health organizations requires that treatment be guided by five specific values (Hernandez et al. 2001): the importance of family, the benefits of individualized care, the right to care that is as unrestrictive as possible, the key role of coordination among services, and cultural competence. Importantly, in published research, the degree to which a treatment plan is reflective of these values can be used to meaningfully distinguish services provided under a system-of-care framework from services provided at organizations that do not follow this framework (Hernandez et al. 2001). Similarly, services in culturally competent organizations must be driven by values that reflect the organizations' commitment to understanding and responding to the needs of the local community. Beyond explicit statements, organizations' values are also reflected in their mission and vision, and in the beliefs and professional activities of staff and administrators (Gruys et al. 2008). The understanding and integration of these values by employees should begin with initial training and orientation efforts (Gruys et al. 2008). These values can then be incorporated into every aspect of human resource management, including hiring, performance appraisal, and rewards or disciplinary actions (Gruys et al. 2008; Wilder et al. 2009).

Although written value statements are an essential and easily accessible declaration of an organization's intentions, they are not sufficient; it is essential to implement organizational practices to ensure that these values guide organizational behavior (Gruys et al. 2008). Organizational behavior management (OBM) interventions can be particularly useful for prompting and reinforcing such value-guided behavior (Wilder et al. 2009). Sample practices include prominently displaying value statements in public areas and workspaces and requiring their incorporation into organizational documents to make these values more salient to service providers. Consistently acting out the organization's values will help reiterate and solidify them among employees, and it will also help increase satisfaction and performance of employees (Gruys et al. 2008), which in turn will lead to a better quality of service for the community. OBM interventions and practices—as well as the dissemination of the organizational values as mentioned earlier—are the responsibility of all members of an organization, but they are largely driven by human resources and leadership personnel, which points to the relation between this organizational function and other functions within the organization (including human resources).

Communication

The sharing of information, both within an organization and among the organization, its clients, and associates, is referred to as its *communication* function (Hernandez et al. 2009). This function includes the content of what is shared (e.g., conceptions of mental health care and child care), the direction of exchange (e.g., community to organization and organization to community), and the format, method, and frequency of exchange (e.g., print media, radio, website, focus groups, community forum, etc.). Culturally competent organizations implement communication in ways that ensure responsiveness to community needs by each of its communication practices. For example, to create a bidirectional information flow, organizations might hold a periodic community forum to gather input on needs and services from clients. Similar information can be obtained by implementing widely announced public comment periods when considering changes to infrastructure or services.

Strategic decisions regarding the method and format of communication from the organization to the community can also enhance cultural competence. In many communities, organizations that wish to increase awareness of their services among Latinos might do well to advertise through smaller-scale ethnic media, such as Spanish-language newspapers or AM radio stations, rather than through mainstream media. Culturally competent organizations develop communication practices based on their understanding of local communities and local cultures. For example, if Latinos in a given community tend to first seek guidance from religious leaders in times of emotional crisis, an organization serving Latinos in this community might consider implementing practices that efficiently communicate information to and from these leaders (e.g., hosting periodic informational events, designating a formal liaison, etc.; Maciak et al. 1999).

Even when methods are strategically chosen in response to local Latino communities, poor content choices can compromise the efficacy of communication. The literature notes case examples where the utilization of carefully developed, culturally competent service was compromised by strategically flawed awareness campaigns. Examples include use of English-language advertising in Spanish-language media, and messages that were crafted to include terms that were unfamiliar to local Latinos (Añez et al. 2005).

Community Participation

Because organizational cultural competence is tantamount to the development of organizational structures, policies, and practices that are responsive to the needs and contexts of the local community, one of the important features of culturally competent organizations is the creation of structures to facilitate community participation in organizational functions (Hernandez et al. 2006, 2009). The regular use of a community forum to gather input, the designation of formal liaisons, and the implementation of public comment periods are all examples of practices that enhance community input. Furthermore, culturally competent organizations often ensure that there is community representation in decision-making bodies (e.g., through designated voting slots on boards and advisory committees). For example, when undertaking efforts to increase access to culturally competent mental health services and programs for the Latino population in Worcester, the Massachusetts Department of Mental Health created a planning council that included representatives from health and education organizations, mental health service consumers, family members of individuals with a behavioral health condition, and members of the community at large (Cardemil et al. 2007). This council chose to begin its work by conducting a community needs assessment, which in turn allowed the council to identify initiatives that would best meet community needs.

Governance

Governance encompasses the processes through which a service organization acts to institute policies, procedures, and goals, including those connected to cultural competence. This includes rules governing organizational practices and the activities of personnel and entities with oversight functions, such as boards of directors and administrators. Effective governance approaches that directly reflect an organizational interest in responding to community needs can be instrumental in the success of efforts to develop culturally competent organizations (e.g., Yee and Tursi 2002). Policies and practices that ensure community representation in organizational decision-making bodies, and that require the explicit alignment of organizational practices with values that are consistent with cultural competence, are two previously discussed examples of approaches to governance that facilitate responsiveness to community and culture (Hernandez et al. 2006, 2009).

The American Society on Aging (ASA) stands as one example of an organization that implemented changes into its governance structure and policies in order to increase cultural competence (Yee and Tursi 2002). In 1983, the ASA established the Minority Concerns Committee as a standing committee within its board of directors. This committee was tasked both with the implementation of efforts to ensure that the organization acted in a manner inclusive of gerontologists from all backgrounds, and with monitoring organizational efforts to remain culturally diverse (Yee and Tursi 2002). In 1994, the ASA also implemented a biannual diversity impact report that monitors diversity in areas such as leadership and staff, number and quality of training sessions related to minority issues, and coverage of minority issues and inclusion of minority authors in ASA publications (Yee and Tursi 2002). The structural and policy changes undertaken by the ASA allow it to assess progress in diversity initiatives and identify steps for strengthening and increasing cultural competence (Yee and Tursi 2002).

Human Resources

Human resource functions ensure that organizations have personnel with the necessary knowledge and skills to ensure that culturally competent services are available, accessible, and utilized (Hernandez et al. 2009). One strategy that organizations might implement to achieve this goal is the recruitment of new personnel who can competently serve target populations. Prior scholarship using the Attraction-Selection-Attrition framework suggests that the long-term success of these recruitment efforts is tied to additional organizational changes (Schneider et al.

2000). Some organizations have facilitated this process by creating opportunities for members of the target service populations to fill professional roles within the organization (e.g., by including educational support within relevant careers as part of employee benefits packages) and by working to ensure that these competent new workers are accepted into and mesh well with the service organization (Schneider et al. 2000).

Another strategy to ensure that human resources adequately support organizational cultural competence involves activities designed to build the individual cultural competence of existing personnel (e.g., Delphin and Rowe 2008). This might involve specialized workshops, seminars, and continuing education opportunities focused on providing employees with the knowledge and skills necessary to respond to the needs and contexts of target populations. Finally, organizations with a commitment to cultural competence will often include criteria regarding demonstrated cultural competence among the other criteria used to make promotion or retention decisions.

Service Array

Service array is an organizational function related to human resources; specifically, it refers to the type and extent of services provided by an organization. A service array is culturally competent to the extent that an organization provides services that directly address the needs of the community (Hernandez et al. 2009). Language services, including bilingual practitioners and translation services, fall into this category (Alegría et al. 2007). Adaptation and location of services may also fall into this category: For example, in communities where the culture is largely steeped in religion and there is strong reliance on religious leaders for guidance and healing, behavioral health service organizations might consider incorporating religious leaders into treatment or providing treatment in religious settings such as churches (Hernandez et al. 2009).

Technical Support

The organizational functions that ensure the availability of critical resources to implement organizational cultural competence efforts, such as technology and financial support, are referred to as *technical support* (Hernandez et al. 2009). Technological resources may be needed to update and maintain client information; to maintain a database of services and tools and data used for planning and evaluation; and to track utilization patterns. Other forms of technical support that overlap with human resources functions might include the retention of consultants or consulting firms that can aid in developing culturally competent services throughout the organization.

Component Four: Direct Service Support

Direct service support, the fourth component included in Hernandez et al.'s (2006, 2009) cultural competence model, refers to three interrelated functions that are directly tied to service provision: availability, accessibility, and utilization. At times, changes to one function will affect another. Each of these functions is described in detail here.

Service Availability

Service availability refers to the structures, policies, and practices that directly lead to the establishment and maintenance of services reflective of the needs of a target population (Hernandez et al. 2009). For instance, if an organization's monitoring of community needs suggests a strong presence of immigrants with limited English-language skills, a culturally competent organization will make changes at structural (e.g., hiring of bilingual personnel), procedural (e.g., requiring that services be provided either in Spanish or through competent interpreters), and policy (e.g., authorizing payments for interpreter services) levels to ensure that services can be made available in Spanish.

Accessibility

Accessibility refers to the structures, policies, and practices that directly facilitate service entry, service use, and service termination by community members (Hernandez et al. 2009). Not all services that are available are accessible. For example, if the economic and working conditions of local Latino populations prevent individuals from using mental health services that are available only during traditional work hours (e.g., Monday through Friday, 9:00 a.m. to 5:00 p.m.), needed services may go unutilized or underutilized (Barrio et al. 2008). Other common obstacles to accessibility include location, cost, complexity of intake procedures, and culturally ascribed stigma associated with mental illness and its treatment. The available literature documents numerous successful solutions to these obstacles, such as the creation of centralized service centers, the provision of home-based services, the implementation of streamlined service procedures, the use of health promoters to aid with system utilization, and the incorporation and use of more culturally acceptable terms and concepts within the organization (Callejas et al. 2009).

A particular organization's choice of strategies to increase accessibility will be largely determined by local contexts (Callejas et al. 2009). For example, in a rural community with an established migrant farm worker health care system, accessibility to behavioral health services might be most immediately affected by making structural, procedural, and policy changes that promote embedding of these services within the established system (Callejas et al. 2009). Doing this successfully might require changes across each of the functions included in the infrastructure domain (e.g., training ambulatory health promoters in behavioral health triage, revising the values of the health care system to include behavioral health).

Utilization

Utilization is defined as an organizational function that involves "the promotion of service use in the community and the facilitation of organizational accountability by tracking [clients'] service use patterns" (Hernandez et al. 2009, p. 1048). Reminder calls for appointments are an example of practices that might directly promote service use (Barrio et al. 2008). Social marketing—making the community aware of services available for use and the benefits associated with these services—is another way in which organizations can promote utilization of services. Organizations can also promote utilization by providing transportation to those who otherwise would be unable to take advantages of the services offered (Barrio et al. 2008) The provision of transportation is also related to *accessibility*. These examples highlight the interrelatedness of all three organizational functions within this component of the model.

To track utilization, culturally competent organizations will collect and use data regarding service characteristics (e.g., type of service, type of provider, location), service use factors (e.g., retention rates, number of service encounters), and service users' characteristics (e.g., demographic data, location). Careful analyses of these data can bring to light strengths and gaps in service provision. For example, results of these analyses can guide the tailoring of services to better meet community needs, can inform strategic planning efforts, and can point to needed service awareness campaigns (Holcomb et al. 1997).

Conclusions

An understanding of cultural competence at the organizational level complements and contextualizes the accounts of cultural competence at the individual and practice levels that dominate behavioral health research and practice (Hernandez et al. 2009). We emphasize that the long-term success of efforts to include culturally competent interventionists and to establish culturally competent practices depends on the success of broader organizational changes.

A conceptualization of organizational cultural competence as compatibility between service environments and the characteristics and culture of the local community (as articulated throughout this chapter) has several important strengths. First, it connects culture directly to services. Second, it facilitates culturally competent services in contexts often overlooked by approaches that rely on broad cultural generalizations (e.g., ethnic groups of local but not regional or national salience, subcultures within larger ethnic groups). Finally, it highlights that cultural competence is an inherent feature of all behavioral health organizations (not only of those serving ethnic minority groups).

Although there have been some exemplary efforts to rigorously examine organizational cultural competence within behavioral service settings, much of the literature in this area is conceptual and descriptive (Harper et al. 2006; Weiner et al. 2008). This suggests that some caution is warranted when incorporating suggestions from the literature into practice settings. To assist practitioners in selecting reliable and useful suggestions, this chapter has highlighted some of the more trustworthy literature sources. Future research and practice would benefit greatly from more careful and systematic documentation and evaluation of efforts, such as exist in other areas of organizational functioning (e.g., Cook et al. 1990; Rogelberg 2005). Likewise, efforts to advance organizational cultural competence practice and scholarship can benefit from the incorporation of empirically supported approaches to assessing and modifying organizational behavior and values. Relevant theories and approaches include, but are not limited to, systems theories (Skyttner 2005), OBM (Wilder et al. 2009), organization development (Gallos 2006), and personnel selection (Cook 2009).

Despite the limitations of some of the organizational cultural competence literature, as a body of work it has served to clearly highlight one important point: Organizational change is required if an organization is to increase the availability, accessibility, and utilization of mental health services to and by Latinos. Only with the support of organizational change are practitioner—and practice-level efforts to decrease the disability burden faced by Latinos likely to experience long-term success. In this regard, it is our sincere hope that this chapter provides a road map on how to understand and bring about organizational cultural competence.

References

Alegría, M., Canino, G., Ríos, R., Vera, M., Calderón, J., Rusch, D., & Ortega, A. N. (2002). Inequalities in use of specialty mental health services among Latinos, African Americans, and non-Latino whites. *Psychiatric Services, 53,* 1547–1555.

Alegría, M., Mulvaney-Day, N., Woo, M., Torres, M., Gao, S., & Oddo, V. (2007). Correlates of past-year mental health service use among Latinos: Results from the National Latino and Asian American Study. *American Journal of Public Health, 97,* 76–83.

Añez, L. M., Paris, M., Bedregal, L. E., Davidson, L., & Grilo, C. M. (2005). Application of cultural constructs in the care of first generation Latino clients in a community mental health setting. *Journal of Psychiatric Practice, 11,* 221–230.

Barrio, C., Palinkas, L. A., Yamada, A., Fuentes, D., Criado, V., Garcia, P., & Jeste, D. V. (2008). Unmet needs for mental health services for Latino older adults: Perspectives from consumers, family members, advocates, and service providers. *Community Mental Health Journal, 44,* 57–74.

Bernal, G., Bonilla, J., & Bellido, C. (1995). Ecological validity and cultural sensitivity for outcome research: Issues for the cultural adaptation and development of psychosocial treatments with Hispanics. *Journal of Abnormal Child Psychology, 23,* 67–82.

Callejas, L. M., Hernandez, M., Nesman, T., & Mowery, D. (2009). Creating a front porch in systems of care: Improving access to behavioral health services for diverse children and families. *Evaluation & Program Planning, 33,* 32–35.

Cardemil, E. V., Adams, S. T., Calista, J. L., Connell, J., Encarnación, J., Esparza, N. K., et al. (2007). The Latino mental health project: A local mental health needs assessment. *Administration & Policy in Mental Health & Mental Health Services Research, 34,* 331–341.

Cook, M. (2009). *Personnel selection: Adding value through people* (5th ed.). Hoboken, NJ: John Wiley & Sons.

Cook, T. D., Campbell, D. T., & Peracchio, L. (1990). *Quasi experimentation.* In M. D. Dunnette & L. M. Hough (Eds.), *Handbook of industrial and organizational psychology* (2nd ed., Vol. 1; pp. 491–576). Palo Alto, CA: Consulting Psychologists Press.

Delphin, M. E., & Rowe, M. (2008). Continuing education in cultural competence for community mental health practitioners. *Professional Psychology: Research & Practice, 39,* 182–191.

Edwards, R. W., Jumper-Thurman, P., Plested, B. A., Oetting, E. R., & Swanson, L. (2000). Community readiness: Research to practice. *Journal of Community Psychology, 28,* 291–307.

Eng, E., & Blanchard, L. (1991). Action-oriented community diagnosis: A health education tool. *International Journal of Community Health Education, 11,* 93–110.

Eng, E., Moore, K. S., Rhodes, S. D., Griffith, D. M., Allison, L. L., Shirah, K., & Mebane, E. M. (2005). Insiders and outsiders assess who is "The Community": Participant observation, key informant interview, focus group interview, and community forum. In B. A. Israel, E. Eng, A. J. Schulz, & E. A. Parker (Eds.), *Methods in community based participatory research for health* (pp. 77–100). San Francisco, CA: Jossey-Bass.

Gallos, J. V (Ed.) (2006). *Organization development: A Jossey-Bass reader.* San Francisco, CA: Jossey-Bass.

Gruys, M. L., Stewart, S. M., Goodstein, J., Bing, M. N., & Wicks, A. C. (2008). Values enactment in organizations: A multi-level examination. *Journal of Management, 34*(4), 806–843.

Guarnaccia, P. J., Lewis-Fernandez, R., & Rivera Marano, M. (2003). Toward a Puerto-Rican popular nosology: *Nervios* and *ataque de nervios. Cultural Medicine & Psychiatry, 27,* 339–366.

Guerrero, M. L., Morrow, R. C., Calva, J. J., Ortega-Gallegos, H., Weller, S. C., Ruiz-Palacios, G. M., & Morrow, A. L. (1999). Rapid ethnographic assessment of breastfeeding practices in periurban Mexico City. *Bulletin of the World Health Organization, 77*(4), 323–330.

Harper, M., Hernandez, M., Nesman, T., Mowery, D., Worthington, J., & Isaccs, M. (2006). *Organizational cultural competence: A review of assessment protocols* (Making Children's Mental Health Services Successful series, FMHI Pub. No. 204-2). Tampa, FL: University of South Florida, Louis de la Parte Florida Mental Health Institute, Research and Training Center for Children's Mental Health.

Hernandez, M., Gomez, A., Lipien, L., Greenbaum, P. E., Armstrong, K., & Gonzalez, P. (2001). Use of the system of care practice review in the national evaluation: Evaluating the fidelity of practice to system of care principles. *Journal of Emotional & Behavioral Disorders, 18,* 19–26.

Hernandez, M., Nesman, T., Isaacs, M., Callejas, L. M., & Mowery, D (Eds.) (2006). *Examining the research base supporting culturally competent children's mental health services.* (Making Children's Mental Health Services Successful series, FMHI Pub. No. 240-1). Tampa, FL: University of South Florida, Louis de la Parte Florida Mental Health Institute, Research and Training Center for Children's Mental Health.

Hernandez, M., Nesman, T., Mowery, D., Acevedo-Polakovich, I. D., & Callejas, L. M. (2009). Cultural competence: A literature review and conceptual model for mental health services. *Psychiatric Services, 60,* 1046–1050.

Holcomb, W. R., Parker, J. C., & Leong, G. B. (1997). Outcomes of inpatients treated on a VA psychiatric unit and a substance abuse treatment unit. *Psychiatric Services, 48,* 699–704.

Hull, P. C., Canedo, J., Aquilera, J., Gracia, E., Lira, I., & Reyes, F. (2008). Assessing community readiness for change in the Nashville Hispanic community through participatory research. *Progress in Community Health Partnerships: Research, Education, & Action, 2,* 185–194.

Isaacs, M. R., Huang, L. N., Hernandez, M., Echo-Hawk, H., Acevedo-Polakovich, I. D., & Martinez, K. (2008). Services for youth and their families in culturally diverse communities. In B. A. Stroul & G. M. Blau (Eds.), *The system of care handbook: Transforming mental health services for children, youth, and families* (pp. 619–639). Baltimore, MD: Paul H. Brookes Publishing.

Lehman, W. E. K., Greener, J. M., & Simpson, D. D. (2002). Assessing organizational readiness for change. *Journal of Substance Abuse Treatment, 22,* 197–209.

Maciak, B. J., Guzman, R., Santiago, A., Villalobos, G., & Israel, B. A. (1999). Establishing La Vida: A community-based partnership to prevent intimate violence against Latina women. *Health Education & Behavior, 26,* 821–840.

McNall, M., & Foster-Fischman, P. G. (2007). Methods of rapid evaluation, assessment, and appraisal. *American Journal of Evaluation, 28,* 151–168.

Newton, F. (1978). The Mexican-American emic system of mental illness: An exploratory study. In J. M. Casas & S. E. Keefe (Eds.), *Family and mental health in the Mexican-American community* (pp. 69–90). Los Angeles, CA: Spanish Speaking Mental Health Research Center.

Oetting, E. R., Jumper-Thurman, P., Plested, B., & Edwards, R. W. (2001). Community readiness and health services. *Substance Use & Misuse, 36,* 825–843.

Office of Minority Health (n.d.). *CLAS Standards Assessment Tool.* Retrieved May 10, 2010, from http://www.qsource.org/uqiosc/CLAS%20Standards%20Assess%20Tool.doc

Ohio Department of Mental Health. (2003). *The Consolidated Culturalogical Assessment Tools.* Columbus, OH: Author.

Piedra, L. M., & Buki, L. P. (2010). Ameliorating mental health disparities in immigrant Latino populations: The application of community readiness theory. *Border-Lines, 14,* 61–94.

Plested, B., Edwards, R. W., & Jumper-Thurman, P. (2006). *Community readiness: A handbook for successful change.* Fort Collins, CO: Tri-Ethnic Center for Prevention Research.

Posavac, E. J., & Carey, R. G. (2007). *Program evaluation: Methods and case studies.* Upper Saddle River, NJ: Pearson Prentice Hall.

Quinn, S. (1999). Teaching community diagnosis: Integrating community experience with meeting graduate standards for health educators. *Health Education Research, 14,* 685–696.

Rogelberg, S. G (Ed.) (2005). *Handbook of research methods in industrial and organizational psychology.* Malden, MA: Blackwell Publishing.

Schneider, B., Smith, D. B., & Goldstein H. W. (2000). Attraction-Selection-Attrition: Toward a person-environment psychology of organizations. In W. B. Walsh, K. H. Craik, & R. H. Price (Eds.), *Person-environment psychology: New directions and perspectives* (pp. 619–639). Mahwah, NJ: Lawrence Erlbaum Associates.

Skyttner, L. (2005). *General systems theory: Problems, perspectives, practice* (2nd ed.). Toh Tuck Link, Singapore: World Scientific Publishing.

Steckler, A. B., Dawson, L., Israel, B. A., & Eng, E. (1993). Community health development: An overview of the works of Guy W. Steuart. *Health Education Quarterly* (Suppl. 1), S3–S20.

Sue, D. W., Bernier, J. E., Durran, A., Feinberg, L., Pedersen, P, Smith, E. J., & Vasquez-Nuttal, E. (1982). Position paper: Cross-cultural counseling competencies. *Counseling Psychologist, 10,* 45–52.

Taplin, D. H., Scheld, S., & Low, S. M. (2002). Rapid ethnographic assessment in urban parks: A case study of Independence National Historical Park. *Human Organization, 61*(1), 80–93.

U.S. Department of Health and Human Services (USDHHS). (2001). *Mental health: Culture, race, and ethnicity.* Rockville, MD: Author.

Valdez, A., Cepeda, A., Negi, N. J., & Kaplan, C. (2009). *Fumando la piedra*: Emerging patterns of crack use among Latino immigrant day laborers in New Orleans. *Journal of Immigrant & Minority Health.* doi:10.1007/s10903-009-9300-5

Weiner, B., Amick, H., & Lee, S. Y. (2008). Conceptualization and measurement of organizational readiness for change: A review of the literature in health service research and other fields. *Medical Care Research & Review, 65,* 379–426.

Weisman, A., Feldman, G., Gruman, C., Rosenberg, R., Chamorro, R., & Belozersky, I. (2005). Improving mental health services for Latino and Asian immigrants. *Professional Psychology: Research & Practice, 36,* 642–648.

Wilder, D. A., Austin, J., & Casella, S. (2009). Applying behavior analysis in organizations: Organizational behavior management. *Psychological Services, 6,* 202–211.

Yee, D., & Tursi, C. (2002). Recognizing diversity and moving toward cultural competence: One organization's effort. *Generations, 26,* 54–58.

Chapter 5
Building Infrastructure Through Training and Interdisciplinary Collaboration

Edward A. Delgado-Romero, Michelle M. Espino, Eckart Werther and Marta J. González

Abstract Establishing and maintaining a mental health infrastructure that accounts for the complexities and diversity within the Latino population provides a unique opportunity to envision culturally appropriate services and training. This chapter introduces the main structural issues present in mental health training, especially with regard to establishing a Latino educational pipeline to the mental health profession, and discusses the specific challenges related to training a bilingual and bicultural workforce. Examples of bilingual and bicultural training programs are highlighted, as well as the importance of promoting interdisciplinary collaborations that can lead to greater resources for education and training. Six recommendations for building infrastructure focused on training bicultural and bilingual mental health providers are offered.

> *Latinos deserve a diverse, multidisciplinary, bilingual and bicultural behavioral workforce.*
> (Chapa and Acosta 2010, p. 4)

The growth of the Latino population and the role it will play in the future labor market demands a reexamination of infrastructures for mental health training. Linguistic competence and culturally appropriate communication skills among mental health providers are key factors that influence client satisfaction and overall quality of physical and mental health care for Latinos (Pérez-Escamilla 2010). However, we are far from meeting the demand for culturally appropriate services. For example, an estimate indicated that in 1999, there were only 20 Latino mental health professionals for every 100,000 US Latinos, and there is no evidence to suggest that this alarming statistic has significantly changed since then (Caldwell et al. n.d.; U.S. Department of Health and Human Services 2001). The need for new infrastructures is clear, yet this need arises within a context that offers many challenges.

Structural barriers for Latinos in mental health treatment include a lack of knowledge about the mental health system, inadequate transportation, high cost of services,

E. A. Delgado-Romero (✉)
College of Education, University of Georgia, GA, USA
e-mail: edelgado@uga.edu

a lack of bilingual providers, and difficulty dealing with the complexities of the US health system (Caldwell et al. n.d.). Latinos, as the largest ethnic minority in the United States, are comprised of new immigrants as well as families that can trace their roots in the United States back for several generations (Chapa and Acosta 2010). They may be monolingual Spanish (typically foreign-born Latinos), bilingual to various degrees, or English monolingual (typically second-generation Latinos and beyond), requiring that service providers have bilingual proficiency as well as an understanding of acculturation issues (Suro 2006). Moreover, the predicted population growth is occurring within a context of heightened social tensions and intense local conflicts over resources. As the Arizona debacle illustrates, inadequate immigration laws and federal neglect for reform have exacerbated negative factors such as prejudice, discrimination, and anti-immigrant sentiment. These add to acculturative stress and contribute to adverse educational, vocational, physical health, and mental health outcomes (Portes and Rumbaut 2001).

Within this context, US mental health providers must confront unprecedented service challenges, create opportunities to promote a greater understanding of the Latino population, and offer culturally responsive treatment (Alegría et al. 2006; Imberti 2007; Martínez Pincay and Guarnaccia 2006). These efforts are hampered by the fact that Latinos are underrepresented in professional organizations such as the American Psychological Association (APA) (2.3%) (Delgado-Romero 2009). Thus, an urgent need exists to create infrastructure, defined by the editors of this volume as "the basic facilities, resources, and human capital needed to provide effective mental health services," that will increase the number of bilingual and bicultural mental health providers. Specifically, in this chapter we focus on the structures and processes needed to train competent bilingual and bicultural mental health service providers. In an effort to make the information widely applicable, we draw from an emerging interdisciplinary literature as well as from our varied experiences as a team of Latino professionals from diverse disciplinary educational backgrounds training in psychology, higher education, counselor education, counseling psychology, social work, and marriage and family therapy.

The chapter is organized as follows. First, we introduce the main structural issues present in mental health training, and discuss the specific challenges related to training a bilingual and bicultural workforce. Next, we highlight some bilingual and bicultural training programs and the learning opportunities they offer. The need to create an infrastructure that promotes interdisciplinary collaborations is then highlighted, followed by a discussion of untapped resources. The chapter closes with six recommendations for infrastructure building for the training of bicultural and bilingual mental health providers.

Structural Issues in Mental Health Service Training

Mental health workers could potentially commit cultural malpractice and become obsolete if they are unable to respond to the rapidly changing demographics in US society (Hall 1997). Within the field of psychology, attention has been directed to the implications of the demographic shifts occurring in the United States, and a significant recommendation is that the field "finds it necessary to include in its ranks *a dramatically enlarged cadre of persons of color* and to ensure that all psychologists demonstrate some level of multicultural competence" (American Psychological Association [APA] 1997; APA Office of Ethnic Minority Affairs [APA OEMA] 2008, p. 22, emphasis added). In the years since the report was published, APA has been unable to significantly increase the number of ethnic minority psychologists across all subfields of psychology. In the case of Latino psychologists, APA was only able to increase the percentage of psychologists by 0.03% between 1999 and 2009 (Delgado-Romero 2009).

Similar trends are observed in other mental health disciplines. The National Association of Social Workers (NASW) and the Council on Social Work Education (CSWE) have both emphasized the need for and importance of having a culturally competent workforce of social workers (National Association of Social Workers [NASW] 2001; Council on Social Work Education [CSWE] 2008). Despite efforts by the NASW, CSWE, and individual social work programs, there continues to be a significant need for social workers who are properly trained to work with the Latino population. Although the number of social work degrees awarded has increased, there continues to be a shortage of social workers with the culturally specific skills and knowledge needed to deliver effective and appropriate services to the Latino population (NASW Center for Workforce Studies 2005; Vidal de Haymes and Kilty 2007). In a report from a national study on licensed social workers, the NASW stated that "the social work profession has not been able to keep pace with population trends in terms of its ability to attract social workers of color" (NASW Center for Workforce Studies 2005, p. 8). In fact, only 3% of those who obtain a graduate degree in social work are Latino (Furman et al. 2009). The lack of progress in Latino mental health training is not unique. Unfortunately, the entire educational system in the United States seems to be failing the Latino population.

Latina scholar Patricia Gándara (2009) termed Latino education a "crisis." Latino participation in higher education declines at every stage of the educational pipeline, resulting in a saturation of Latinos at less selective or open-door institutions and in a troubling absence of Latino influence at the highest levels in flagship academic institutions (Delgado-Romero 2009). Latino undergraduates, in comparison with their non-Latino White counterparts, are more likely to attend two-year colleges (Arbona and Nora 2007), go to school part-time, work during college, be first generation, be independent with dependents, and have low rates of graduate school enrollment (Carter 1997; Fry 2002, 2004; Nora and Rendón 1996; Solórzano et al. 2005). A constricted pipeline results in very few Latino students enrolling in doctoral programs and even fewer (just over half) finishing their doctorates within 10 years (Council of Graduate Schools 2008).

Problems with Latino education are made worse by the fact that the Latino population is growing at a fast pace and the majority of this growth is coming from children and adolescents who drop out of school disproportionately. For example, in the state of Georgia, the Latino population increased by 300% from 1990–2000, and many school systems were transformed into majority Latino school systems seemingly overnight; this trend was coupled with some of the highest dropout rates in the nation (Delgado-Romero et al. 2007). Consequently, Latino youth are taking paths toward low-skill, nontechnical, and low-paying careers, as the attainment gap worsens (Portes et al. in press).

There are many competing hypotheses as to why Latino students do not thrive in the profession of psychology despite their interest in the discipline. The reasons range from a lack of academic preparation, admissions criteria based on culturally biased tests, devaluation or lack of interest in diversity on the part of training programs, a lack of Latino role models, overt or covert discrimination, and the fact that many psychology training programs are geographically located in rural areas. Much of the higher education retention literature focuses on individual students as solely responsible for their own retention, rather than assessing how institutional environments contribute to attrition (Hernández 2002; Richardson and Skinner 1990). In addition, an issue that has not received much attention is the mentoring or advice that Latino students receive. For example, Latino students who have a passionate commitment to Latino issues may be receiving mentoring from advisors who foreclose (intentionally or inadvertently) science-oriented roles (Delgado-Romero et al. 2007). Similar to the important role of secondary school teachers in mentoring Latino children and encouraging them to consider college (Arellano and Padilla 1996) research has brought to light the important role that faculty of color can play in helping Latino students persist (Gloria and Robinson Kurpius 1996). However, only 2.9% of all full-time faculty and 3% of administrators on college campuses are Latino, which creates limited opportunities for Latino students to connect with potential Latino mentors (Castellanos and Jones 2003). Nevertheless, it should be noted that faculty and administrators of all ethnic backgrounds can and should help mentor Latino students.

The limited availability of mentors is concerning because mentors contribute to students' socialization processes in graduate school. Successful socialization processes occur when there are opportunities for formal and informal interactions between faculty and graduate students, faculty have a genuine interest in graduate students' success, there is an environment in which responsibilities and roles between faculty and graduate students are articulated and clear, the environment is not competitive, and there is a balance between identifying as a student and as a future researcher/faculty member (Weidman and Stein 2003). However, graduate socialization processes seldom display those characteristics. For Latino doctoral students, issues of race, class, and gender compound the struggles as they contend with a limited Latino presence in graduate programs. In addition, self-doubt, changing relationships with family (brought about by the physical distance from the institution to home), and adjustments to the academic rigor of a program may prompt early dropout (Figueroa et al. 2001; Herrera 2003; Solórzano and Yosso 2001). The limited infrastructures available in colleges and universities make it difficult to track and disaggregate graduate student populations that leave. Administrators' lack of commitment to learn more about graduate student attrition is based on beliefs that students' behavior is directly related to lack of ability, rather than the result of any possible structural, cultural, and/or psychological barriers within graduate schools and programs (Deem and Brehony 2000; Ferreira 2003; Lovitts 2001). Therefore, the constricted pipeline for Latinos is troubling. Unprecedented efforts are needed to dramatically increase the number of Latino students who are prepared to enter graduate school, who success-fully complete their graduate programs in mental health fields, and who are prepared to offer culturally appropriate bilingual and bicultural services. With more efforts to open the pipeline, we can narrow the gap between Latinos' growing need for cultur-ally appropriate services and the mental health professions' ability to meet that need.

Working with Latinos, in fact, has been part of the training experience for many psychologists. For example, in 2009, 11% of predoctoral internships offered a ma-jor rotation with Spanish-speaking clients, and 59% offered minor rotations. Among postdoctoral fellowships, 44% offered training with Spanish speakers (Association of Psychology Postdoctoral and Internship Centers 2009). Moreover, a 2007 workforce analysis of 20,000 APA members found that psychologists reported working with ethnic minority clients more frequently than with other clients in areas such as sub-stance abuse or severe mental illness (Delgado-Romero 2009). These statistics reflect a growing need to expand mental health services for Latinos—yet we must still con-tend with a limited multidisciplinary bilingual and bicultural workforce (Bernal and Castro 1994; Chapa and Acosta 2010), culturally insensitive or ineffective treatments (Tucker et al. 2007), and the exclusion of the Latino population as participants in the knowledge base of mainstream mental health (Carter et al. 1998; Delgado-Romero et al. 2005; Ponterotto 1988; Shelton et al. 2009). These structural issues interfere with the training of mental health practitioners who can effectively work with the Latino population. Moreover, unaddressed structural issues may negatively affect the entire Latino population by producing low levels of satisfaction, noncompliance with treatment, and poor outcomes among consumers (Chapa and Acosta 2010). These consequences run counter to the ethical imperative of "do no harm," included in most major mental health organizations' ethics codes (see Gibson and Mitchell 2007).

Based on our working knowledge, we envision an educated, community-based workforce that has the necessary clinical, research, and theoretical training to work effectively with the Latino population across various levels of language proficiency and other contextual concerns (e.g., social class, ethnicity, race, immigration sta-tus). This workforce would also focus on the strengths of the Latino population and work toward addressing the systemic barriers that Latinos face. Such a work-force does not currently exist; Latinos are underrepresented in the fields of medicine (3%), clinical psychology (1%), social work (4.3%), and registered nursing (1.7%) (Chapa and Acosta 2010). Ruiz (2002, p. 87) asserted that it is "very important" to have a higher representation of Latinos in the mental health professional workforce to decrease the adverse effects of insufficient representation. Thus, it is important to review the challenges in creating a well-prepared cadre of professionals.

Challenges Related to Training a Bicultural and Bilingual Workforce

Cultural competence among mental health practitioners has been a long-standing concern (Worthington et al. 2007). However, the literature on effective interven-tions with bilingual Latinos is still developing. One critical distinction is that bilingual and bicultural therapists are either "born" or "made" through rigorous training programs (Clouse and Delgado-Romero 2008). Providers in the "born" group tend to be of Latino heritage and have conversational language skills that they learned from speaking Spanish at home, though they may not have received formal Spanish-language training (Biever et al. 2004). Such workers struggle with an unfamiliar professional vocabulary as they utilize mental health concepts in Spanish. Frequently, because these workers have been trained in English and possess conversational language skills, they are assumed by their monolingual colleagues to have a facility with the technical mental health terminology needed to conduct therapy in Spanish. They are often pressed into service with Spanish-speaking clients who present a variety of personal and professional dilemmas (Castaño et al. 2007; Engstrom and Min 2004; Verdinelli and Biever 2009a, b). Although these providers are able to deliver services in Spanish and often point to the benefits of their cultural connections as buffers against burnout, many report feeling like they live in two worlds, being frustrated by their lack of training, feeling isolated, and experiencing emotional exhaustion from working in two languages (Clouse and Delgado-Romero 2008; Engstrom and Min 2004).

In addition to working on cases that are known to be more complex, tiring, and demanding because of language barriers, bilingual workers may face additional challenges when working in insensitive work environments (Engstrom et al. 2009). Although being bilingual can be an asset during the hiring process, it can become a liability in terms of workload, as well as in attaining raises or promotions (Engstrom et al. 2009). Commonly, bilingual workers must take on additional job responsibilities as translators or interpreters for monolingual colleagues, often without additional compensation. Misunderstandings of the complexities of working in two languages fuel such expectations (Piedra 2010). Agency and health care administrators need to identify and test for the language skill set that bilingual workers should possess and address issues of retention and equity by advocating for pay differentials and workload adjustments (Engstrom et al. 2009).

In an innovative study, Elderkin-Thompson et al. (2001) empirically investigated the accuracy of untrained bilingual nurses who were translating medical information for patients. They found that in one-half of the encounters, serious miscommunication problems altered the physician's understanding of the symptoms or the credibility of the patient concerns. They identified common processes in translational miscommunication that could be avoided either by providing extensive training or by using trained interpreters. As this example illustrates, individuals who lack training and who do not have qualified bilingual and bicultural supervisors run the risk of providing inadequate services. For example, the first author of this chapter was the only bilingual and Latino person in his graduate program. He was the only person who could see Spanish-speaking clients in the department training clinic, despite his lack of formal Spanish-language training and the absence of bilingual supervision. He had lingering concerns about the adequacy of his therapy in Spanish, and upon years of reflection realized that he lacked the power to adequately address the issue with monolingual English-speaking supervisors. Therefore, bilingual therapists may encounter a double bind, in that they are often the only provider for a vulnerable population and at the same time feel overwhelmed and overextended (Rivas et al. 2004; Verdinelli and Biever 2009a, 2009b). Thus, the potential for professional burnout and turnover may intensify.

An understanding of the challenges faced by bilingual mental health workers signals inadequate training, lack of resources, lack of accreditation criteria, outdated agency policies, and exploitation (Rivas et al. 2004). Increasingly, there is a need for ongoing training in bilingual assessment, cultural competency, and methods for conducting bilingual therapy (Biever et al. 2004). Without this training, the mental health field will continue to face attrition of bilingual workers (Furman et al. 2009).

Opportunities Offered through Bilingual Training Programs

The majority of bilingual and bicultural trainees are being schooled in generalist mental health programs that often have very few Latino faculty (Broussard and Delgado-Romero 2008; Delgado-Romero et al. 2003). Accredited programs usually have a multicultural commitment that is codified by an accrediting agency (e.g., APA 2003), but the operationalization of that commitment varies by program in coursework, clinical training, and evaluation. Formal bilingual training programs in psychology and social work can offer the kind of coursework, field experience, and clinical supervision that will prepare students to work with Latino populations (Clouse and Delgado-Romero 2008; Vidal de Haymes and Kilty 2007). In this section, we review some of the bilingual programs that are available and their key features. The existence and success of these programs indicate that there is both a need and a market for bilingual training for mental health practitioners. For example, the Psychological Services for Spanish Speaking Populations (PSSSP) program at Our Lady of the Lake University (OLLU) in San Antonio, Texas, is an APA-accredited program designed to assist bilingual mental health providers in becoming equally competent at providing services in English and Spanish (Biever et al. 2002). The program includes coursework in the following areas: professional and technical Spanish, language and psychological variables in interviews and assessments with Latinos, Spanish-language professional communication skills, sociocultural foundations of counseling Mexicans and Mexican Americans, normal family development processes across cultures, theories of multicultural counseling, and Latino psychology. The program also offers a cultural immersion component in Mexico during the summer. Implemented in 1997, the program has trained many OLLU students and bilingual service providers. In a forthcoming paper, OLLU faculty will discuss the various outcome measures they use to evaluate their program (Biever et al. under review).

In California, several colleges offer training experiences with Latino populations as part of their program, such as at Pacific Oaks College in Pasadena, which offers a master's degree in Marriage and Family Therapy (MFT): Latina/o Family Studies Specialization, with an educational emphasis on the diverse mental health needs of Latino children and families. This program offers a bilingual language component that focuses on educating and developing mental health professionals who possess the linguistic ability to serve monolingual Spanish-speaking clients and their families. The program coursework includes areas of study in Latino history, psychology, and family systems in the context of immigration, acculturation, trauma, and advocacy (for more information, see http://www.pacificoaks.edu/programs/marital-family-therapy). Similarly, the Phillips Graduate Institute offers a pre-master's traineeship in the Latino Family Therapy program, in which students are required to know conversational Spanish because supervision and therapy are conducted in Spanish (http://pgi.edu/ca_27.aspx).

Similarly, in an effort to increase the number of culturally competent social workers who are capable of responding to the needs of the Latino population, some schools of social work have implemented curricular programs that focus on Latino issues and provide cultural and language experiences (see Vidal de Haymes and Kilty 2007). Examples of these efforts include an international track that emphasizes immigrant and refugee issues; language and cultural immersion and interchange programs between US, Mexican, and Latin American universities; and collaborative graduate social work programs between US and Puerto Rican universities, as well as the development of a bicultural and bilingual undergraduate social work curriculum (Vidal de Haymes and Kilty 2007). A specific effort to increase the number of bilingual social workers is a collaborative tuition assistance program established by the state of Illinois. This program involves a collaboration between public and private institutions of higher education and the Illinois Department of Children and Family Services. Through the program, bilingual individuals who pursue a BSW or MSW degree receive tuition and stipend assistance (see Vidal de Haymes and Kilty 2007). Although this program has been discontinued for funding reasons, it is a noteworthy effort to increase the representation of Spanish-speaking social workers.

The Imperative for Interdisciplinary Work

It is vital that an "aggressive, integrated, and national strategy" within mental health be implemented to appropriately address the mental health needs of the Latino population (Vega and Lopez 2001). Interdisciplinary collaboration, therefore, is essential, as many Latinos receive services from different sectors of the health industry and interact with different service providers (Vega and Lopez 2001). It is not uncommon for Latinos to access services via nontraditional mental health settings and providers (e.g., family doctors or clergy) rather than through traditional mental health settings and providers (e.g., psychologists, social workers, counselors) (Vega and Lopez 2001). Latinos who require health services often suffer from a complex interaction of medical and mental health needs that necessitates a multifaceted approach to intervention (Banks et al. 2007; Carillo and de la Cancela 1992). Given these factors, it seems imperative that professionals in the fields of medicine, psychology, social work, counseling, and nursing, as well as clergy members, work together in a collaborative manner to appropriately address Latino mental health issues.

One example of a Latino professional collaboration is the formation of the National Hispanic Health Professionals Leadership Network by the National Hispanic Medical Association (NHMA). The Network was created to provide a forum for interdisciplinary collaboration, as well as to address the fact that Latino patients access the mental health system through a variety of means (Martínez Pincay and Guarnaccia 2006). In 2010, this network consisted of (1) NHMA, (2) Association of Hispanic Mental Health Professionals, (3) *Hablamos Juntos* (a project designed to build connections and communication between health care providers and Latino patients), (4) Hispanic American Allergy and Asthma Association, (5) Hispanic Dental Association, (6) The Latino Caucus of the American Public Health Association, (g) Latino Health Communications, (7) Latinos and Hispanics in Dietetics and Nutrition, (8) National Association of Hispanic Nurses, (9) National Forum for Latino Healthcare Executives, (10) National Latino Behavioral Health Association, (11) the U.S. Department of Health and Human Services Regional Minority Health Consultants, and (12) the National Latina/o Psychological Association. The Network meets during the annual NHMA conference and provides training, networking, and recognition (e.g., awards) of leadership by national Latino health care leaders.

Another example of a successful interdisciplinary collaboration is the multidisciplinary team under the direction of the Office of Minority Health and National Resource Center for Hispanic Mental Health (Chapa and Acosta 2010). This group gathered to create five consensus statements in response to the underrepresentation of Latinos as health care professionals and the lack of attention given to Latino health issues. Through their consensus statements, the team aspires to assist in the development of a diverse workforce, with the goal of providing Latinos meaningful access to behavioral health services. These documents are seen as a multidisciplinary effort to improve the Latino behavioral health condition. The five consensus statements (Chapa and Acosta 2010; p. 4) are:

1. The Latino population in the USA is facing a public health crisis due to poor or unmet behavioral health needs.
2. The lack of bilingual and bicultural behavioral health workforce plays a significant role in disparities across all three areas of behavioral health care service delivery (i.e., availability, access, and quality care).
3. Meaningful access to behavioral health care for Latinos in the USA is a social justice issue.
4. Latinos deserve a diverse, multidisciplinary, bilingual, and bicultural behavioral health workforce.
5. The time for action is NOW!

In this effort, there are successful models that can be replicated. An example of a multidisciplinary approach in addressing the health needs of Latinos at the provider level is the Cambridge Hospital Latino Health Clinic (see Carillo and de la Cancela 1992). This clinic, which was established in 1981, brings together specialists from many disciplines (e.g., occupational medicine, primary care, psychiatry, psychology, and social medicine). These specialists focus on understanding the many issues faced by the Latino community. Their multidisciplinary approach to service delivery enhances interagency collaboration, centralized case coordination, flexibility and adaptability of services, continuity of care, and mutual support for professionals (Carillo and de la Cancela 1992). As a result, the Cambridge Hospital Latino Health Clinic provides a systemic approach to bicultural and bilingual health care for Latinos. It has a long-standing commitment to training and service provision that has both produced culturally and linguistically competent practitioners and served the immediate needs of the Latino population in an integrated and culturally sensitive manner.

Despite the availability of such programs, the need to develop infrastructure continues to be great. Next, we turn our attention to resources yet untapped that may promote development of a bilingual and bicultural workforce.

Untapped Resources for Latino Mental Health

There are several untapped resources for Latino mental health. In this section, we identify three major groups: (a) students, faculty, and staff at Hispanic-serving institutions (HSIs), (b) international Latino mental health workers, and (c) non-Latino mental health workers. This section introduces each group and the links to Latino mental health.

Half of Latino undergraduates can be found at those institutions known collectively as Hispanic-serving institutions (Santiago 2008). These are institutions that have approximately 25% Latino enrollment. However, the designation of HSI is not a federal one, and the designation is somewhat fluid given changes in enrollment; several institutions are on the verge of becoming HSIs (Santiago and Andrade 2010). Currently, there are more than 225 such colleges (including community colleges) in Puerto Rico and states such as Arizona, California, Colorado, Florida, Illinois, Kansas, New Jersey, New Mexico, New York, and Texas, with 70% of the institutions in California, Puerto Rico, and Texas being HSIs (Santiago 2008). HSIs are emerging as areas of interest for researchers (Crisp and Cruz 2010; De Los Santos, Jr., and De Los Santos 2010; Gonyea 2010; González 2008; Santiago and Andrade 2010), as half of Latino students in the United States are educated at 8% of the colleges and universities in the United States (Santiago 2008). Accredited mental health training programs are usually not as prevalent at HSIs as they are in predominantly White institutions (Brown 2010), and only one-third of HSIs offer graduate degrees (Santiago 2008). Therefore, efforts to increase the number of training programs at these institutions, and efforts to form collaborations with such programs, would be a promising area to explore.

Another untapped resource is mental health professionals in Latin America and the Caribbean. For example, in Argentina, seeking therapy is an accepted social practice; the country has 34 universities offering degrees in psychology (Gómez 2007). At 133 psychologists for 100,000 inhabitants, the availability of psychologists there is more than 6.5 times greater than the availability of Latino psychologists in the United States (Gómez 2007). Also, though Brazil is not a Spanish-speaking country, it is interesting that it is predicted that in coming years there will be more psychologists in Brazil than in the United States (Hutz et al. 2004). Traditionally, due to the provinciality of American psychology (Arnett 2008), concerns about English fluency, and issues regarding incompatible models of training, international Latino mental health workers have not been seen as a resource for US clients. We contend that the profession may be unable to maintain these views much longer.

Another untapped resource is the pool of non-Latino trainees. The issue of how best to train non-Latino monolingual students to be multiculturally competent has become an increasingly popular topic over the past 20 years (Worthington et al. 2007). It is clear that the need for multiculturally competent services exceeds the available Latino workforce in the short term, and that individuals of other ethnicities will increasingly serve the Latino population. Therefore, bicultural and bilingual non-Latinos must be involved in such service provision. In developing a bicultural and bilingual workforce, there should be clear efforts to provide multicultural training to all mental health service providers, including training on how to access and use translation services (Hsieh 2006).

In light of the challenges and opportunities in creating a mental health services infrastructure, we provide a broad range of recommendations that can be implemented in various settings. These are discussed next.

Recommendations for Building Infrastructure

Based on the literature we have reviewed, and the great need to address the shortage of bilingual and bicultural mental health service providers, we present several recommendations:

1. Immediate and dramatic action is needed to enhance the retention and success of Latino, as well as bilingual and bicultural, graduate students, faculty, and practitioners in the mental health field.
2. Training programs must recruit faculty and graduate students based on meaningful criteria.
3. Training programs must regularly evaluate their programs and services.
4. We must increase collaborations in order to build infrastructure.
5. Collaborations are needed among people with various levels of education, not just those with graduate degrees.
6. Infrastructure must be built in specific places for specific populations.

Immediate and dramatic action is needed to enhance the retention and success of Latino, as well as bilingual and bicultural, graduate students, faculty, and practitioners in the mental health field. Facing a demographic and social justice imperative, the mental health profession must respond with a dramatic change. The word *dramatic* is used intentionally to reflect the APA report that stated "psychology finds it necessary to include in its ranks a *dramatically enlarged cadre of persons of color*" (APA OEMA 2008, p. 22, emphasis added). A dramatic solution will mean a departure from the status quo. We have suggested that engaging HSIs as partners in graduate education could produce a dramatic change. This partnership would involve developing more mental health training programs within HSIs, and creating pipelines from HSIs to existing mental health training program (e.g., faculty exchange programs, grant partnerships, and shared practicum sites).

Another possible way to enlarge the cadre of ethnic minority psychologists is to promote collaboration with Latin American psychologists. Although most training programs in the United States have dropped second-language requirements as part of their training, this is not the case in Latin America. Many bilingual psychologists in Latin America know English and have obtained doctoral degrees abroad in such countries as Canada, the United States, and Europe. Many of them have taught courses in Latin American countries, contributing to the exchange of knowledge and skills (Sánchez-Sosa and Valderrama-Iturbe 2001). We propose the idea of a bilateral working agreement through consultation and collaboration with bilingual Latin American psychologists in regards to bilingual training, concepts, techniques, and terminology that would best meet the mental health needs of the US Latino population. Through organizations like the Interamerican Society of Psychology, mental health training programs could have reciprocal training agreements to add both demographic diversity and new theoretical perspectives to US psychology, while bringing in new perspectives about the experiences of Latinos in the United States to Latin America (Suro 2006). We note that the official languages of the Interamerican Society of Psychology are English, Portuguese, and Spanish, which means that there is already a strong foundation for bilingual collaborations.

Training programs must recruit faculty and graduate students based on meaningful criteria. The selection of faculty and graduate students in mental health programs is key to achieving effective bilingual and bicultural service provision. For mental health training programs to have maximum impact in the future, they must train, hire, and retain mental health professionals who are committed to multicultural competence, regardless of their ethnic background. These individuals should be selected based on openness to experience, multicultural and bilingual interest and ability, and personal and professional commitment to Latino issues (Delgado-Romero et al. 2007).

Training programs must regularly evaluate their programs and services. Currently, several programs offer certifications, courses, clinical experience, and extensive training in working with Latino populations. However, we do not know what the long-term educational and practice outcomes of these programs are. Do these training programs result in more culturally and linguistically competent practitioners? What types of training and experience are the key components in effective training? Research indicates that the foundation of an effective bilingual program is accurate assessment of language ability before commencement of employment or language training (Biever et al. under review; Elderkin-Thompson et al. 2001; Engstrom et al. 2009). The concept that bicultural and bilingual competence is a lifelong endeavor (see APA 2003) must undergird training programs. This competence should be evaluated and developed in a standardized way through periodic assessment. The evaluation process should include definable and measurable outcomes related to both the provider and the client (Biever et al. under review). Training programs and accrediting boards must also revisit what they require as minimal standards of bicultural and bilingual competence to reflect the reality of the growing Latino population.

We must increase collaborations in order to build infrastructure. Infrastructure can best be built through collaboration across and within disciplines and professional affiliations. There are many multicultural, ethnic minority and Latino professional organizations. To better build infrastructure, there must be purposeful collaboration among these organizations. For example, in psychology, the president of the National Latina/o Psychological Association meets twice yearly with the presidents of the Asian American Psychological Association, the Association of Black Psychologists, the Society of Indian Psychologists, the Society for the Psychological Study of Ethnic Minority Issues, and representatives of APA OEMA. The group, which is collectively known as the Council of National Psychology Associations for the Advancement of Ethnic Minority Interests, works to create a national agenda on ethnic minority issues. Similar structures both within and across professions (e.g., National Hispanic Health Professionals Leadership Network) that provide opportunities for interdisciplinary dialogue are sorely needed.

Collaborations are needed among people with various levels of education, not just those with graduate degrees. Although our focus in this paper has been on graduate training programs, graduate-level mental health professionals rely on a variety of support staff (e.g., interpreters, administrative assistants, accountants, insurance workers, clergy, probation offers, technology support personnel) to provide effective treatment to Latino populations. Latino clients will most likely interact with a variety of support personnel before they ever set foot in a therapy office. The bicultural and bilingual competence of these personnel may play a significant role in mental health outcomes (Tucker et al. 2007). To engage competent individuals at all levels of service within a system (e.g., from receptionists to medical doctors) shows respect for both the issue and everyone involved in the provision of services.

Infrastructure must be built in specific places for specific populations. As Morales (2009) pointed out, the demographic growth of the Latino population will occur primarily in the West and Southwest of the United States; states like California and Texas already have Latino populations that constitute more than 50% of the state population. At the same time that these Latino populations are getting larger, Latinos are also making inroads into states where they have not traditionally lived (e.g., Georgia; see Delgado-Romero et al. 2007). Hence, the challenges in infrastructure building may be different in the various regions. For example, in California the challenge may be the expansion of existing services, whereas in Georgia it may be the development of services from the ground up, with a special emphasis on high school student retention.

Beyond a regional approach, psychologists need to be prepared to work with specific populations while paying attention to the relevant context. For example,

Mexican Americans constitute around three-fourths of all US Latinos. However, in some areas, Mexican Americans are not the majority population; for example, Cubans are the majority in Miami, and Puerto Ricans the majority in New York. One impediment to service access is undocumented status, which is more likely to be an impediment for the population of Mexican ancestry than that of Puerto Rican ancestry. Therefore, mental health service providers in regions with large concentrations of Mexican individuals need to be prepared to address undocumented status as a barrier to service provision. Furthermore, although salient differences in Latino populations and individuals are important (country of origin, foreign- versus US-born, documented versus undocumented), the reality of an emerging panethnic identification for consequent generations of Latinos should also be kept in mind (Diaz-McConnell and Delgado-Romero 2004). As Suro (2006) stated, Latino identity in the United States is a fluid process that is a work in progress. Therefore, mental health professionals must be flexible in balancing differences versus commonalities (e.g., cultural values; see Santiago-Rivera et al. 2002).

Conclusions

In this chapter we have identified many challenges and potential avenues to address these challenges. The demographic, cultural, and ethical imperative to address these issues is clear. We hope that the mental health professions and allied health professionals can find the will (*ganas*) to address the need for infrastructure in a comprehensive and coordinated way. We feel that the future depends on it—and, as Chapa and Acosta (2010) stated, Latinos deserve such a workforce.

References

Alegría, J. M., Mulvaney-Day, N., Woo, M., Torres, M., Gao, S., & Oddo, V. (2006). Correlates of past-year mental health service use among Latinos: Results from a National Latino and Asian American Study. *American Journal of Public Health, 97*, 68–75.

American Psychological Association (APA). (2003). Guidelines on multicultural education, training, research, practice and organizational change for psychologists. *American Psychologist, 58*, 377–402.

American Psychological Association (APA). (1997). *Visions & transformations: The final report of the APA Commission on ethnic minority recruitment, retention, and training in psychology.* Washington, DC: Author.

American Psychological Association, Office of Ethnic Minority Affairs (APA OEMA). (2008). *A portrait of success and challenge—Progress report: 1997–2005.* Washington, DC: Author. Retrieved from www.apa.org/pi/oema/cemrrat_report.html

Arbona, C., & Nora, A. (2007). The influence of academic and environmental factors on Hispanic college degree attainment. *Review of Higher Education, 30*, 247–269.

Arellano, A. R., & Padílla, A. M. (1996). Academic invulnerability among a select group of Latino university students. *Hispanic Journal of Behavioral Sciences, 18*(4), 485–507.

Arnett, J. J. (2008). The neglected 95%: Why American psychology needs to become less American. *American Psychologist, 63,* 602–614.

Association of Psychology Postdoctoral and Internship Centers. (2009). *APPIC online directory.* Retrieved from www.appic.org/directory/4_1_directory_online.asp

Banks, M. E., Buki, L. P., Gallardo, M. E., & Yee, B. W. K. (2007). Integrative healthcare and marginalized populations. In I. Serlin (Series Ed.), *Humanizing healthcare: A handbook for healthcare integration: Vol I. Mind-body medicine* (pp. 147–173). Westport, CT: Greenwood Publishing.

Bernal, M. E., & Castro, F. G. (1994). Are clinical psychologists prepared for service and research with ethnic minorities? Report of a decade of progress. *American Psychologist, 49,* 797–805.

Biever, J. L., Castaño, M. T., de la Fuentes, C., González, C., Servín-López, S., Sprowls, C., & Tripp, C. G. (2002). The role of language in training psychologists to work with Hispanic clients. *Professional Psychology: Research and Practice, 33,* 330–336.

Biever, J. L., Castaño, M. T., González, C., Levy Navarro, R., Sprowls, C., & Verdinelli, S. (2004). Spanish-language psychotherapy: Therapists' experiences and needs. *Advances in Psychology Research, 29,* 157–182.

Biever, J. L., Gómez, J. P., González, C. G. & Patrizio, N. (under review). Psychological services to Spanish-speaking populations: A model curriculum for training competent professionals.

Broussard, D., & Delgado-Romero, E. A. (2008). Identifying Latina/o psychology faculty. El Boletin Online. Retrieved from http://nlpaboletin.blogspot.com/2008/11/identifying-latinao-psychology-faculty_12.html

Brown, A. (2010). *Hispanic serving institutions and psychology.* Unpublished manuscript.

Caldwell, A., Couture, A., & Nowotny, H. (n.d.). *Closing the mental health gap: Eliminating disparities in treatment for Latinos.* Kansas City, MO: Mattie Rhodes Center. Retrieved from http://mattierhodes.org/UserFiles/File/SAMHSA_full_report.pdf

Carillo, J. E., & de la Cancela, V. (1992). The Cambridge Hospital Latino Health Clinic: A model for interagency integration of health services for Latinos at the provider level. *Journal of the National Medical Association, 84,* 513–519.

Carter, D. F. (1997). College student degree aspirations: A theoretical model and literature review with a focus on African American and Latino students. In J. C. Smart (Ed.), *Higher education: Handbook of theory and research, 12* (pp. 129–171). New York: Agathon Press.

Carter, J. A., Akinsulure-Smith, A. M., Smailes, E. M., & Clauss, C. S. (1998). The status of racial/ethnic research in counseling psychology: Committed or complacent? *Journal of Black Psychology, 24,* 322–334.

Castaño, M. T., Biever, J. L., González, C. G., & Anderson, K. B. (2007). Challenges of providing mental health services in Spanish. *Professional Psychology: Research and Practice, 38,* 667–673.

Castellanos, J., & Jones, L. (Eds.). (2003). *The majority in the minority: Expanding the representation of Latina/o faculty, administrators, and students in higher education.* Sterling, VA: Stylus.

Chapa, T., & Acosta, H. (2010). *Movilizandonos por nuestro futuro*: Strategic development of mental health workforce for Latinos. Retrieved from http://minorityhealth.hhs.gov/Assets/pdf/Checked/1/MOVILIZANDONOS_POR_NUESTRO_FUTURO_CONSENSUS_REPORT2010.pdf

Clouse, S., & Delgado-Romero, E. (2008). *Language, training, and burnout experiences of Spanish speaking therapists.* Poster session presented at the Cultural Competency Conference, Georgia State University, Atlanta, GA.

Council of Graduate Schools. (2008). *Ph.D. completion and attrition: Analysis of baseline demographic data from the Ph.D. completion project.* Washington, DC: CGS Publications.

Council on Social Work Education (CSWE). (2008). *Educational policy and accreditation standards.* Alexandria, VA: Author. Retrieved from http://www.cswe.org/File.aspx?id=13780

Crisp, G., & Cruz, I. (2010). Confirmatory factor analysis of a measure of "mentoring" among undergraduate students attending a Hispanic serving institution. *Journal of Hispanic Higher Education, 9,* 232–244.

Deem, R., & Brehony, K. J. (2000). Doctoral students' access to research cultures—Are some more equal than others? *Studies in Higher Education, 25*(2), 149–165.

Delgado-Romero, E. A. (2009). *Latinos and Higher Education: The case of psychology.* Invited address presented at Cross-Cultural Winter Roundtable conference for Psychology and Education at Teachers College, New York, NY.

Delgado-Romero, E. A., Flores, L., Gloria, A., Arredondo, P., & Castellanos, J. (2003). The majority in the minority: Developmental career challenges for Latino and Latina psychology faculty. In L. Jones & J. Castellanos (Eds.), *The majority in the minority: Retaining Latina/o faculty, administrators, and students in the 21st century* (pp. 257–283). Sterling, VA: Stylus Books.

Delgado-Romero, E. A., Galván, N., Maschino, P., & Rowland, M. (2005). Race and ethnicity: Ten years of counseling research. *Counseling Psychologist, 33,* 419–448.

Delgado-Romero, E. A., Manlove, A., Manlove, J., & Hernandez, C. A. (2007). Controversial issues in the recruitment and retention of Latino/a faculty. *Journal of Hispanic Higher Education, 6,* 1–18.

Delgado-Romero, E. A., Matthews, P. H., & Paisley, P. O. (2007). A school counseling conference focused on the emerging Latino/a populations: A model in the state of Georgia. *Journal of Hispanic Higher Education, 6,* 209–221.

De Los Santos, Jr., A. G., & De Los Santos, G. E. (2010). Hispanic-serving institutions in the 21st century: Overview, challenges, and opportunities. *Journal of Hispanic Higher Education, 2,* 377–391.

Diaz-McConnell, E., & Delgado-Romero, E. A. (2004). Panethnic options and Latinos: Reality or methodological construction? *Sociological Focus, 4,* 297–312.

Elderkin-Thompson, V., Silver, R. C., & Waitzkin, H. (2001). When nurses double as interpreters: A study of Spanish-speaking patients in a U.S. primary care setting. *Social Science & Medicine, 52,* 1343–1358.

Engstrom, D. W., & Min, J. W. (2004). Perspectives of bilingual social workers: "You just have to do a lot more for them." *Journal of Ethnic & Cultural Diversity in Social Work, 13,* 59–82.

Engstrom, D. W., Piedra, L. M., & Min, J. W. (2009). Bilingual social workers: Language and service complexities. *Administration in Social Work, 33,* 167–185.

Ferreira, M. M. (2003). Gender issues related to graduate student attrition in two science departments. *International Journal of Science Education, 25*(8), 969–989.

Figueroa, M. A., González, K. P., Marin, P., Moreno, J. F., Navia, C. N., & Pérez, L. X. (2001). Understanding the nature and context of Latina/o doctoral student experiences. *Journal of College Student Development, 42,* 563–580.

Fry, R. (2002). *Latinos in higher education: Many enroll, too few graduate.* Washington, DC: Pew Hispanic Center.

Fry, R. (2004). *Latino youth finishing college: The role of selective pathways.* Washington, DC: Pew Hispanic Center.

Furman, R., Negi, N. J., Iwamoto, D. K., Rowan, D., Shukraft, A., & Gragg, J. (2009). Social work practice with Latinos: Key issues for social workers. *Social Work, 54,* 167–174.

Gándara, P. (2009). *Rescatando sueños*—Rescuing dreams. In P. Gándara & F. Contreras (Eds.), *The Latino education crisis: The consequences of failed social policies* (pp. 304–334). Cambridge, MA: Harvard University Press.

Gibson, R. L., & Mitchell, M. (2007). *Introduction to counseling and guidance* (7th ed.). Englewood Cliffs, NJ: Prentice Hall.

Gloria, A. M., & Robinson Kurpius, S. E. (1996). The validation of the cultural congruity scale and the university environment scale with Chicana/o students. *Hispanic Journal of Behavioral Sciences, 18*(4), 533–549.

Gómez, B. (2007). Psychotherapy in Argentina: A clinical case from an integrative perspective. *Journal of clinical Psychology: In session, 63*(8), pp. 713–723.

Gonyea, N. E. (2010). The impact of acculturation on Hispanic students' learning styles. *Journal of Hispanic Higher Education, 9.* 73–81.

González, R. G. (2008). College student civic development and engagement at a Hispanic serving institution. *Journal of Hispanic Higher Education. 7,* 287–300.

Hall, C. C. I. (1997). Cultural malpractice: The growing obsolescence of psychology with the changing U.S. population. *American Psychologist, 52,* 642–651.

Hernández, J.C. (2002). A qualitative exploration of the first-year experience of Latino college students. *NASPA Journal, 40*(1), 69–84.

Herrera, R. (2003). Notes from a Latino graduate student at a predominately White university. In J. Castellanos & L. Jones (Eds.), *The majority in the minority: Expanding the representation of Latina/o faculty, administrators and students in higher education* (pp. 111–125). Sterling, VA: Stylus.

Hsieh, E. (2006). Understanding medical interpreters: Reconceptualizing bilingual health communication. *Health Communication, 20,* 177–186.

Hutz, C. S., McCarthy, S., & Gomes, W. (2004). Psychology in Brazil: The road behind and the road ahead. In M. J. Stevens & D. Wedding (Eds.), *Handbook of international psychology* (pp. 151–168). New York, NY: Taylor & Francis Books.

Imberti, P. (2007). Who resides behind the words? Exploring and understanding the language experience of the non-English-speaking immigrant. *Families in Society: The Journal of Contemporary Social Services, 88,* 67–73.

Lovitts, B. E. (2001). *Leaving the ivory tower: The causes and consequences of departure from doctoral study.* Lanham, MD: Rowman & Littlefield.

Martínez Pincay, I., & Guarnaccia, P. J. (2006). "It's like going through an earthquake": Anthropological perspectives on depression among Latino immigrants. *Journal of Immigrant Minority Health, 9,* 17–28.

Morales, E. (2009). *Psychology's preparedness in science and practice amid changing multicultural demographics.* Paper presented at the annual meeting of the American Psychological Association, Toronto, Canada.

National Association of Social Workers (NASW). (2001). *NASW standards for cultural competence in social work practice.* Retrieved from http://www.socialworkers.org/practice/standards/NASWCulturalStandards.pdf

National Association of Social Workers (NASW) Center for Workforce Studies. (2005). *Assuring the sufficiency of a frontline workforce: A national study of licensed social workers.* Retrieved from http://workforce.socialworkers.org/studies/nasw_06_execsummary.pdf

Nora, A., & Rendón, L.I. (1996). Hispanic student retention in community colleges: Reconciling access with outcomes. In C. Turner, M. Garcia, A. Nora, & L.I. Rendón (Eds.), *Racial & ethnic diversity in higher education* (pp. 269–280). Needham Heights, MA: Simon & Schuster Custom Publishing.

Pérez-Escamilla, R. (2010). Health care access among Latinos: Implications for social and health care reform. *Journal of Hispanic Higher Education, 9,* 43–60.

Piedra, L. M. (2010). Latinos & Spanish: The awkwardness of language in social work practice. In R. Furman & N. Negi (Eds.), *Social work practice with Latinos* (pp. 262–281). Chicago: Lyceum Books.

Ponterotto, J. G. (1988). Racial/ethnic minority research in the *Journal of Counseling Psychology:* A content analysis and methodological critique. *Journal of Counseling Psychology, 35,* 410–418.

Portes, A., & Rumbaut, R. G. (2001). Not everyone is chosen: Segmented assimilation and its determinants. In *Legacies: The Story of the Immigrant Second Generation* (pp. 44–69). Berkeley & Los Angeles, CA: University of California Press.

Portes, P., Delgado-Romero, E. A., & Salas, S. (in press). Latinos (not) in higher education, and the continuum of group based inequality: A cultural-historical perspective. In D. S. Sandhu, J. B. Hudson, & M. Taylor-Archer (Eds.), *Handbook of diversity in higher education.* Huntington, NY: Nova Science Publishers.

Richardson, R. C., Jr., & Skinner, E. F. (1990). Adapting to diversity: Organizational influences on student achievement. *Journal of Higher Education, 61*(5), 485–511.

Rivas, L., Delgado-Romero, E. A., & Ozambela, K. R. (2004). Our stories: Convergence of the language, professional, and personal identities of three Latino therapists. In L. Weiling & M.

Rastogi (Eds.) *Voices of color: First-person accounts of ethnic minority therapists* (pp. 23–41). Thousand Oaks, CA: Sage Publications.

Ruiz, P. (2002). Hispanic access to health/mental health services. *Psychiatric Quarterly, 73,* 85–91.

Sánchez-Sosa, J. J., & Valderrama-Iturbe, P. (2001). Psychology in Latin America: Historical reflections and perspectives. *International Journal of Psychology, 36,* 384–394.

Santiago, D. A. (2008). *Hispanic serving institutions.* Retrieved from http://www.edexcelencia. org/research/hispanic-serving-institutions-hsis

Santiago, D. A., & Andrade, S. J. (2010). Emerging Hispanic-serving institutions (HSIs): Serving Latino students. Washington, DC: *Excelencia* in Education Publications.

Santiago-Rivera, A. L., Arredondo, P., & Gallardo-Cooper, M. (2002). *Counseling Latinos and la familia: A guide for practitioners.* Thousand Oaks, CA: Sage Publications.

Shelton, K. L., Delgado-Romero, E. A., & Wells, E. M. (2009). Race and ethnicity in empirical research: An 18-year review. *Journal of Multicultural Counseling and Development, 37,* 130–140.

Solórzano, D. G., & Yosso, T. J. (2001). Critical race and LatCrit theory and method: Counterstorytelling. *Qualitative Studies in Education, 14*(4), 471–495.

Solórzano, D.G., Rivas, M.A., & Vélez, V.N. (2005, June). Community college as a pathway to Chicana/o doctoral production. *Latino Policy & Issues Brief* (11). Los Angeles: UCLA Chicana/o Studies Research Center.

Suro, R. (2006). A developing identity: Hispanics in the United States. *Carnegie Reporter, 3,* 22–31.

Tucker, C. M., Ferdinand, L. A., Mirsu-Paun, A., Herman, K. C., Delgado-Romero, E. A., van den Berg, J. J., & Jones, J. D. (2007). The roles of counseling psychologists in reducing health disparities. *Counseling Psychologist, 35,* 650–678.

U.S. Department of Health and Human Services. (2001). Mental health: culture, race, and ethnicity—a supplement to mental health: A report of the surgeon general. Retrieved from http://www.surgeongeneral.gov/library/mentalhealth/cre/sma-01-3613.pdf

Vega, W. A., & Lopez, S. R. (2001). Priority issues in Latino mental health service research. *Mental Health Services Research, 3,* 189–200.

Verdinelli, S., & Biever, J. L. (2009a). Experiences of Spanish/English bilingual supervisees. *Psychotherapy, 46,* 158–170.

Verdinelli, S., & Biever, J. L. (2009b). Spanish-English bilingual psychotherapists: Personal and professional language development and use. *Cultural Diversity & Ethnic Minority Psychology, 15,* 230–242.

Vidal de Haymes, M., & Kilty, K. M. (2007). Latino population growth, characteristics and settlement trends: Implications for social work education in a dynamic political climate. *Journal of Social Work Education. 43,* 101-116.

Weidman, J. C., & Stein, E. L. (2003). Socialization of doctoral students to academic norms. *Research in Higher Education, 44*(6), 641–656.

Worthington, R. L., Soth-McNett, A. M., & Moreno, M. V. (2007). Multicultural counseling competencies research: A 20-year content analysis. *Journal of Counseling Psychology, 5*(4), 351–361.

In a book about building infrastructures for Latino mental health, a chapter focused on access to higher education seems like an anomaly. Yet, throughout the book numerous scholars point to a serious shortage of bilingual service providers and the intersecting problems of poverty, language, and low levels of education and their effects on Latino mental health (see Chaps. 1, 2, 3, 5, 11, and 13). Indeed, the extent to which we experience our lives through complex institutions distinguishes modern life from the past (Mettler 1998; Klinenberg 2002; Piedra 2006). Highly-specialized institutions and complex models of service-delivery systems characterize our technologically advanced society, creating especially challenging problems for marginalized populations (Klinenberg 2002; Piedra 2006). Therefore, institutional access facilitates social inclusion, a fact underscored in early 20th century life first by the women's suffrage movement and later by the civil rights movement.

In this new millennium, access to educational institutions has come to the fore as critical to public health. As researchers turned their attention to the role of poverty and education in health disparities, they find that those who are poor and least educated generally experience the worst health (Braveman et al. 2010). However, even those with intermediate levels of income and education are less healthy than the wealthiest and most educated (Braveman et al. 2010). Within this context, we must consider access to high education as a cornerstone of Latino mental health.

The benefits of a college education are well documented. Those who attain at least a bachelor's degree earn more in median lifetime earnings than high-school graduates (Barrow and Rouse 2005; Institute for Higher Education Policy [IHEP] 2005). They also have better health outcomes, increased civic participation, and higher social capital (Institute for Higher Education Policy [IHEP] 2005). At the societal level, college graduates contribute to higher overall earnings, lower rates of unemployment, and higher tax revenues to local, state, and federal governments (Baum and Ma 2007; Trostel 2010). In light of the economic and social benefits attached to postsecondary education, it is not surprising that education beyond high school is now considered a natural continuation of the schooling process, particularly in developed societies such as the United States. As a result, colleges and universities increasingly serve a diverse student body and must strive to ensure the academic success of all students, regardless of ethnic or class backgrounds.

The fact that Latinos lag in terms of college enrollment and degree completion underscores the urgency of addressing their educational needs (Gándara and Contreras 2009). The underrepresentation of Latinos in higher education is particularly troubling because the Latino youth population has grown exponentially in recent years. From 1990 to 2006, the number of Latino students in the nation's public schools nearly doubled (Fry and Gonzales 2008). This increase represents 60% of the total growth in the nation's public school enrollments over the past 15 years (Fry and Gonzales 2008). Among preschoolers, Latino representation is even higher. In 2010, Latinos accounted for one in four of the cohort of kindergartners who will graduate from high school in 2023 (Nasser and Overberg 2010). In the context of an aging society, these numbers call attention to the important role of Latino youth in future labor markets (Tienda forthcoming). However, if US society is to reap benefits from these demographic trends, we must give special consideration to and, arguably, make a larger public investment in their education (Fry and Gonzales 2008; Morales and Bonilla 1993; Ridings et al. 2011; Sullivan 2006; Tienda forthcoming).

Although programs and policies exist that facilitate the academic achievement of the Latino population, in this chapter we argue that because so many of current and future Latino college students are the first in their families to attend college, understanding both the academic and psychological needs of first-generation college students is critical. Therefore, this chapter has several goals. First, we describe the barriers that Latino first-generation college students encounter in the pursuit of higher education. Next, we present information on enrollment patterns and the psychological factors associated with the educational experience of first-generation students. Using these sections as a foundation, we show how the creation of infrastructures to increase the number of Latino students in higher education must rest on three foundational strategies to facilitate recruitment, retention, and successful degree completion for this population. Throughout our discussion, we reflect on meeting both the concrete and psychological needs of first-generation college students.

Educational Barriers for First-Generation Latino Students

Many of today's Latino students will be the first in their families to complete a high school degree and attend an institution of higher education. As first-generation students, they must overcome numerous academic, financial, cultural, and social obstacles in the pursuit of a postsecondary education. Some scholars describe the challenges that Latino students face as "accumulated disadvantage" (Schneider et al. 2006, p. 179). Although this is true for all first-generation students, four central factors contribute to the particular heightened disadvantage for Latino students.

First, many Latino students are unprepared for school—as early as the first grade. Because many come from immigrant families with low levels of formal education, even before starting school their educational experiences will differ from those of their peers (Brown et al. 2003; Castellanos and Jones 2003). For example, compared to non-Latino parents, Latino parents are less likely to read to their children and enroll them in early education programs (Schneider et al. 2006).

Second, Latino students frequently do not take courses perceived as preparation for college (Schneider et al. 2006). These students, in fact, are less likely to be placed in these courses, because of "tracking" policies, because they are identified as English-language learners, or due to their teachers' biased perception of their potential (Lopez 2009). Without this preparation, they are more likely to need remedial coursework (55%) compared to non-Latino students (27%; Engle et al. 2006). Their academic disadvantage is reflected in lower scores on standardized college entrance examination tests (ACT, SAT) (Warburton et al. 2001) and poorer performance on reading, math, and critical-thinking examinations than non-Latino students (Reid and Moore 2008).

Third, because many Latino parents did not attend college, they fail to understand the responsibilities, mindset, and behaviors associated with postsecondary matriculation and the collegiate experience. Consequently, first-generation Latino college students tend to have a limited network of well-educated adults who can help prepare them for the transition from high school to college, creating an information gap (Brown et al. 2003; Reid and Moore 2008; Tym et al. 2004). Although Latino parents clearly value education (Brown et al. 2003; Zalaquett 2006), their own experiences reflect expectations of full-time employment and/or marriage in young adulthood. Given this background, Latino parents have a difficult time understanding the purpose of the prolonged adolescence that may extend through the third decade of life—often referred to as *emergent adulthood*—that is characteristic of middle-class young adults in contemporary society (Arnett 2000; Henig 2010).

Finally, because so many US-born Latino students come from economically disadvantaged households, they are more likely to attend ethnically segregated, under-resourced schools (Chapa 2005; Schneider et al. 2006; Tienda forthcoming; Tienda and Sullivan 2009). These underresourced schools are known for overcrowded classrooms, low-quality textbooks, and marginal instructional quality (Gloria et al. 2006). Furthermore, at all levels of education, limited family resources for enrichment experiences, books, exam preparatory courses, and computers have a widening effect on the achievement gap (Schneider et al. 2006; Zalaquett 2006). The cumulative effect of these complex factors contributes to Latino students' low rates of four-year college enrollment, and even lower rates of degree completion.

Major Hurdles: Undergraduate Admissions, Retention, and Graduation

Although variations exist, as a whole Latinos tend to have low levels of college enrollment. Only 13% of all Latinos have a bachelor's degree, the lowest among all ethnic groups in the United States (U.S. Census Bureau 2010). Although college enrollment for Latinos increased from 6% in 1990 to 11% in 2005 (Santiago 2007), the enrollment gap between Latino students and students from other ethnic groups has increased as well (Fry 2005). In 2005, the college enrollment rate—the percent of high school completers who enrolled in college the fall immediately after graduation—was 54% for Latino students and 73% for non-Latino White students (Santiago 2007). A number of factors contribute to these low rates of college enrollments.

The Two-Year College Preference

First-generation college students, in comparison to those with one college-educated parent, are more likely to enroll at two-year institutions (Tym et al. 2004). Specifically, 58% of all Latino students nationwide, and 75% of Latino students in California, attend a two-year institution (Contreras and Gándara 2006). This choice to favor community college over four-year institutions reflects a number of needs: (a) financial concerns, (b) flexible class scheduling, (c) part-time attendance, and (d) proximity to family (Pryor et al. 2005; Zell 2010).

Regardless of their reasons for attending a two-year institution, the initial investment in higher education pays off upon the completion of a four-year degree. Unfortunately, few actually achieve the goal of transferring to a four-year institution (Long and Kurlaender 2009). Because many two-year institutions lack structures to facilitate transfers, 97% of Latinos who enroll in community colleges never make it to four-year institutions (Brown et al. 2003; Contreras and Gándara 2006).

Challenges in Applying to Four-Year Institutions

The process of applying to four-year institutions is filled with obstacles for those unfamiliar with the process. Obtaining letters of recommendation and transcripts, filling out applications, and writing coherent applications essays challenge even the average high school student (Bornstein 2004; Douthat 2005). However, for many first-generation students, this process occurs within a context where there is minimal adult guidance for completing applications, proofreading essays, and providing help in deciding where to apply and whether to apply for early admission (Bornstein 2004). Early-admissions programs, for example, offer many benefits to applicants, but they almost exclusively help students whose parents and guidance counselors are more likely to have the resources to take advantage of them (Douthat 2005; Fallows 2001). In addition, each application requires an application fee and scores from standardized tests (ACT, SAT), which also have their own application processes and associated fees. Moreover, numerous deadlines pervade the process: To apply for college, to apply for early admission, to apply for a fee waiver, to register to take a standardized test, to take the test, to apply for financial aid.

Students from low-income households are also less likely to know about the availability of financial aid, and thus are more likely to let the high cost of attending college keep them from applying in the first place (Douthat 2005; O'Connor et al. 2010). Although each year thousands of students successfully complete college applications, the complexities of actually applying put Latino first-generation students at a decisive disadvantage. For those with few resources who manage to complete an application process, the victory is in actually applying.

Administrators lament that applications from low-income students are unfortunately weak (Bornstein 2004). For example, first-generation college students' average score on the SAT college entrance examination was 858 points, compared with 1011 points for students whose parents had completed college (Warburton et al. 2001). They also tend to earn lower scores on reading, math, and critical-thinking examinations while in college (Reid and Moore 2008). These scores often reflect institutional disparities in academic preparation rather than innate ability or even differences in student motivation.

Questions on college applications often fail to capture another critical ingredient for academic success: Persistence in the face of early-life obstacles (Bornstein

2004). Interestingly, scholars report that motivation to attend college, based on personal interest, intellectual curiosity, and the desire to attain a rewarding career, predicts college adjustment (Dennis et al. 2005). Although most high school students engage in leadership and community service activities, athletic programs, and part-time employment to pay for extras, economically disadvantaged students might forgo such experiences to care for younger siblings and/or engage in work that contributes to the financial well-being of the family. Successfully shouldering these responsibilities while remaining in school indicates a level of maturity and leadership in the young person. However, because college applications are tailored to assess the skills of middle-class students, application questions frequently fail to pick up on the assets of the first generation. Moreover, without savvy adults to help students tailor their college essays to highlight these assets, most first-generation students fail to convey nonacademic qualities such as persistence, maturity, and character that translate well to the higher-education environment (Bornstein 2004).

Legal Status: The Plight of Undocumented Students

Legal status plays a small but significant role in the enrollment patterns of Latinos. The vast majority of Latino students who attend college are US citizens (86%), followed by legal residents (12%) and undocumented students (2%; Santiago 2007). However, researchers estimate that 2.1 million people could potentially benefit from legislation that creates a pathway for status legalization based on obtaining a higher education degree or through military service (Batalova and McHugh 2010; Immigration Policy Center 2010). Of this group, 1.6 million are of Latino origin.

Undocumented students—many of whom came to the United States as children and know no other country—encounter profound obstacles to higher education. In addition to the usual obstacles confronting first-generation students, undocumented students live with the fear of being "discovered" and deported if they fill out official forms or are otherwise identified in the course of their studies (Jones 2010; Perez 2010).

Although no federal laws require a person to have US citizenship to attend college, various schools around the country have policies that require a Social Security number or legal residency as a prerequisite for enrollment. Georgia and South Carolina have both passed legislation banning undocumented students from attending their top state universities (Brown 2010). Only 10 states permit eligible undocumented students to attend public universities at in-state tuition rates: California, Illinois, Kansas, Nebraska, New Mexico, New York, Oklahoma, Texas, Utah, and Washington. However, opponents to illegal immigration are currently contesting this privilege in the California Supreme Court as a possible violation of federal immigration law (Brown 2010).

Unfortunately, even for those who benefit from in-state tuition, undocumented students remain ineligible for federal and state financial aid, including student loans, and therefore must finance their education up front (Jones 2010). Even when the most determined manage to graduate, without legal status they are still unable to work in the United States (Perez 2010). The daunting obstacles facing undocumented students lead many to question the merits of embarking on a long, financially costly, and emotionally draining process that may not have a significant payoff at the end.

Psychological Challenges to Educational Success

Despite all these obstacles to degree attainment, among Latinos who graduate, nearly half are first-generation students (Santiago 2007). Even so, many first-generation Latino students encounter formidable psychological challenges that can affect degree attainment. Many struggle with a lower sense of self-efficacy and self-esteem than those with at least one college-educated parent (Hottinger and Rose 2006). For many, the transition from the largely nonacademic home and community environment into a predominantly academically focused environment can overwhelm and discourage students (Hottinger and Rose 2006). Moreover, without adequate social support, these students may suffer a loss of self-worth and self-efficacy (Thayer 2000). Indeed, one study found that peer support was directly related to academic performance (Dennis et al. 2005). Unfortunately, friends and family who have not attended college may be more likely to criticize students for devoting time to school responsibilities that take them away from family or community activities (Pryor et al. 2005).

Nevertheless, for families that are able to support their children, researchers have uncovered several protective factors that facilitate educational success. Parental support and encouragement were found to exert a positive influence in helping students persist in their studies (Nora et al. 2006). Parents who are successful in supporting their child share inspirational stories, help in ways that conserve the student's time to study, and facilitate the student's motivations to stay focused (Auerbach 2006; Ceja 2004). A qualitative analysis of successful Latino students' narratives (Zalaquett 2006) found eight factors that positively influenced their pursuit of a college education: (a) the need for family support and encouragement, (b) the belief that a quality education and good grades are important, (c) a sense that academic and career success honors family, (d) a desire to have a positive impact through accomplishment, (e) the need for the support and encouragement of friends, (f) obtaining adequate financial aid, (g) experiencing community support, and (h) perceiving teachers and other school personnel as positive influences.

Social support on campus also plays a critical role for this group. Latino students who are most likely to graduate report a connection to groups on campus (Nora et al. 2006).

Financial Needs

Another major concern for first-generation Latino students centers on how to navigate the financial assistance process to pay for a college education (Nunez and Cuccaro-Alamin 1998). Many Latino families do not know the actual cost of a college education and often fail to take into account additional fees and expenses (e.g., the cost of books), which adds to the economic stress of attending college. Moreover, many in the Latino community are leery of debt and prefer grants and scholarships to taking out student loans (Schmidt 2003). Instead of taking out loans, many students meet their financial needs by holding jobs while in college. In one study, more than half of the first-generation college students surveyed (55%) stated that they would seek a job to help pay for expenses, and 36% planned to work full time while in college (Pryor et al. 2005). Although most college students work to meet extra needs, the use of work to pay for significant portions of college expenses has mental health consequences. Managing a full work schedule while attending school limits class selection, reduces available study time, and lowers the quality of the educational experience (Hottinger and Rose 2006). In such a context, the stress of attending might lead students to question their motivation and may contribute to attrition (Longerbeam et al. 2004).

The Sociopolitical Context of Higher Education

The larger sociopolitical context in which Latino enrollment patterns arise warrants closer attention. There has been increased scrutiny of equity in college admission criteria, especially at elite public institutions (Chapa 2005; Jaschik 2010; Tienda and Sullivan 2009). Across the nation, affirmative action programs in higher education have drawn both criticism and lawsuits, and have generally raised the question as to whether such programs are necessary in contemporary society. Arizona, California, Michigan, Nebraska, and Washington state currently ban the consideration of race, ethnicity, or gender by units of state government, including public colleges and universities (Jaschik 2010).

More problematic, but garnering much less public scrutiny, is the fact that in states with high Latino populations—most notably states such as Texas and California—public investments in higher education have not kept pace with the demand (Tienda and Sullivan 2009; Trostel 2010). Trostel (2010) wrote that, nationwide, over the past two decades, state expenditures for higher education have fallen. Using data from the US Census Bureau's State and Local Government Finances database, he calculated that in fiscal year 1984, nationwide net state funding for higher education was 4.1% of total state government spending (Trostel 2010). In 1994, this proportion was 2.4%, and in 2004 it was 1.8% (Trostel 2010).

Indeed, much of the backlash against affirmative action programs—institution-specific programs used to diversify a school—coincide with what Tienda and Sullivan (2009) called a "college squeeze," in which college-age population growth outpaced the expansion of four-year institutions and created intense competition for access to the most selective four-year public institutions. Tienda and Sullivan (2009) pointed out that because affirmative action is a widely discussed and controversial issue, it provides an easier target for public ire than the demographic changes driving the "academic crunch," which are more subtle and rarely noticed. Consequently, we have entered an era suspicious of affirmative action programs and inclined toward race-blind selection processes.

Within this contentious context, Chapa (2005) reminds us of the two core functions of affirmative action programs in higher education. First, these programs operate on the premise that for the purposes of diversifying an institution, the elimination of discrimination practices is a necessary but insufficient measure. Second, whereas affirmative action programs vary in scale and scope, all these programs address institutional homogeneity by explicitly focusing on key characteristics—race, ethnicity, gender—in bestowing individual benefits. The justification for affirmative action rests on historical inequalities in access to public education resources for racial and ethnic groups (Chapa 2005). Unfortunately, these conditions persist for many Latino students today (Chapa 2005; Schneider et al. 2006; Tienda forthcoming; Tienda and Sullivan 2009), especially in states with large Latino populations such as California and Texas, where educational disparities are particularly pronounced (Chapa 2005). Hence, without institutional programs such as affirmative action, Latinos' chances for participation in higher education are reduced. Instead, nonrace-based percentage programs have emerged as vehicles for achieving educational parity.

Race-Neutral Percentage Programs

California, Florida, and Texas have implemented a type of percentage program in lieu of affirmative action (Tienda and Sullivan 2009). Although there are significant variations among the programs for all three states, they have shown a positive effect in increasing Latino participation at the state's most selective universities (Chapa 2005; Tienda and Sullivan 2009). The most controversial is the Top 10% plan in Texas, which guaranteed those students who graduate in the top 10 percentile of their senior class admission to their choice of state universities, regardless of ethnic or racial identification and test scores (Alon and Tienda 2007; Chapa 2005). Administrators use test scores only to determine class placement and financial aid eligibility (Tienda and Sullivan 2009). Because standardized tests measure developed ability rather than motivation, imagination, and intellectual curiosity, these exams are biased against low-income students whose preparation reflects the stark educational disparities endemic in the United States (Alon and Tienda 2007; Tienda and Sullivan 2009).

Even so, precisely because Texas has a number of poor-quality high schools with overwhelmingly minority enrollments, this plan created a way to diversify campuses by increasing the number of feeder schools that send minority students to its flagship campus (Tienda and Sullivan 2009). However, the plan has serious drawbacks. Although the segregated school systems in Texas facilitated the diversification of top-ranking state institutions, the plan does not resolve the issue of socioeconomic class (O'Connor et al. 2010; Tienda and Sullivan 2009; Tienda forthcoming). Among those eligible to attend top-ranking institutions, students from low-income families are less likely to attend flagship four-year institutions compared to students coming from middle-class families (Tienda and Sullivan 2009). Moreover, the 10% plan had the effect of turning an informal practice of accepting top 10 candidates into a de facto policy (Tienda and Sullivan 2009). Black and Latino candidates who fell outside the top tier actually fared worse under this policy (Cortes forthcoming).

Moreover, like its predecessor—affirmative action—the 10% plan has come under scrutiny for using only one factor in admissions. Indeed, programs that rely on a narrow range of variables, such as test scores or class ranking, do little to address a striking disparity between low-income and middle-income communities: The capacity to launch their second- and third-tier students on a pathway to college (Bornstein 2004). For Latinos coming from families with low levels of education and from communities and schools without a culture of sending its youth to college, outreach and support must begin early and persist throughout their educational career. Pre-college programs exist (see Appendix A for information about these programs), but must be expanded to keep up with the rising demand. The infrastructures needed to build and expand these programs are the focus of the next section.

Strategies to Increase Enrollment

The creation of infrastructures to increase the number of Latino students in higher education must rest on three foundational strategies: (a) expand existing national and state policies to facilitate access to higher education through stronger financial aid packages and support programs; (b) pass legislation to address the educational needs of undocumented youth; and (c) develop institutional practices that facilitate retention. In the following paragraphs, we specifically discuss each of these core strategies.

Strategy 1: Expand TRIO

The federal government has long recognized its role in facilitating access to higher education. The history of TRIO reflects an evolution of legislation since 1964 designed to support disadvantaged students by enhancing college preparation, facilitating admissions, and assisting in retention (U.S. Department of Education, Office of Postsecondary Education [USDE-OPE] 2008). Upward Bound, the first of the

TRIO programs, began as a pilot project authorized by the Economic Opportunity Act of 1964 to encourage low-income youths to complete high school and prepare for college. A year later, the landmark Higher Education Act of 1965 authorized federal financial aid for postsecondary education and created Talent Search to help students in applying for newly available aid. Four years later, legislators amended the Higher Education Act of 1965 to include a third program—Special Services for Disadvantaged Students program, now called Student Support Services (SSS)—and the TRIO name was born (U.S. Department of Education, Office of Postsecondary Education [USDE-OPE] 2008).

Since 1968, lawmakers have expanded the TRIO programs to provide a wider range of services (U.S. Department of Education, Office of Postsecondary Education [USDE-OPE] 2008). Today, nine programs are funded under the TRIO umbrella. Seven of these TRIO programs offer direct services to program participants. In addition to these seven programs, the US Congress also authorizes two programs focused specifically on improving the design and administration of TRIO services. The most recent addition is the Child Care Access Means Parents in School (CCAMPIS) program to assist institutions in providing campus-based child-care services for low-income student parents (U.S. Department of Education, Office of Postsecondary Education [USDE-OPE] 2008). All of these initiatives are critical in providing Latino students with increased access to higher education (Brown et al. 2003). (For more information about TRIO, see http://www2.ed.gov/about/offices/list/ope/trio/index.html.)

With the addition of CCAMPIS, TRIO signaled the need for targeted support services. Given TRIO's history of expanding its programs, this legislation could arguably serve as a mechanism for adding support programs throughout the educational pipeline. Under TRIO, one could envision an amendment to fund a nationwide Hispanic Pre-school College Bound Program, to establish in the minds of the community, teachers, parents, and children the idea that college preparation begins in preschool (S. Maldonado, personal communication, November 14, 2010). Such a program would be critical for communities with schools that do not have strong traditions of sending their youth to college. One could also envision targeted programs for states with high youth populations, many of which are also those states with large Latino population. States with large Latino youth populations, such as California, Florida, New York, and Texas, must expand the institutional capacity of their flagship schools. By increasing the number of faculty and staff and coupling that expansion with intensive outreach and reasonable financial supports, these states will go far in facilitating enrollment of Latinos and quelling public tensions that arise from the "academic church" (Tienda forthcoming; Tienda and Sullivan 2009).

Although one could argue that expanding programs through TRIO would be prohibitively expensive, in the following section we will show how investments in higher education reap substantial economic returns for American society. We begin, however, by turning to the DREAM Act and discussing the fact that, although its passage could assist many individuals, the nation would ultimately be its greatest beneficiary.

Strategy 2: The DREAM Act

The Development, Relief, and Education for Alien Minors (DREAM) Act seeks to provide a path to legalization for unauthorized youth and young adults by allowing them to apply for legal permanent resident status on a *conditional* basis (Batalova and McHugh 2010). Eligibility is based on whether, upon enactment of the law, they are under the age of 35, arrived in the United States before the age of 16, have lived in the United States for at least the last five years, and have obtained a US high school diploma or equivalent (Batalova and McHugh 2010). The conditional basis of their status is removed in six years if they successfully complete at least two years of postsecondary education or military service and if they maintain good moral character during that time.

Researchers estimate that enactment of this law would immediately make 726,000 unauthorized young adults eligible for conditional legal status; of these, roughly 114,000 would be eligible for permanent legal status after the six-year wait because they already have at least an associate's degree (Batalova and McHugh 2010). Another 934,000 potential beneficiaries are children under 18 who will age into conditional-status eligibility in the future, if they earn a US high school diploma or obtain a General Education Diploma. If passed, the DREAM Act would enable states to offer the in-state tuition rate to undocumented students (Abaddon 2010; National Council of La Raza 2010) by repealing a section of the 1996 Illegal Immigration Reform and Immigrant Responsibility Act that penalized states for offering in-state tuition rates to unauthorized youth (Batalova and McHugh 2010). However, passage of the DREAM Act bill remains contentious. Opponents of the Act argue that it provides a back door for immigration reform by providing a form of amnesty and therefore encourages illegal immigration (The Editorial Board 2010).

The opposition's charge that the DREAM Act would serve as an amnesty program of sorts merits careful analysis. On the one hand, opponents have a point: The proposed legislation does provide an alternative pathway to citizenship for a select group of people who are in the country illegally. On the other hand, the criteria for eligibility are stringent; not all who are technically eligible will be able to meet the requirements. The same researchers who estimated that 2.1 million people would be eligible for conditional legal status under the DREAM Act qualify their estimates with a notable caution: "[H]istorical trends indicate that far fewer are likely to actually gain permanent (or even conditional) status, due primarily to the bill's education attainment requirements" (Batalova and McHugh 2010, p. 1). By their estimates, roughly 38% of potential beneficiaries—825,000 people—would likely obtain permanent legal status and as many as 62% would likely fail to do so (Batalova and McHugh 2010). These estimates suggest that the DREAM Act would hardly open any floodgate in sanctioning illegal immigration. Rather, this piece of legislation would help US society recoup its initial investments in the public education of undocumented youth who were reared and educated in the United States and exhibit the skills and motivation to make a substantial contribution to society as college graduates or military officers. As Batalova and McHugh (2010) pointed out, "In an age when human capital is the ultimate resource both for individuals and societies, the legislation would provide stability and opportunity to these young all-but-Americans whose education and career prospects are otherwise extremely limited" (p. 18).

The gains for society are quite significant. One researcher estimated that the extra tax revenues from college graduates alone (roughly $471,000 per degree over a lifetime) are more than six times the gross government cost per college degree (Trostel 2010). Trostel (2010) conservatively estimated the average real fiscal internal rate of return on government investment in college students to be 10.3%.

Strategy 3: Institutional Practices That Facilitate Retention

Once students enter college, many find that the cultural universe of campus life differs vastly from their own home and community. First-generation students are particularly vulnerable to experiencing cultural and social isolation, which may compound other stressors such as low expectations from teachers and peers, family tensions, and financial concerns, all of which can affect their academic performance and desire to persist in their studies (Oseguera et al. 2009). Hottinger and Rose (2006) found that Latino students who perceive a hostile campus climate and experience a lower sense of belonging are more likely to drop out than students who feel more accepted and welcome in school. Therefore, campus-specific programs that help students feel more connected to the campus community, and that can foster a sense of belonging and acceptance, are critical to the success of first-generation students. In this section, we begin by discussing campus-specific programs that promote student well-being and academic success while in college. To illustrate the potential for such programs, we describe two programs instituted at the University of Illinois at Urbana Champaign (UIUC) and University of Central Florida (UCF), both of which are designed to help Latino students and their families feel welcome. Next, we highlight the important role of counseling and outreach for first-generation Latino students. Finally, we discuss the role of the Internet in assisting with recruitment and retention.

Latino Family Visit Day

Since 2003, UIUC has collaborated with Bank One/JP Morgan Chase to host a Latino Family Visit Day (LFVD), when Latino students and their families are invited for a day on campus free of charge. Faculty and staff present a series of workshops in English and Spanish that address the multifaceted college experience. Parents especially appreciate the emphasis on fostering interpersonal relationships throughout the program. Specific activities that create a sense of belonging for students and parents include hosting a resource fair, providing them with a directory of campus resources, engaging them in academic dialogues, facilitating a student-parent panel discussion, and introducing them to alumni. In addition to these resources and activities, transportation, child care, and recreational opportunities are offered throughout the day.

Parents report that LFVD helps them build relationships with university staff, faculty, and students as well as other Latino parents (Rodriguez et al. 2007). One exciting and unexpected outcome of LFVD is that many younger siblings of the students who accompanied the family to LFVD ultimately decided to pursue higher education as well, many enrolling at UIUC (Rodriguez et al. 2007). Thus, this program succeeds at addressing both recruitment and retention issues.

First-Generation College Student Program at UCF

UCF's Multicultural Academic and Support Services offers the First-Generation College Student Program to retain and increase graduation rates of first-generation students by providing guidance and resources to promote their self-esteem, confidence, and academic achievement (see http://www.mass.ucf.edu/firstgeneration. php). The program offers a structured approach to help students transition to college by providing them with an academic home, demystifying the college experience, and helping them navigate the university landscape. In doing so, the program helps students connect to different resources on campus, serving much like an embassy would for a citizen in a foreign country (E. Range, personal communication, August 2010).

However, the program also acts as a bridge for families to maintain positive relationships with the student, through outreach and by offering workshops. For many students, the challenges of adjusting to college life, the financial pressures, and a difficult transition from dependence to independence create an emotional gap and distancing from their families, who often have difficulty understanding the students' experiences.

Ideally, the program seeks to foster a positive identification with the university community that facilitates students' motivation to develop morally, intellectually, and socially throughout their studies. Specialized workshops that pair students with campus resources and seminars on topics relevant to college success (e.g., developing academic skills, adjusting to college, managing relationships) focus on building such an identification.

Fostering Support Networks through Counseling, Outreach, and the Internet

In almost all spheres of campus life, first-generation students need guidance. Beyond helping them adjust psychologically to a new environment, counselors also serve as potential mentors and role models. Emotional support through counseling services can help students normalize stressors related to academic life and develop coping skills that foster self-efficacy. Because finding their way in this new environment creates much anxiety, counselors who work with college students must consider the students' psychological, social, cultural, and environmental contexts

(Gloria and Rodriguez 2000). In addition to addressing the presenting problem, counselors should include in their assessments an understanding of the student's university environment, ethnic identity, acculturation, and social support systems (Gloria and Rodriguez 2000).

Although faculty, staff, and administrators often see emotional support as the purview of the counseling department, such support can also come in the form of outreach from various departments and offices on campus. Within the student community, the presence of faculty, staff, and administrators as familiar faces conveys the message that the educational leadership cares about their well-being. The demonstration of "presence" reflects an interest in students' everyday lives, and results in students reaching out for services and assistance when they are in academic or emotional need.

Informal exposure to faculty, staff, and administrators can be accomplished through their attendance at students' milestone events, such as welcome fairs, orientations, graduations, and congratulatory parties. Faculty can also engage with students at informal mixers, sharing personal and professional stories that validate students' experiences, encouraging them to succeed, and providing guidance on how students can advocate for themselves throughout their academic experience. Although Latino students especially benefit from outreach by Latino faculty, staff, or administrators, engaging a broad spectrum of individuals from the university community underscores a collective process to care for vulnerable students. Whereas the importance of Latino role models and mentors cannot be underestimated— the mere presence of Latino faculty and staff demonstrates that they can succeed academically as well (Gloria and Rodriguez 2000; Reyes 2009)—there are still far too few Latino faculty for them alone to fill that role.

Moreover, the well-being of students is the responsibility of the entire staff and faculty, not just those who happen to be Latino. For example, at UIUC, the Counseling Center staff offer an orientation program to new incoming first-generation students. As part of the program, students attend a presentation by another first-generation student and receive a resource guide for navigating college life. The resource guide includes a list of acronyms of college terms to help students navigate common jargon that can pose challenges for newcomers to campus life. In addition, students are included in a listserv designed for first-generation students, where they can share information about campus resources, ask questions, and learn from each other (J. Thome, personal communication, July 2010).

In an era of accelerated technological advancement, the Internet plays a critical role for college students. The Internet enables greater access to professors, offers more research possibilities, facilitates collaborations with fellow students, and provides an incredible wealth of information on academic-oriented email services (Jones 2002). Most institutions of higher education assume that their students have access to and communicate via the Internet, but this may not be the case for all Latino students. Latinos, particularly those who are from low-income families, are the most digitally underserved population in the United States (Ginossar and Nelson 2010; Lorence et al. 2006). Factors that contribute to this digital divide include the cost of owning a computer, the recurring expense of paying for Internet access (Fox and Livingston

2007; Slate et al. 2002), and the lack of Internet access in communities where many Latinos live (Mossberger et al. 2006). Lack of access to the Internet—the preferred medium through which colleges communicate with potential students—thus stands as a major barrier for first-generation Latino students (Vargas 2004).

The National Latina/o Psychological Association (NLPA) illustrates the networking benefits for students. NLPA operates a listserv specifically for students. This digital space offers students the opportunity to connect with others, share information, and develop relationships with potential mentors within the Latino psychology community at the local and national levels. In the past, students have posted queries ranging from how to deal with diversity issues in their workplaces to how to locate the Spanish version of a given psychological assessment. Much like the listserv developed for first-generation students at the University of Illinois, this medium enhances students' sense of belonging, their social support, and their ability to complete their academic programs successfully.

Conclusion

During times of fiscal austerity, federal and state governments hesitate to invest in higher education. Yet, the failure to provide educational support for Latino students and their families will prove in the end to be shortsighted and unwise. As Dr. Vasquez writes in the foreword of this book, "Indeed, the link between what society can do to advance the well-being of individuals, families, and communities and how this contributes to mental health outcomes must become a central part of our current discourse" (p. viii). The most coordinated, comprehensive mental health system will be always constrained by its mandate. In the future, schools will play a decisive role in determining access to high-paying jobs and high quality of life. The size of the Latino youth population and the role they will play in future labor markets warrants a larger public investment in their education.

The future is hardly bleak. Despite serious obstacles, Latino families place a high value on education. With appropriate supports, Latino students can succeed. An investment in their higher education today represents an investment in the nation's ability to respond to rapid changing demographics and ultimately, the development of our future labor force—including the mental health and health care sectors.

Appendix A

Pre-College Programs

Pre-college programs provide first-generation Latino college students with a plethora of benefits. Such programs help students become better prepared for college, facilitate the transition to college, and help them find ways to balance their social and academic lives (Engle et al. 2006). The following is a list of select programs designed to help students gain admission into college.

Posse. Founded in 1989, Posse identifies public high school students with great academic and leadership potential that may be otherwise overlooked by traditional college selection processes. Colleges and universities that collaborate with Posse award Posse Scholars four-year, full-tuition leadership scholarships. Students selected to participate in the program are granted the opportunity to attend college at various universities across the nation. At any of these universities, students are placed in supportive, multicultural teams known as "Posses." The presence of a multicultural team of students from diverse backgrounds fosters a campus environment that is more welcoming and supportive for all. Moreover, students' multicultural leadership skills are fostered and supported through workshops, campus events, and individual mentorship.

Additional goals of the program include helping the collaborating institutions build more interactive campus environments so that they are welcoming to people of all backgrounds, and ensuring that Posse Scholars excel academically and continue with their studies through graduation. Posse has served more than 1,850 students since its inception (Gándara & Contreras 2009), providing critically important support to students both before and after college enrollment. For more information about Posse, see http://www.possefoundation.org/.

Summer Bridge. The Summer Bridge program exists in various participating universities across the nation and is intended to help students transition successfully into college. Specifically, this program helps students make academic, social, and personal adjustments to the university. The program typically consists of rigorous academic residential programs, cultivating a diverse group of scholars who engage actively with the university community. The program supports students by providing a stimulating and challenging academic experience, personalized advising and counseling, and an intellectually and socially enriching residential experience. Specifically, the program helps students develop study skills and time management strategies, and it supports students as they navigate college life, formulate their career aspirations, and develop relationships with potential mentors. Students also receive academic support to develop strong writing, mathematics, and reading skills. Many Summer Bridge programs are now developing a parent involvement component as well (Oseguera et al. 2009).

Puente Program. The Puente program was launched as a grassroots initiative to address the low rate of academic achievement among Latino students in California. Originally, Puente was created for Latino students, but it is now open to all students (Oseguera et al. 2009). Its mission is to increase the number of educationally disadvantaged students who enroll in four-year colleges and universities, earn college degrees, and return to their communities as mentors to and leaders of future generations. The program includes writing, counseling, and mentoring components. Currently, Puente operates in 56 community colleges and 32 high schools in California. For more information, see http://www.puente.net/about/.

ENLACE. In Spanish, *enlace* means "link or a weaving together" in such a way that the new entity is stronger than its component parts. ENLACE is a W.K. Kellogg Foundation multiyear higher education initiative designed to strengthen educational attainment and increase opportunities for Latinos to enter and complete college (Oseguera et al. 2009). ENLACE consists of 13 partnerships in 7 states (Arizona, California, Florida, Illinois, New Mexico, New York, and Texas) that are working to increase the number of Latina/o graduates from high school and college. Specifically, the program's objectives are: (a) to strengthen selected Hispanic Serving Institutions (HSIs), public schools, and community-based organizations to serve as catalysts and models for systemic change in education; (b) to support partnerships between higher education and local communities that increase community involvement and educational success by Latino students; (c) to support the creation and implementation of education models based on best practices that improve enrollment, academic performance, and graduation of Latino high school and college students; (d) to facilitate the expansion and sustainability of successful programs through strategic planning, networking, leadership development, and policy; and (e) to disseminate information about successful models to key stakeholders in order to stimulate changes in policies and practices related to the education of Latinos. For more information, see http://www.edpartnerships.org/Template.cfm?Section=ENLACE.

References

Abaddon, A. P. (2010). *Basic information about the DREAM Act legislation.* Retrieved from http://dreamact.info/students

Alon, S., & Tienda, M. (2007). Diversity, opportunity, and the shifting meritocracy in higher education. *American Sociological Review, 72,* 487–511.

Arnett, J. J. (2000). Emerging adulthood: A theory of development from the late teens through the twenties. *American Psychologist, 55*(5), 469–480.

Auerbach, S. (2006). "If the student is good, let him fly": Moral support for college among Latino immigrant parents. *Journal of Latinos & Education, 5*(4), 275–292.

Barrow, L., & Rouse, C. (2005). Does college still pay? *Economists' Voice, 2*(4). Retrieved from http://www.transad.pop.upenn.edu/downloads/barrow-rouse.pdf

Batalova, J., & McHugh, M. (2010). DREAM vs. reality: An analysis of potential DREAM Act beneficiaries. *Migration Policy Institute.* Retrieved from http://www.migrationpolicy.org/pubs/DREAM-Insight-July2010.pdf

Baum, S., & Ma, J. (2007). *Education pays: The benefits of higher education for individuals and society.* Washington, DC: The College Board.

Bornstein, D. (2004). *How to change the world: Social entrepreneurs and the power of new ideas* (pp. 164–182). New York: Oxford University Press.

Braveman, P. A., Cubbin, C., Egerter, S., Williams, D. R., & Pamuk, E. (2010). Socioeconomic disparities in health in the United States: What the patterns tell us. *American Journal of Public Health, 100*(S1), S186–S196.

Brown, R. (2010). Five public colleges in Georgia ban illegal-immigrant students. *New York Times.* Retrieved from http://www.nytimes.com/2010/10/14/us/14georgia.html

Brown, S., Santiago, D., & Lopez, E. (2003). Latinos in higher education: Today and tomorrow. *Change: The Magazine of Higher Learning, 35*(2), 40-46.

Castellanos, J., & Jones, L. (2003). Latina/o undergraduate experiences in American higher educa-tion. In J. Castellanos & L. Jones (Eds.), *The majority in the minority: Expanding the represen-tation of Latina/o faculty, administrators and students in higher education* (pp. 1–13). Sterling, VA: Stylus.

Ceja, M. (2004). Chicana college aspirations and the role of parents: Developing educational resil-iency. *Journal of Hispanic Higher Education, 3*(4), 338–362.

Chapa, J. (2005). Affirmative action and percent plans as alternatives for increasing successful participation of minorities in higher education. *Journal of Hispanic Higher Education, 4,* 181–196.

Contreras, F. E., & Gándara, P. (2006). The Latina/o PhD pipeline: A case of historical and con-temporary under-representation. In J. Castellanos, A. M. Gloria, & M. Kamimura (Eds.), *The Latina/o pathway to the PhD: Abriendocaminos* (pp. 91–111). Sterling, VA: Stylus.

Cortes, K. E. (forthcoming). Do bans on affirmative action hurt minority students? Evidence from the Texas Top 10% Plan. *Economics of Education Review.* Retrieved from http://ftp.iza.org/dp5021.pdf

Dennis, J. M., Phinney, J. S., & Chuateco, L. I. (2005). The role of motivation, parental support, and peer support in the academic success of ethnic minority first-generation college students. *Journal of College Student Development, 46*(3), 223–236. doi:10.1353/csd.2005.0023

Douthat, R. (2005). Does meritocracy work? *Atlantic Monthly.* Retrieved from http://www.the-atlantic.com/magazine/archive/2005/11/does-meritocracy-work/4305/

Engle, J., Bermeo, A., & O'Brien, C. (2006). *Straight from the source: What works for first gen-eration college students.* Washington, DC: The Pell Institute for the Study of Opportunity in Higher Education.

Fallows, J. (2001). The early-decision racket. *Atlantic Monthly.* Retrieved from http://www.the-atlantic.com/magazine/archive/2001/09/the-early-decision-racket/2280/

Fox, S., & Livingston, G. (2007). *Latinos online: Hispanics with lower levels of education and English proficiency remain largely disconnected from the internet.* Retrieved from http://www.pewinternet.org/PPF/r/204/report display.as.

Fry, R. (2005). *The higher dropout rate of foreign-born teens: The role of schooling abroad.* Wash-ington, DC: Pew Hispanic Center.

Fry, R., & Gonzales, F. (2008). *One-in-five and growing fast: A profile of Hispanic public school students.* Washington, DC: Pew Hispanic Center. Retrieved from http://pewhispanic.org/re-ports/report.php?ReportID=92

Gándara, P., & Contreras, F. (2009). *The Latino education crisis: The consequences of failed social policies.* Cambridge, MA: Harvard University Press.

Ginossar, T., & Nelson, S. (2010). Reducing the health and digital divides: A model for using com-munity based participatory research approach to e-health intervention in low income Hispanic communities. *Journal of Computer-Mediated Communication, 15,* 530–551.

Gloria, A. M., & Rodriguez, E. R. (2000). Counseling Latino university students: Psychosociocul-tural issues for consideration. *Journal of Counseling & Development, 78,* 145–154.

Gloria, A. M., Castellanos, J., & Kamimura, M. (2006). Understanding the history of Latina/os on the road to the university: Education for la RazaCosmica. In J. Castellanos, A. M. Gloria, & M. Kamimura (Eds.), *The Latina/o pathway to the PhD: Abriendocaminos* (pp. xxiii–xxxv). Sterling, VA: Stylus.

Henig, R. M. (2010). What is it about 20-somethings? Retrieved from http://www.nytimes.com/2010/08/22/magazine/22Adulthood-t.html?sq=emergent%20adulthood&st=cse&scp=1&pagewanted=print

Hottinger, J. A., & Rose, C. B. (2006). First generation college students. In L. A. Gohn, G. R. Al-bin, & G. R. Albin (Eds.), *Understanding college student subpopulations: A guide for student affairs professionals* (pp. 115–134). Washington, DC: National Association of Student Person-nel Administrators.

Immigration Policy Center. (2010). The DREAM Act: Creating economic opportunities. Retrieved from http://www.immigrationpolicy.org/sites/default/files/docs/DREAM_Act_Economic_Fact_Sheet_091610_2.pdf

Institute for Higher Education Policy [IHEP]. (2005). The investment payoff: A 50-state analysis of the private and public benefits of higher education. Retrieved from http://www.ihep.org/assets/files/publications/g-l/InvestmentPayoff.pdf

Jaschik, S. (2010). Arizona bans affirmative action. *Inside High Ed*. Retrieved from http://www.insidehighered.com/news/2010/11/03/arizona

Jones, M. (2010). Coming out illegal. *New York Times*. Retrieved from http://www.nytimes.com/2010/10/24/magazine/24DreamTeam-t.html?ref=magazine&pagewanted=print

Jones, S. (2002). *The Internet goes to college*. Washington, DC: Pew Internet & American Life Project.

Klinenberg, E. (2002). *Heatwave: A social autopsy of disaster in Chicago*. Chicago: University of Chicago Press.

Long, B. T., & Kurlaender, M. (2009). Do community colleges provide a viable pathway to a baccalaureate degree? *Educational Evaluation and Policy Analysis, 31*(1), 30–53. doi:10.3102/0162373708327756

Longerbeam, S. D., Sedlacek, W. E., & Alatorre, H. M. (2004). In their own voices: Latino student retention. *NASPA Journal, 41*(3), 538–550.

Lopez, M. H. (2009). *Latinos and education: Explaining the attainment gap*. Washington, DC: Pew Hispanic Center.

Lorence, D. P., Park, H., & Fox, S. (2006). Racial disparities in health information access: Resilience of the digital divide. *Journal Medical Systems, 30*(4), 241–249.

Mettler, S. (1998). *Dividing citizens: Gender and federalism in New Deal public policy*. Ithaca, NY: Cornell University Press.

Morales, R., & Bonilla, F. (1993). *Latinos in a changing U.S. economy: Comparative perspectives on growing inequality* (Vol. 7). Newbury Park, CA: Sage.

Mossberger, K., Tolbert, C. J., & Gilbert, M. (2006). Race, place and information technology. *Urban Affairs Review, 41*(5), 583–620.

Nasser, H. E., & Overberg, P. (2010). Kindergartens see more Hispanic, Asian students. *USA Today*. Retrieved from http://www.usatoday.com/news/nation/census/2010-08-27-1Akindergarten27_ST_N.htm

National Council of La Raza.(2010). *Dream Act*. Retrieved from http://www.nclr.org/index.php/issues_and_programs/immigration/dream_act/

Nora, A., Barlow, L., & Crisp, G. (2006). An assessment of Hispanic students in four-year institutions of higher education. In J. Castellanos, A. M. Gloria, & M. Kamimura (Eds.), *The Latina/o pathway to the PhD: Abriendocaminos* (pp. 55–77). Sterling, VA: Stylus.

Nunez, A. M., & Cuccaro-Alamin, S. (1998). *First generation students: Undergraduates whose parents never enrolled in postsecondary education*. Washington, DC: U.S. Department of Education, National Center for Education Statistics.

O'Connor, N., Hammack, F. M., & Scott, M. A. (2010). Social capital, financial knowledge, and Hispanic student college choices. *Research in Higher Education, 51*, 195–219.

Oseguera, L., Locks, A. M., & Vega, I. I. (2009). Increasing Latina/o students' baccalaureate attainment: A focus on retention. *Journal of Hispanic Higher Education, 8*(1), 23–53.

Perez, W. (2010, Winter). Higher education access for undocumented students: Recommendations for counseling professionals. *Journal of College Admission, 32–35*.

Pew Hispanic Center. (2009). Between two worlds: How young Latinos come of age in America. Retrieved from http://pewhispanic.org/files/reports/117.pdf

Piedra, L. M. (2006). *Facets of caring: An organizational case study of Interfaith House, residential program for homeless mentally ill adults*. Doctoral dissertation. The University of Chicago, Chicago, Illinois.

Pryor, J. H., Hurtado, S., Saenz, V. B., Lindholm, J. A., Korn, W. S., & Mahoney, K. M. (2005). *The American freshman: National norms for fall 2005*. Los Angeles: Higher Education Research Institute.

Reid, M. J., & Moore, III, J. L. (2008). College readiness and academic preparation for post-secondary education: Oral histories of first-generation urban college students. *Urban Education, 43*(2), 240–261.

Reyes, R., .III (2009). "Key interactions" as agency and empowerment: Providing a sense of the possible to marginalized, Mexican-descent students. *Journal of Latinos & Education, 8*(2), 105–118.

Ridings, J. W., Piedra, L. M., Capeles, J., Rodríguez, R., Freier, F., & Byoun, S.-J. (2011). Building a Latino youth program: Using concept mapping to identify community-based strategies for success. *Journal of Social Service Research, 37*(1), 34–49.

Rodriguez, A. P., Carrillo, I. Y., Kann, V. M., & Acevedo, L. C. (2007, April). *Latino parents and students exposing the structural inequalities of a university.* Paper presented at the annual meeting of the American Educational Research Association, Chicago, IL.

Santiago, D. A. (2007). *Voces (Voices): A profile of today's Latino college students.* Washington, DC: Excelencia in Education.

Schmidt, P. (2003). Academe's Hispanic future: The nation's largest minority group faces big obstacles in higher education, and colleges struggle to find the right ways to help. *Chronicle of Higher Education, 50*(14), A8.

Schneider, B., Martinez, S., & Owens, A. (2006). Barriers to educational opportunities for Hispanics in the United States. In M. Tienda & F. Mitchell (Eds.), *Hispanics and the future of America* (pp. 179–227). Washington, DC: National Academies Press.

Slate, J. R., Manuel, M., & Brinson, J. R. (2002). The "digital divide": Hispanic college students' views of educational uses of the Internet. *Assessment & Evaluation in Higher Education, 27,* 75–93.

Sullivan, T. A. (2006). Demography, the demand for social services, and the potential for civic conflict. In D. W. Engstrom & L. M. Piedra (Eds.), *Our diverse society: Race and ethnicity—Implications for 21st century American society* (pp. 9–18). Washington, DC: NASW Press.

Thayer, P. B. (2000, May). Retention of students from first generation and low income backgrounds. *Opportunity Outlook, 2*–8.

The Editorial Board. (2010). Tired politics: Dream Act opponents rely on resentment to block fairness. Retrieved from http://www.stltoday.com/news/opinion/columns/the-platform/article_83ddbf38-c695-11df-9f570017a4a78c22.html.

Tienda, M. (forthcoming). Hispanics and U.S. schools: Problems, puzzles and possibilities. In M. T. Hallinan (Ed.), *Frontiers in sociology of education.* Retrieved from http://theop.princeton.edu/reports/forthcoming/FrontiersChapter_final.pdf

Tienda, M., & Sullivan, T. A. (2009). The promise and peril of the Texas uniform admission law. In M. Hall, M. Krislov, & D. L. Featherman (Eds.), *The next twenty-five years? Affirmative action and higher education in the United States and South Africa* (pp. 155–174). Ann Arbor: University of Michigan Press.

Trostel, P. A. (2010). The fiscal impacts of college attainment. *Research in Higher Education, 51,* 220–247. doi:10.1007/s11162-009-9156-5

Tym, C., McMillion, R., Barone, S., & Webster, J. (2004). *First-generation college students: A literature review.* Texas Guaranteed Student Loan Corporation. Retrieved from http://www.tgslc.org/pdf/first_generation.pdf

U.S. Census Bureau. (2010). *The 2010 statistical abstract: Educational attainment.* Retrieved from http://www.census.gov/compendia/statab/2010/tables/10s0224.pdf

U.S. Department of Education, Office of Postsecondary Education [USDE-OPE]. (2008). *A profile of the federal TRIO programs and child care access means parents in school program.* Retrieved from http://www2.ed.gov/about/offices/list/ope/trio/trioprofile2008.pdf

Vargas, J. H. (2004). *College knowledge: Addressing information barriers to college.* Boston: Education Resources Institute.

Warburton, E. C., Bugarin, R., & Nunez, A. (2001). *Bridging the gap: Academic preparation and postsecondary success of first-generation students.* Washington, DC: National Center for Education Statistics.

Zalaquett, C. P. (2006). Study of successful Latina/o students. *Journal of Hispanics in Higher Education, 5,* 35–47.

Zell, M. C. (2010). Achieving a college education: The psychological experiences of Latina/o community college students. *Journal of Hispanic Higher Education, 9*(2), 167–186.

Chapter 7
Putting Students to Work: Spanish Community Service Learning as a Countervailing Force

Annie R. Abbott

Abstract Linguistic and cultural competence are essential components of mental health infrastructures for US Latinos, many of whom are monolingual Spanish speakers or have limited English proficiency. However, few human service providers are bilingual, and they are overtaxed. To fill this gap, agencies can look toward the Spanish program at their nearest college or university. Traditionally, Spanish students learned mostly about literature in a classroom or in study abroad. Today, Spanish community service learning (CSL) connects language students with local Spanish-speakers in order to form mutually beneficial relationships. This chapter defines Spanish CSL and offers human service providers guidelines for creating effective community—university relationships. When done well, Latinos benefit when Spanish CSL students support the work of mental health professionals.

The demographic data tell the story: In the first decade of this new century, the Latino population increased, often dramatically, in 49 out of 50 states (Pew Hispanic Center 2010). Latinos settled in destinations previously unaccustomed to Latino immigrants (Johnson and Lichter 2008), creating new infrastructure needs. Of the foreign-born Latinos who arrived during that time period, a majority of both youth and adults either only speak Spanish at home or speak English less than very well (Pew Hispanic Center 2010). This situation creates both challenges and opportunities. Educators and human service providers are challenged by the new linguistic and cultural needs, especially in geographical areas that do not have a traditional Latino base that can serve as a support system to the newcomers. For example, teachers encountering Latino children in the classroom for the first time may misinterpret cultural cues. Students may avoid direct eye contact with the teacher not as a sign of disrespect or insouciance, but rather as a sign of respect from their own cultural perspective and practices. Professionals working with Central American women who have recently given birth may be surprised by the bracelets worn by

A. R. Abbott (✉)
University of Illinois, Urbana-Champaign, IL, USA
e-mail: arabbott@illinois.edu

babies and the girdles worn by the mothers, each practice imbued with cultural significance. Language and culture, then, can be seen as barriers to overcome.

On the other hand, Spanish community service learning (CSL) is a teaching methodology that prizes community assets such as languages and cultures. Spanish CSL takes students out of the classroom and puts them in the community to use and improve their Spanish by working side-by-side with Spanish-speakers. In this way, human service providers who need to connect across languages and cultures with Latino immigrants can use these Spanish CSL students to bridge that divide. Although Spanish CSL can be done with students of all age groups, because I have been teaching and supervising Spanish CSL courses at the University of Illinois, Urbana-Champaign (UIUC) for six years, I will concentrate on how mental health providers can partner with a Spanish CSL program in higher education to utilize the range of auxiliary services those students can provide. This partnership, in turn, can facilitate the provision of mental health services to Latinos. The examples are numerous. Spanish CSL students can provide detailed directions, in Spanish, for finding an agency. They can provide child care—a frequent service barrier—in Spanish while the parent receives mental health services. They can serve as a scribe for adults with poor literacy skills in Spanish. Because language barriers complicate even the most mundane tasks, in the absence of these Spanish CSL students, many of these tasks fall to an overburdened service provider or completely through the cracks. Therefore, Spanish CSL, through its supportive functions, can play a critical role in reducing mental health disparities among Spanish-speakers. It is imperative, though, that this partnership with university Spanish CSL students and human service providers be well designed, and throughout this chapter I will detail how to accomplish that.

Spanish Community Service Learning: An Example of a Mutually Beneficial Partnership

As the local Latino immigrant community in Central Illinois rapidly increased during the late 1990s and 2000s, the counselors at the East Central Illinois Refugee Mutual Assistance Center (ECIRMAC) found that they lacked the linguistic skills and cultural know-how to work effectively with this new group of service recipients. In response, they hired one full-time Spanish-speaking counselor, and by 2004 she attended to the myriad needs of hundreds of Spanish-speaking clients—translating official documents, accompanying them to court dates, guiding families through the school system, settling lease disputes, procuring winter clothes for children and more. When that counselor faced a major health crisis due, in part, to work-related stress, the not-for-profit agency struggled to find a solution that would be tenable for their limited staff yet still allow them to fulfill their mission: To aid in the resettlement of refugees and immigrants, regardless of country or origin, in the East-Central Illinois area and to aid in the exchange and preservation of their respective cultures.

That same year, less than one mile away at my university, UIUC, I was teaching an advanced Spanish conversation course. Many of the students had studied abroad in a Spanish-speaking country and were taking the elective course in order to maintain their fluency and broaden the cultural knowledge they had acquired. Others were preparing to study abroad and were excited about the prospect of soon using their Spanish with native speakers and immersing themselves in a Latino culture. By chance, I learned about ECIRMAC's work and their need for Spanish-speakers, and the course was changed so that students spent half their time in the classroom and half their time volunteering at ECIRMAC.

This pedagogical method, CSL, brought that social service agency and these Spanish students together, allowing both sides to meet their goals. During the first semester, ECIRMAC gained 12 students of Spanish who each volunteered 28 hours in their office, answering phones, receiving clients, taking messages, translating documents and eventually handling some low-risk tasks such as calling the power company to sort out a mistake in a client's bill. Students earned course credit for communicating with native speakers, thereby improving their Spanish and deepening their knowledge of Latino cultures (Abbott and Lear 2010; Lear and Abbott 2008). Today, each semester, an average of 100 UIUC Spanish students provide a total of 2,800 volunteer hours to a dozen local schools and social service agencies that need the university students' Spanish language skills in order to better meet the needs of their Latino students, service recipients and stakeholders. Several years after we forged a CSL partnership, that original bilingual counselor at ECIRMAC said, "I cannot imagine my life without my volunteers … They really get involved. They have a chance to really practice the language, be close to the culture and see what kind of problems an immigrant can run into." (Kossler Dutton 2007). The same bilingual counselor still provides the direct services that she alone is professionally equipped to give, but the students' assistance with office tasks, client preparation, transportation, and inter-agency phone calls gives her more time to do the job for which she was trained.

Whereas this particular partnership began by chance, human service providers who struggle to meet the needs of their Spanish-speaking clients can purposefully seek the support of a nearby Spanish department. This chapter points out both challenges and solutions for establishing and maintaining effective university-community partnerships that meet the dual goals of fostering linguistic and cultural development among students and also ensuring that Spanish-speaking clients are well served. With the proper program design, Spanish CSL can be the axis of a mutually beneficial relationship that helps human service providers overcome language barriers and at the same time creates opportunities for university Spanish students to improve their Spanish and develop transcultural competence. These partnerships can serve as an important cornerstone in a culturally and linguistically responsive infrastructure that can effectively address Latino mental health.

This chapter, then, details why and how partnerships between human service providers and a Spanish CSL program can be a part of the solution. First, I contextualize how the rapid increase of Spanish-speakers in the United States has created parallel shifts in human service infrastructure needs and university Spanish studies' curricular designs. I then describe the UIUC Spanish CSL program model, but because each campus and community partner is unique, I also offer ideas for variations on that model. Specifically, I concentrate on four fundamentals for a successful community–campus partnership that take into account important issues that might not be readily apparent to community partners in human services: How to ensure that students receive academic credit and faculty oversight in the design and execution of their work in the community; how to forge a community–campus partnership so that everyone's expectations are clear and achievable; how to incorporate teaching materials that help students be successful in a professional context, not just the classroom; and how to incorporate technology to meet the needs of human service providers who are located far from a university campus or serve Spanish-speakers infrequently. Finally, the chapter concludes with an example of one student's experience doing her CSL work in a mental health program for Latinas. The description of her Spanish CSL work shows that, although it is true that more bilingual professionals are needed to increase Spanish-speakers' access to care, students with language skills but no mental health background can still play an important, supportive role to the experts who provide direct services.

Spanish: Challenges and Solutions for Mental Health Providers and Foreign-Language Educators

The literature shows that the lack of infrastructure for Latino mental health in the United States leads to at least two problems. First, linguistic and cultural barriers prevent or complicate Spanish-speakers' access to care. Second, the bilingual service providers who do serve them end up doing different and additional work compared to their monolingual colleagues.

Sentell et al. (2007) found that individuals who did not speak English were less likely to receive needed services than those who spoke only English. They concluded that limited English proficiency (LEP) "is associated with lower use of mental health care" and, in their sample, "[s]ince LEP is concentrated among Asian/ [Pacific Islanders] and Latinos, it appears to contribute to racial/ethnic disparities in mental health care." (p. 289). Gregg and Saha (2007) add another complicating element to the general picture of language barriers for non-English speakers. They differentiate between the correct translation of words (*parole*) in a clinical setting versus the communicative competence required to correctly translate the meaning behind those words (*langue*). If few Spanish-speaking mental health providers are currently in the system, even fewer have been fully trained in communicative competence. For example, the word (*parole*) "*susto*" in Spanish is easily translated to "fright" or "scare," and someone who reports to have had "*un susto*," has had "a fright" or "a scare." However, it has been well established that the cultural meaning (*langue*) of "*susto*" goes much deeper (Rubel et al. 1984). In a medical and mental health context, "*susto*" is more closely related to what the dominant North American culture denominates as post-traumatic stress disorder (Joyce and Berger 2007), and "*susto*" is an integral part of some Latino groups' syncretic beliefs about the causes of Type-2 diabetes (Poss and Jezeweski 2002).

When LEP service recipients do find a bilingual human service provider with whom to work, their particular circumstances (e.g., limited acculturation, anxieties surrounding immigration status, lack of familiarity with the service system) increase the workload of their provider (Engstrom and Min 2004). In the end, bilingual social workers have, according to Engstrom et al. (2009, p. 181) "more work demands and work consequences than do monolingual workers." Not only do specific tasks take additional time and effort to accomplish for an LEP client than for an acculturated English speaker, bilingual social workers also grapple with unique issues such as "language fatigue" from constantly switching between languages (Engstrom et al. 2009, p. 176). In sum, it is clear that current human service infrastructures for Spanish-speakers are both limited and strained.

The rapid increase in the number of Spanish-speakers in the United States has not only created a lack of infrastructure for Latino mental health, it has also precipitated a sea-change in the field of Spanish studies. In fact, Carlos Alonso, while Chair of the Department of Spanish and Portuguese at Columbia University, asserted that, "Spanish should no longer be regarded as a foreign language in this country; and, consequently, we should undertake an institutional rethinking and reshaping of the place occupied by Spanish language and culture in the US academic world." (Alonso 2006, p. 17). Indeed, the profession has been impelled toward deep-seated change by a recent report on foreign languages and higher education by the Modern Languages Association (2007, n.p.) that clearly states that "The language major should be structured to produce a specific outcome: Educated speakers who have deep translingual and transcultural competence." Although these outcomes may seem obvious, universities' foreign language curricula have traditionally dedicated themselves to the study of literature and, more recently, linguistics. Headlines are made when the department head of a prestigious university makes a bold statement and when our national professional organization sends out press releases regarding their call for change in foreign language studies, but a quieter voice is also urging Spanish departments to change: Our alumni. When they graduate and enter the professional world, they are often called upon to translate, interpret and help Spanish-speakers while on and off the job, simply because no one else can. Yet the traditional Spanish major better equips them to analyze a poem than to translate agency documents or advocate for a family whose utilities have been mistakenly cut off. Colomer and Harklau (2009, p. 658) describe the situation of high school Spanish teachers in ways that parallel that of bilingual human service providers: "Spanish teachers, as some of the few Spanish-speaking educators in new immigrant communities, are bearing an especially heavy burden as impromptu, unofficial translators and school representatives." That burden is described as disruptive, unappreciated and coercive even though it can also be deeply satisfying in human terms. Thus, it would seem that now more than ever, Spanish departments and human service providers are working toward similar goals: Language skills and cultural know-how for a globalized world.

CSL, then, provides the bridge between human service providers' infrastructure needs and trends in university Spanish studies. At its essence, CSL consists of three fundamental elements. First, students must perform a service that meets a community need. Second, that service must connect to and enhance the academic content of the course. Finally, students must reflect upon their experiences in the community. The result is a "meaningful community service that is linked to students' academic experience through related course materials and reflective activities." (Zlotkowski 1998, p. 3). Studies show that CSL does have a positive effect on students' learning, especially within a well-designed course or program (Eyler and Giles 1999), even fostering a sense of engaged citizenship and social justice among students (Benigni Cipolle 2010; Jones and Abes 2004; Perry and Katula 2001). The literature specifically on Spanish CSL is also clear: When students both serve and learn in the community, their advancement toward deep translingual and transcultural competence occurs in ways that cannot be achieved solely within the confines of a classroom (Abbott and Lear 2010; Beebe and DeCosta 1993; Hellebrandt et al. 2003; Hellebrandt and Varona 1999; Lear and Abbott 2008; Long and Macián 2008; Plann 2002; Weldon 2003). Students, however, are not the only beneficiaries in CSL. As the students work in the community, they are helping to create missing pieces in the infrastructure for Latino human services. This creates a truly mutually beneficial relationship—students' learning increases and Latinos' access to human service providers grows. Finally, the same demographics with which human service providers struggle—the rapid increase of Spanish-speakers in the United States that live in cities and non-urban areas where they previously did not live—actually facilitate the implementation of a Spanish CSL program. Human services' challenge is Spanish's opportunity.

A Spanish Community Service Learning Model: The University of Illinois, Urbana-Champaign

Building a successful community–campus partnership is challenging but doable. According to Jacoby (2003, p. xviii), "Service learning partnerships are complex, interdependent, fluid, dynamic, and delicate." As such, much has been written about how to forge, assess, and sustain successful partnerships (Carter 2004; Clarke 2003; Gugerty and Swezey 1996; Jacoby and Associates 2003; Kesler Gilbert et al. 2009; Schaffer et al. 2003). However, almost all the literature on partnerships assumes that English is the common language of all stakeholders or that the issues and best practices remain the same if another language (or languages) is used within the partnership. Instead, Spanish CSL partnerships require more and different work to align expectations, clarify underlying community needs, define appropriate tasks for students and assess the outcomes (Lear and Abbott 2009).

Despite the challenges, successful Spanish CSL partnerships are achievable, especially when everyone involved commits to working out the kinks in the short-term in order to attain long-term success. In its first semester during the fall of 2004, the Spanish CSL course in UIUC's Department of Spanish, Italian, and Portuguese involved just twelve students working with one community partner. In the 2009–2010 academic year, approximately 200 students each worked 28 hours with one of a dozen community partners. That represents 5,600 volunteer hours dedicated to serving the local Spanish-speaking community—a very significant number alone, but even more important when considering the value of the students' Spanish language skills.

Human service providers can tap this potential at any nearby university or college that teaches Spanish, especially those that offer a Spanish major. However, navigating the campus and understanding CSL's place in it can be confusing (Carmichael Strong et al. 2009). The conversation may be approached from two directions. The Spanish program itself is the place to begin. It may be housed in its own department or combined with other languages (e.g., the Department of Spanish, Italian, and Portuguese; Modern Languages; Romance Languages; World Languages; or Humanities). Not all Spanish programs have an existing CSL structure, so the next step is to approach a campus-level entity. Patience and persistence are key at this stage because many campuses, especially large ones, are decentralized. UIUC, for example, has no central CSL office. However, CSL is a part of the oversight of several campus units: The Office of the Vice Chancellor for Public Engagement, the Center for Teaching Excellence, and the Office of Volunteer Programs. The conversation may wind through many units, departments, and people before yielding fruit.

Precisely because all Spanish programs are potential CSL partners, but not all of them have an established CSL program, I offer the following description of the UIUC Spanish CSL model as a resource for human service providers as they broach a conversation with a Spanish department with no existing CSL infrastructure. Many Spanish programs or faculty are eager to institute a CSL program but are unsure of the work it involves. Many resources are available to those academics who wish to prepare a high-quality Spanish CSL course (Abbott 2010; Hellebrandt et al. 2003; Hellebrandt and Varona 1999; Lear and Abbott 2009). However, the following suggestions take into consideration the perspectives and needs of the community entity that needs students with knowledge of the Spanish language and Latino cultures combined with the professional skills necessary to navigate within a human services context.

Recommendations for the Development of a Spanish CSL Program

Ensure that Students Receive Academic Oversight and Credit for their CSL Work

At UIUC, students may take two fully-integrated Spanish CSL courses. The first, "Spanish in the Community," is a sixth-semester course that introduces students to the theory and practice of CSL and to the local Latino community. Each semester, we offer four sections capped at 20 students each; the class fills quickly and many students request overrides. Each week, students spend two hours in class and two hours working with the community partner of their choice (for a total of 28 hours in the community). Course requirements include a series of reflective essays, on-line quizzes, two exams, and active participation in both the classroom and community. After that course, students may enroll in "Spanish & Entrepreneurship: Languages, Cultures & Communities," an upper-level course that retains the same CSL structure (28 hours in class and 28 hours working with a community partner) but introduces a different course content: Social entrepreneurship. Thus, students' service remains the same, but their learning shifts toward comparing the theory of social entrepreneurship against the challenges non-profits face in creating economic sustainability alongside culturally appropriate programming. Course requirements include reflective essays, on-line quizzes, two exams, community participation, and a team project that benefits the community partners (fund raising, grant writing, market research, marketing, etc.).

Although a fully integrated Spanish CSL course is the ideal, other possibilities do exist. A Spanish department may take an already existing course (e.g., conversation, composition) and insert a CSL requirement into it. This may require some rearrangement of course assignments and changes in a few lesson plans, but it can be an easy entry point for a Spanish department just starting CSL. Additionally, CSL can fit well within an honors program. Individual students may elect to do CSL work for honors credit within a traditional class, or a faculty-advised honors club may use CSL for their service project. At UIUC, our honors students may do CSL work for any fifth-semester or higher Spanish course. In all these cases, it is important that the three essential elements of CSL are still in place; if not fully integrated into the course, students may perceive their CSL work as disconnected from the class content and opportunities for reflection may be non-existent or one-shot with little opportunity for growth (such as only requiring a final paper about the CSL experience).

Although the introductory and intermediate UIUC Spanish courses (that is, first and second year basic language classes) do not include CSL, other Spanish programs do. Many campuses require foreign language study, so there is a large pool of students to draw from at this level. However, any CSL work must take into account their more limited language skills. It is then necessary to manipulate the following variables to make the CSL work successful: Level of Spanish required, the stakes of the task at hand, and the amount of supervision necessitated. So, for example, if a human services agency plans to participate in a local health fair and wants to encourage Spanish-speakers to attend, a Spanish 101 student may go to a local community or workplace that employs Spanish-speakers and hand out a detailed Spanish-language flyer about the event. The language requirements are appropriate for several reasons. While passing out the flyer, the student can use the simple greetings and social niceties that even Spanish 101 students have learned. The flyer explains the event's details so that the student does not have to struggle to do so with limited Spanish. If someone does need to hear the information orally (because of low vision, illiteracy, etc.), the student will have had time to look up words and compose a response ahead of time. The stakes are low because an unsuccessful communicative exchange will simply result in one less person attending a potentially helpful but non-essential event. And finally, the level of supervision is minimal because the language demands and the stakes are both low. A number of successful scenarios are plausible: In the office, students can supervise the children that accompany service recipients while the service provider consults, uninterrupted, with the adult; at the front desk, students could greet clients and fill in part or all of a standard intake form before the counselor meets with the client to tackle the weightier issues; at the end of a session, the client and student can work out the details of scheduling a follow-up visit while the counselor returns to more substantial work tasks. However, with beginning and intermediate Spanish students, a high level of supervision for the students is necessary if both the language demands and the stakes are high.

Build Community–Campus Partnerships That Are Mutually Beneficial

At UIUC, we currently work with around a dozen community partners. With our social service agency partners, students do office work, translate, interpret, accompany clients to meetings, make phone calls on their behalf, help fill out forms, update the website, etc. With our school partners, our students serve as classroom aids in Spanish-language bilingual classrooms, tutors in a high school ESL center, and some students have even worked with newly arrived Spanish-speaking children at a Head Start. Our students also work with youth organizations (e.g., Boy Scouts), civic groups and other organizations that do outreach to the Latino community.

Forming the partnerships requires several initial conversations and then frequent contact with all parties in order to ensure that everyone clearly defines their expectations and reaches them. Frequent pitfalls include overestimating the students' language proficiency and cultural competence, underpreparing students for routine office tasks that may, in fact, be new to them, and underestimating the small efforts that an agency can do to help establish students' "authority" in clients' eyes, to name just a few (Lear and Abbott 2009). Ideally, once expectations have been aligned, one side will draft a project description or list of volunteer duties, and the other side will edit and confirm the document. That contract is then signed by the community partner, Spanish instructor or program director and the students. Given the unpredictable nature of the work involved in human services, flexibility must be worked into the contracts. However, many university students have highly structured lives (many take classes, hold a job, and participate in numerous extracurricular activities) and limited transportation (students in traditional campuses sometimes have no car), so big shifts in their work duties and hours can cause problems for all involved.

It is essential that human service providers clearly define both what they would like the Spanish CSL students to do (within the confines of their linguistic and professional capabilities) and what projects and/or tasks they can feasibly support. In general, community partners' requests for students' help falls on two extremes of the spectrum. On one end, many human service providers simply want help with the variety of tasks that typically emerge during the workday. This fits the Spanish CSL model well when the stream of Spanish-speaking clients is steady (students are disappointed if their skills are not put to use at all during their CSL work hours) and the type of tasks requires high levels of human contact (e.g., greeting and guiding clients, answering the phone, asking questions in order to fill out a form), not deskwork that could be done anywhere (e.g., translating documents, creating web content). This, in fact, is the case with our original community partner, ECIRMAC. When asked if they would like our students to work on any special programs or long-term projects, they have reiterated that what they really need is someone to answer the door, take messages, fill out forms and help clients with simple but time-consuming tasks. Tackling new projects and supervising the students working on them would pull the under-resourced staff too far away from the constant flow of services that must be provided each day. On the other end of the spectrum, some community partners want help with a clearly delineated project. For example, one of our partners organizes an annual visit to our community by the Mexican Mobile Consulate, and they need students to help with that undertaking. The tasks, deadlines, and contacts are complex yet carefully delineated, and Spanish CSL students easily follow clear instructions and then feel a real sense of accomplishment when the event takes place and many local Mexican immigrants have been helped. Students often go beyond our partners' expectations as well, bringing their own fresh perspectives to an organizations' processes and skills (e.g., technology, social media) that may be less developed within the organizations' staff. In sum, a successful CSL partnership will combine careful planning, flexibility, and openness to new ideas on all sides.

Use Teaching Materials That Build the Specific Skills Students Need in the Community and Strengthen Their Critical Thinking

Spanish studies is lucky to have many good textbooks at all levels of instruction, but the publishing industry has only recently begun to address the emergence of CSL in Spanish courses. Only *Temas: Spanish for the Global Community* (Cubillos and Lamboy 2007) introduces service learning features at the introductory level. Each chapter suggests small ways for students to access information from the community ("*En tu comunidad*"), and each unit ends with a suggested service activity ("*Servicio comunitario*"). At the intermediate level, both *Diálogos: Hacia una comunidad global* (Taceloski et al. 2010) and *En comunidad: comunicación y conexión* (Nichols et al. 2009) seek to put in a global context the immigration issues that students encounter when working in the local Latino community. These books do a very good job of presenting students with tools for critical analysis within the framework of traditional textbooks' emphasis on academic reading and writing skills.

Ideally, though, the textbook will guide students through the nuts and bolts of the CSL work as well as the broader socio-cultural analysis. *Comunidades: Más allá del aula* (Abbott 2010) attempts to do just that. Although designed as a textbook for more advanced students, when paired with a grammar review book, *Comuni-dades* could also be used at the intermediate and fifth-semester level. Most impor-tantly, the content of the textbook tackles only the struggles, questions, and gaps that CSL students themselves describe and the community partners' frustrations with students' few but disruptive shortcomings—linguistic, cultural, and profes-sional. Surprisingly, it is not the technical or profession-specific vocabulary that students need most; they can pick that up on the job and with a quick search on an internet browser. Instead, undervalued tasks that require the utmost precision and thoroughness cause students and community partners the most problems. Although textbook choice and curricular materials may seem to fall solely within the purview of the Spanish faculty teaching the CSL course, the community partner wants to ensure that the materials used in class enhance the students' performance within the organization. Furthermore, most Spanish instructors have never worked in human services, so the textbook needs to introduce students to the everyday work tasks of that setting. In that way, Spanish instructors can concentrate on what they do best—helping students acquire linguistic, cultural, and critical thinking skills.

Numbers, for example, are taught in the first days of every Spanish 101 course, and students and faculty alike often assume they have mastered them. Nonetheless, the most common complaint I received about my students in the early days was about the poor quality of the telephone messages they would leave for the bilingual counselor at ECIRMAC. The partnership came close to collapsing when yet another student left a cryptic message—and this time with a six-digit telephone number. Consequently, *Comunidades* includes two complete lessons on the telephone and message-taking.

First, in a surprisingly difficult task, students practice listening and producing numbers in small then progressively larger combinations in order to hone their lan-guage skills. Students then examine cultural information about telephone numbers. Whereas English speakers tend to say telephone numbers one number at a time (3-5-5-2-3-3-1), Spanish-speakers usually group the numbers (3-55-23-31). Speaking in a foreign language on the telephone is, by itself, challenging. When the information over the phone comes to you in a format that is different than what your cultural background leads you to expect, getting a correct telephone number on the message pad becomes even more difficult. To further complicate matters, many students have no previous experience taking messages in a professional context and therefore are unaware of professional strategies for effective phone communication. *"Repita, por favor"* may be the only phrase students know to say when they don't understand something, but if used too often, the caller may give up and hang up in frustration. This textbook, then, asks students to analyze alternative responses and find more effective strategies they can use when in the community (asking the speaker to re-peat only the specific, missing information—*Repita el último número, por favor*; asking the speaker to repeat the same information in a different way—*Dígame su número un número a la vez, por favor*; and asking the speaker to confirm the infor-mation—*¿3-55-23-31 es correcto?*). In the bigger picture, part of transcultural com-petence requires students to recognize their own, usually unexamined, cultural perspectives. Therefore, activities in the textbook invite students to explore their uses of the telephone and other communication devices and, ultimately, conclude that their cultural relationship with the telephone (e.g., unlimited telephone plans, frequent phone calls to their parents, and numerous texts to their friends) may be quite different than that of the Latino clients with whom they are speaking in their CSL work.

Filing, in many students' estimation, is busywork. However, filing is an essential task in all human services offices. Dealing with names, like numbers, seems to be a skill students master very early in their Spanish studies. Nevertheless, our human service community partners also complained that students misfiled documents. As a result, another lesson within *Comunidades* reviews the alphabet, Hispanic names, forms, and filing. Again, the information is presented in terms of language skills, cultural knowledge, and professional abilities. Students practice listening to names, writing names, spelling names, and asking questions to clarify the correct spelling (students realize that it is important to confirm whether a name is Rivera with a "v" or Ribera with a "b"; Vázquez with two "z's" or Vásquez with one "s" and one "z"). Cultural knowledge surrounding names is also essential in order for CSL students to fill out and file forms correctly. A client may go by the first name of Marisa even though her legal name is María Luisa. If her papers end up in two separate files, serious problems could occur for both the agency and the client. One activity, then, asks students to put a series of Hispanic names in alphabetical order. They quickly realize how difficult this task is because the number and combinations of first, middle, and last names are not always the same, yet identifying the first last name is essential to correct filing. Moreover, two different names from the list—Dra. Mª Garcia and María Luisa García Méndez—could potentially be the same person. Finally, students are asked to contrast their perception of filing ("boring") with the import it has in the professional realm. Clients' misfiled forms can wreak havoc with an organization's record-keeping, internal and external audits, and clients' cases.

In the end, no textbook can ever fully anticipate the linguistic, cultural, and professional needs of all CSL students. The nature of the human interactions outside of the classroom and the specificities of each human service agency are simply too variable. Moreover, no textbook can teach students every cultural difference in the meaning of words (for example, *susto*). However, good communication about shortfalls and problems will allow the Spanish instructor or program director to create teaching materials that address an organization's unique needs, instill within students a mindset of actively searching for transcultural differences and provide them with strategies for handling those differences.

Leverage Technology to Facilitate CSL Administration and Build Sustainable Solutions to Human Service Needs

To be honest, although Spanish CSL holds great promise for both human service providers and Spanish students, it takes work to get right. Spanish faculty often find themselves brokering the needs of all parties and attending to time-consuming details that never come up in a traditional classroom. In addition, some human service providers are too far away from campus for college Spanish students to reach by bus or bike. Thankfully, technology can help address both problems.

Our UIUC Spanish CSL program uses a wiki to make the program's administration collaborative and accessible. The wiki's front page introduces students and community partners to the program set-up and rules. From there, each community partner's own page describes their organization, the nature of the CSL work, contact information, and schedule openings. Because the wiki is open to the public, community partners can edit their information at any time, and students can sign up for a specific partner and time slots on a first-come first-served basis. At the very beginning of our Spanish CSL program, when only one class, 12 students and 1 community partner were involved, I, as the course professor, was at the center of all communication and scheduling. As the program grew, each stakeholder needed to share in those tasks. Thus, the wiki has allowed us to create work processes (such as student-centered self-scheduling) that are standardized and that can be implemented by me or any student assistant. I edit the information for our community partners who do not have the technical expertise, access, or time to contribute to the wiki themselves.

Currently, the model of our Spanish CSL program only allows us to partner with schools and human service agencies that are within a roughly five-mile radius of our university campus and that serve Spanish-speakers every day, all day (or at every pre-determined meeting time). The partnership is not mutually beneficial if students spend their time in the community and never or very rarely use their Spanish. Consequently, there are human service providers we cannot currently serve: Those that are more than a few miles from campus and those that need urgent but infrequent help with Spanish-speakers. Our next stage of program growth will use technology to build mutually beneficial partnerships with distant partners and those with infrequent needs.

The possible scenarios using technology in Spanish CSL are myriad and more project-based. For example, the director of a local women's shelter told me that on the very few occasions that Latinas did arrive at the shelter, they left when no one could communicate with them. Spanish CSL students cannot work each week at the shelter if there are rarely Spanish-speaking residents and visits and calls from Spanish-speakers are sporadic. They can, however, consult with shelter employees in order to write a "welcome" statement, script it in Spanish, produce a short video that concludes by asking the listener to wait while a Spanish-speaker is sought and upload it to a video-sharing site, such as YouTube, for the shelter's easy access. Employees can play the video then immediately contact Spanish CSL students via a social-networking site (such as Facebook) so that the soonest available student visits, calls or Skypes the shelter, and communicates in Spanish with the visitor. In addition to creating the shelter's signage in Spanish, students could create a podcast of a walking tour of the facilities. Just getting to the shelter can be challenge for some people, so students could visually document the bus trip from a Latino community to the shelter using Flickr (to create a set of photos with captions and tags) or Google Maps (to make a map with pinpoints, videos, and text). Furthermore, students could create a screencast (using, e.g., Jing) that guides Spanish-speakers through the information to fill in on an agency's commonly-used forms. Even basic technology can connect Spanish CSL students with community partners who are far away. For example, if students can access an agency's library of forms, perhaps through a password-protected wiki, they can talk to a client over the phone, fill out a form with the client's information then fax the form to the agency for approval and any necessary signatures.

As of now, these technology-based Spanish CSL projects are untested, but they do hold promise for remote human service providers or those who serve Spanish-speakers infrequently. They are not a cure-all though. A well-designed but unused Google map, for example, helps no one, and a recent report shows that only 51% of foreign-born Latinos use the internet (Livingston 2010). Obviously, a mixed strategy of technology-based Spanish CSL projects and face-to-face contact holds the greatest potential.

Transportation: A Specific Case of a Spanish CSL Student's Supporting Role

As stated in the introduction, Spanish students with no background in human services can still play a vital role in building infrastructures for Latino mental health. They can help human service professionals by unburdening them of some of the "extra" tasks that Spanish-speaking clients bring to the provider-recipient relationship. The reflective essay below was written by a Spanish CSL honors student. It details how her work allowed her to serve and learn and at the same time unburden the mental health service provider of the clients' transportation issue:

> Over the past few weeks I have experienced a new service learning opportunity … volunteering with the School of Social Work. When I initially signed up to work with the School of Social Work, I thought that I would be babysitting children while their mothers attended a weekly seminar about depression. Once I arrived however, I found that I had been recruited for a different task. The director of the group sessions found that during the course of the semester many women were unable to make it to the weekly group meetings because their carpool driver had other commitments and no other transportation was available to them. Champaign-Urbana has one of the best bus systems in the state, but many of the women were intimidated to utilize the bus as a method of travel because the schedules, buses and signs are all in English. My new project for the School of Social Work is to meet women without transportation at their homes and teach them how to use the [bus system] to get to their group meetings on campus.

> At first, I was very nervous about this volunteer project. I was not concerned so much about speaking Spanish with the women; I was more worried about trying to find my way around parts of Urbana that I had never been to before to meet the woman I was working with. These feelings however helped me empathize with how the women trying to use the buses to come to campus must feel. If it was this stressful for me to use the bus to get to a new part of Urbana, it must be much more difficult for someone who doesn't speak English to work up the courage to take a bus and not know they will be able to get directions if they need to.

After catching the Gold route bus, I successfully arrived at Perkins Road and Cunningham Avenue to meet with the woman and her children. I found it was difficult to explain the idea of a transfer because the woman had never used the bus before. Even though I did not know the word in Spanish for transfer, I explained [that] the woman could get off the bus at a central bus terminal and then change to any other route which would take her anywhere she wanted to go in the Champaign-Urbana area.

Overall this service project has left me feeling like I made a positive impact on someone's life. The woman that I was working with had never ridden the bus before in her life, which meant that she was dependent on her mother or brother to drive her and her daughters wherever she needed to go. Now that someone took the time to show her how to use the bus she can be more independent. This will help her greatly in feeling like she has more control over her own life. Instead of depending on a family member to take her to work, she can now take the bus which stops almost directly in front of her place of employment. Riding the bus will open up many opportunities for all of the women who attend the group and are dependent on others for transportation. The women can now feel free to schedule appointments at their convenience, shop whenever they like and set their own work schedules. While many of the women signed up for group sessions with the School of Social Work to learn about depression, some of the women have learned how to become more independent by riding the bus (Kern 2010).

As this student's reflective essay demonstrates, all parties can meet their goals through a well-designed Spanish CSL partnership. In this particular example, by delegating the transportation problem to the CSL student, the mental health service provider was able to concentrate on the mental health issue at hand: Providing weekly seminars about depression. The student learned from her CSL work: Her bus rides and conversations with Latinas improved her knowledge of the Spanish language and furthered her cultural knowledge. She even showed concrete signs of transcultural competence by articulating her own culturally informed reaction to the bus system, comparing that to the cultural context of the Latina woman she accompanied and using this understanding in her interactions with the woman. Finally, one seemingly insignificant task—showing Latinas how to ride the bus—enhances the women's lives and increases their access to the rare yet vital Spanish-language mental health infrastructure provided in their community. And that, after all, is the outcome all human service providers desire.

References

Abbott, A. (2010). *Comunidades: Más allá del aula*. Upper Saddle River, NJ: Prentice Hall.

Abbott, A., & Lear, D. (2010). The connections goal area in Spanish community service-learning: Possibilities and limitations. *Foreign Language Annals, 43,* 231–245.

Alonso, C. J. (2006). Spanish: The foreign national language. *ADFL Bulletin, 37*(2–3), 15–20.

Beebe, R. M., & DeCosta, E. M. (1993). Teaching beyond the university: The Santa Clara University Eastside Project: Community service and the Spanish classroom. *Hispania, 76,* 884–891.

Benigni Cipolle, S. (2010). *Service learning and social justice: Engaging students in social change*. Lanham, MD: Rowman & Littlefield.

Carmichael Strong, E., Green, P. M., Meyer, M., & Post, M. A. (2009). Future directions in campus-community partnerships: Location of service-learning offices and activities in higher education. In J. R. Strait & M. Lima (Eds.), *The future of service-learning: New solutions for sustaining and improving practice* (pp. 9–32). Sterling, VA: Stylus.

Carter, R. (2004). The Michigan Community Scholars program and its community partners: Developing a service strategy as a volunteer organization. In J. A. Galura, P. A. Pasque, D. Schoem, & J. Howard (Eds.), *Engaging the whole of service-learning, diversity, and learning communities* (pp. 177–183). Ann Arbor, MI: The OCSL Press at the University of Michigan.

Clarke, M. (2003). Finding the community in service-learning research: The 3-"I" model. In S. H. Billig & J. Eyler (Eds.), *Deconstructing service-learning: Research exploring context, participation, and impacts* (pp. 125–146). Greenwich, CT: Information Age.

Colomer, S. E., & Harklau, L. (2009). Spanish teachers as impromptu translators and liaisons in new Latino communities. *Foreign Language Annals, 42,* 658–672.

Cubillos, J. H., & Lamboy, E. M. (2007). *Temas: Spanish for the global community* (2nd ed.). Boston, ma: Thomson Heinle.

Engstrom, D., & Min, J. W. (2004). Perspectives of bilingual social workers: "You just have to do a lot more for them." *Journal of Ethnic & Cultural Diversity in Social Work, 13,* 59–82.

Engstrom, D., Piedra, L. W., & Min, J. W. (2009). Bilingual social workers: Language and service complexities. *Administration in Social Work, 33,* 167–185.

Eyler, J., & Giles, D. (1999). *Where's the learning in service-learning?* San Francisco: Jossey-Bass.

Gregg, J., & Saha, S. (2007). Communicative competence: A framework for understanding language barriers in health care. *Journal of General Internal Medicine, 22* (Suppl. 2), 368–370.

Gugerty, C. R., & Swezey, E. D. (1996). Developing campus-community relationships. In B. Jacoby & Associates (Eds.), *Service-learning in higher education* (pp. 92–108). San Francisco, CA: Jossey-Bass.

Hellebrandt, J., & Varona, L. T. (1999). Introduction. In E. Zlotkowski (Series Ed.) & J. Hellebrandt & L. T. Varona (Vol. Eds.) *Construyendo puentes (Building bridges): Concepts and models for service-learning in Spanish* (American Association for Higher Education Series on Service-Learning in the Disciplines, pp. 1–7). Washington, DC: American Association for Higher Education.

Hellebrandt, J., Arries, J., & Varona, L. (Vol. Eds.). (2003). In C. Klein (Series Ed.), *Juntos: Community partnerships in Spanish and Portuguese* (American Association of Teachers of Spanish and Portuguese Professional Development Series handbook, Vol. 5). Boston, MA: Thompson Heinle.

Jacoby, B. (2003). Preface. In B. Jacoby & Associates (Eds.), *Building partnerships for service-learning* (pp. xvii–xxii). San Francisco, CA: Jossey-Bass.

Jacoby, B., & Associates. (2003). *Building partnerships for service-learning.* San Francisco, CA: Jossey-Bass.

Johnson, K. M., & Lichter, D. T. (2008). *Population growth in new Hispanic destinations.* Retrieved from http://www.carseyinstitute.unh.edu/publications/PB-HispanicPopulation08.pdf

Jones, S., & Abes, E. (2004). Enduring influences of service-learning on college students' identity development. *Journal of College Student Development, 45,* 149–165.

Joyce, P. A., & Berger, R. (2007). Which language does PTSD speak? The "Westernization" of Mr. Sánchez. *Journal of Trauma Practice, 5,* 53–67.

Kern, B. (2010, March 30). Student reflection. Retrieved from http://spanishandillinois.blogspot.com/2010/03/student-reflection_30.html

Kesler Gilbert, M., Johnson, M., & Plaut, J. (2009). Cultivating interdependent partnerships for community change and civic education. In J. R. Strait & M. Lima (Eds.), *The future of service-learning: New solutions for sustaining and improving practice* (pp. 33–51). Sterling, VA: Stylus Publishing.

Kossler Dutton, M. (2007, July 14). Spanish-language students build skills, insights by working with local communities. *Madera Tribune.* Retrieved from http://www.maderatribune.com/news/newsview.asp?c=219845

Lear, D., & Abbott, A. (2008). Foreign language professional standards and CSL: Achieving the 5 C's. *Michigan Journal of Community Service Learning, 14,* 76–86.

Lear, D., & Abbott, A. (2009). Aligning expectations for mutually beneficial community service-learning: The case of Spanish language proficiency, cultural knowledge, and professional skills. *Hispania, 92,* 312–323.

Livingston, G. (2010, July 28). The Latino digital divide: The native born versus the foreign born. Retrieved from http://pewhispanic.org/reports/report.php?ReportID=123

Long, D., & Macián, J. (2008). Preparing Spanish majors for volunteer service: Training and simulations in an experiential course. *Hispania, 91,* 167–175.

Modern Language Association, Ad Hoc Committee on Foreign Languages. (2007). Foreign languages and higher education: New structures for a changed world. *Profession 2007.* Retrieved September 12, 2010, from http://www.mla.org/flreport

Nichols, P. A., Johnson, J. A., Lemley, L. R., & Osa-Melero, L. (2009). *En comunidad: Comunicación y conexión.* New York, NY: McGraw-Hill.

Perry, J., & Katula, M. (2001). Does service affect citizenship? *Administration & Society, 33,* 330–365.

Pew Hispanic Center. (2010). *Statistical Portrait of Hispanics in the United States, 2008:* Table of change in the hispanic population, by state: 2000 and 2008. Retrieved from http://pewhispanic.org/files/factsheets/hispanics2008/Table%2014.pdf

Plann, S. J. (2002). Latinos and literacy: An upper-division Spanish course with service learning. *Hispania, 85,* 330–338.

Poss, J., & Jezeweski, M. A. (2002). The role and meaning of *susto* in Mexican Americans' explanatory model of type 2 diabetes. *Medical Anthropology Quarterly, 16,* 360–377.

Rubel, A. J., O'Nell, C. W., & Collado-Ardón, R. (1984). *Susto, a folk illness.* Berkeley, CA: University of California Press.

Schaffer, M. A., Williams Paris, J., & Vogel, K. (2003). Ethical relationships in service-learning partnerships. In S. H. Billig & J. Eyler (Eds.), *Deconstructing service-learning: Research exploring context, participation, and impacts* (pp. 147–168). Greenwich, CT: Information Age.

Sentell, T., Shumway, M., & Snowden, L. (2007). Access to mental health treatment by English language proficiency and race/ethnicity. *Journal of General Internal Medicine, 22* (Suppl. 2), 289–293.

Taceloski, K., Kauffman, R. A., & Overfield, D. M. (2010). *Diálogos: Hacia una comunidad global.* Upper Saddle River, NJ: Prentice Hall.

Weldon, A. (2003). Spanish and service-learning: Pedagogy and praxis. *Hispania, 86,* 574–583.

Zlotkowski, E. (1998). A new model of excellence. In E. Zlotkowski (Ed.), *Successful service learning programs. New models of excellence in higher education* (pp. 1–14). Bolton, MA: Anker.

Part III
Priority Contexts for Infrastructure Development: Vulnerable Populations

Chapter 8
Serving Latino Families Caring for a Person with Serious Mental Illness

Concepción Barrio, Mercedes Hernández and Armando Barragán

Abstract What do mental health practitioners need to know about providing culturally relevant services for Latino families dealing with severe mental illness in a loved one? In this chapter, we will review salient sociocultural issues that practitioners and program managers need to consider in the design and delivery of quality care for Latino families with a member diagnosed with schizophrenia and other related disorders. We will examine pertinent research and practice areas on: the caregiving ideology characteristic of Latino families, cultural issues that affect Latino family participation in services, family involvement in services in the early stages of the illness, and psychoeducational approaches with Latino families. We will draw from our experience in the development of a culturally based psychoeducational intervention for Spanish-speaking families and discuss the applicability of a cultural exchange framework for increasing the cultural fit between family and provider cultures. Finally, the practice implications of an approach that prospectively takes into account the cultural strengths and resources that families bring into treatment are addressed.

The emergence of a serious and persistent mental illness, such as schizophrenia, affects not only the individual but the family as well. Because mental illness tends to affect young people, family members often find themselves faced with their loved one's denial of the illness and treatment resistance, while both grappling with their understanding of the mental illness and facing the challenges of finding appropriate care and services. Ethnic disparities in mental health care are well documented, and especially pronounced among immigrant Latinos (Barrio et al. 2003b; United States Department of Health and Human Services [USDHHS] 2001). Latino families confront multiple barriers in accessing comprehensive and culturally relevant services for their loved one and for themselves. By default, Latino families compen-

This work was supported, in part, by the National Institute of Mental Health grants K01 MH-01954 and R34 MH-076087

C. Barrio (✉)
University of Southern California, Los Angeles, CA, USA
e-mail: cbarrio@usc.edu

sate for service disparities by providing essential care to their affected relative, and most continue to provide invaluable support long after the person finally receives services. Although not unique to Latinos, family caregiving is particularly salient among Latino families. Logically, without the informal care that Latino families provide, formal health and mental health systems of care would likely be inundated with demands for services (Biegel et al. 1991).

In this chapter, we examine several sociocultural issues that program managers and practitioners need to consider in serving Latino families caring for a member diagnosed with schizophrenia or a related psychotic disorder (i.e., schizophrenia, schizoaffective disorder, schizophreniform, and psychotic disorder not otherwise specified) or other serious mental disorders (i.e., bipolar disorders and major depressive disorder with psychosis). Such disorders are often characterized by an illness course that is debilitating, persistent, and overwhelming for family and others involved. These families represent a critical and often unrecognized resource in the care of Latinos living with mental illness. As such, engaging family caregivers in treatment and supporting them must be a central component of any mental health infrastructure for Latinos. Toward this goal, we focus on pertinent research and practice literature regarding: (a) the caregiving ideology characteristic of Latino families, (b) the way that culture shapes the treatment expectations of family members and service providers, (c) the need for family involvement in services during the early stages of illness, and (d) the usefulness of psychoeducational approaches in helping Latino families. In addition to the literature, we draw from our practice and research experience in community-based mental health settings and our experience developing a culturally based psychoeducational intervention for Spanish-speaking families. Although many of the lessons learned can be applied more broadly to other immigrant groups, our work primarily focuses on Spanish-speaking Mexican immigrants with low levels of acculturation. Finally, we address several areas, including the way services are reimbursed, that require further consideration if we are to build a mental health services infrastructure that can truly provide culturally relevant services to Latino families.

The Caregiving Ideology Characteristic of Latino Families

Latino culture has consistently been characterized as highly familistic with an interdependent orientation and values that reflect strong emotional commitments to the family collective and family life (Hall 2001; Vega 1995). When addressing the serious mental illness of a loved one, familistic values are exemplified in the caregiving patterns and practices of Latino families. Specifically, research studies show that Latino clients diagnosed with a serious mental disorder are more likely to live with family members than their European American counterparts (Barrio et al. 2003a; Guarnaccia 1998). An estimated 70% to 90% of Latino adults with serious mental illnesses live with family members (Guarnaccia 1998; Kopelowicz 1998; Ramirez García et al. 2009). By comparison, approximately 30% to 65% of the non-Latino

White client population with serious mental illnesses live with family members (Murray-Swank and Dixon 2004). These ethnic differences in living situation reflect the strong cultural expectations and preferences of the Latino family to care for a loved one with a mental illness (Guarnaccia 1998; Pickett et al. 1998). Latino families are more likely to express greater hope, optimism, and faith regarding long-term outcomes of the affected member's mental illness than non-Latino White families (Guarnaccia 1998). From our ethnographic work, we learned that Latino families with low levels of acculturation reported a positive sense of obligation to care for their loved one; many family members considered institutional placement of their son or daughter unthinkable and tantamount to abandonment (Barrio and Yamada 2010). Latino family members regarded the provision of care at home as a permanent and culturally sanctioned living situation. Because a supportive living arrangement serves as a protective factor against the disruptive effects of a serious mental illness, incorporating families into treatment services has positive implications for the care of persons with a mental illness (Kopelowicz 1998).

Although many variations in family structure exist, Latino families have been recognized for their extensive social support patterns and kinship networks (Barrio and Hughes 2000; Vega 1995). When it comes to caring for a family member with a serious mental illness, women typically take responsibility for the provision of in-home care and interfacing with the service system. From our research in community-based settings, we observed that mothers, grandmothers, wives, daughters, and sisters occupied the role of the primary caregiver for a loved one with mental illness. Often, Latino clients were accompanied to their appointments by a family member. When the primary caregiver was Spanish-language dominant, a bilingual family member with a higher level of education would often accompany her. Interestingly, when family group psychoeducational services were offered in Spanish and in the evening, we observed a greater representation of male family members—especially fathers, husbands, and brothers—who actively participated along with the primary caregiver. Many male family members have inflexible work schedules that do not permit them to attend during the day, but are ready and willing to attend program services held in the evening; this shows their support for the woman relative and demonstrates their interest in learning about the mental illness. Clearly, this suggests that increased involvement in services by key family members can be achieved by making structural modifications (such as accommodating the scheduling needs of family members) that increase the accessibility of services.

Cultural Issues that Affect Latino Family Participation in Services

Despite the willingness of family members to support the care of their loved one, several cultural issues complicate the involvement of Latino families in treatment services. Studies have highlighted several barriers that negatively influence the participation of Latinos and other ethnic minority families in services. Low socioeconomic status and low levels of educational attainment are associated with inadequate knowledge of mental illness and a lack of familiarity with formal support groups (Cook and Knox 1993; Guarnaccia 1998; Medvene et al. 1995). The stigma attached to mental illness, coupled with ethnic minority status, can contribute to family members' reluctance to ask for help outside the immediate family (Cook and Knox 1993). As a source of shame, stigma has been found to significantly increase caregivers' subjective burden and psychological distress (Magaña et al. 2007). Additionally, family members' attitudes toward the provider system vary. Some family members distrust professionals and are reluctant to access services, whereas others show great deference toward professionals (Guarnaccia 1998; Pickett et al. 1998). These issues underscore how poverty, education, stigma, and attitudes can shape the interface between Latino culture and the culture of the service provider system (Barrio 2000; Solomon 1998).

Self-help and advocacy organizations, such as the National Alliance on Mental Illness (NAMI), have encountered difficulties in engaging Latino families to join or form affiliate groups. Consequently, NAMI has made concerted efforts to improve its outreach particularly to Spanish-speaking families (NAMI 2008). Even so, language barriers remain a persistent impediment for Latino family involvement in such advocacy groups. For example, when NAMI and other consumer advocacy meetings are not tailored to Latino families, Spanish-speaking family members are by default excluded from the discussion and often appear confused trying to keep up with the content and process of the meeting, even when translators are available. Clearly, the sole presence of a translator is insufficient for overcoming language and cultural barriers.

In one study of ethnic family participation in support and self-help groups, we found marked differences in how the groups originated as well as in the nature of the groups (Barrio et al. 2000). Spanish-speaking groups began in response to the need for linguistically accessible psychosocial services for families. Notably, these groups were started and facilitated by mental health professionals. By comparison, African American and Native American groups were started and facilitated by family members or consumer advocates. Such differences in group origins reflect the difficulties families have in overcoming cultural and language barriers on their own. Among the successful groups, mental health providers engaged in active and sustained outreach well beyond mailings or posting of group meeting announcements in predominantly immigrant communities. Strategies for engagement included identifying and engaging families during their first contact with the provider system. Groups were scheduled in the evening to accommodate work schedules and transportation constraints and thereby maximize group participation. Facilitators of Spanish-speaking groups emphasized the importance of a psychoeducational approach that accommodates the range of literacy levels among Spanish-speaking families when meeting their needs for information and engaging them in a shared decision-making process (Barrio and Dixon, in press). Group discussions often addressed psychiatric disorders, spirituality, faith, hope, and meaning-making. Other issues discussed in group included addressing causal attributions and cultural beliefs about mental illness, and perceived stigma of mental illness. Group facilitators indicated that Latino Spanish-speaking families lacked an awareness of the potential advocacy and activism roles they could play in the treatment of their loved ones. Assuming these roles should not be an expected outcome of group participation. Similar to other studies (Medvene et al. 1995), group facilitators reported that Latino families preferred that mental health professionals lead the support groups (Barrio et al. 2000). The complexity of addressing cultural and language issues seem to require professional expertise.

The practice principles underlying most psychiatric rehabilitation programs emphasize increasing levels of independence of the clients they serve (Stroul 1989). Yet, treatment goals that prioritize independent living skills and hold high expectations for individual self-sufficiency conflict with Latino cultural norms that value interdependence and mutual reliance among family members (Barrio 2000). Within Latino families, interdependence and the centrality of the family are closely aligned (Behnke et al. 2008; Hall 2001; Ramirez García et al. 2009). The value placed on interdependence within a family context is underscored when one considers that the predominant living arrangement for adult Latinos with serious mental illness is indeed the family. In contrast, providers may view interdependent relationships within the Latino family as dysfunctional overinvolvement antithetical to the goal of independence. However, it is important to keep in mind that studies have found that people diagnosed with schizophrenia who come from cultures that foster interdependence present more benign clinical profiles and better outcomes than individuals from cultures that value individualism and independence from family (Brekke and Barrio 1997; Hooper 2004; Jablensky et al. 1992). The acceptance and care conveyed within a family context may protect the family members living with mental illness from feeling isolated and blamed for their illness (Guarnaccia and Parra 1996).

As such, by understanding the value of interdependence, Latino caregivers can help providers improve service delivery. Clients and their families may find that traditional treatment approaches or recommendations fail to correspond with their own cultural views and expectations (Barrio 2000; Solomon 1998; Sue et al. 2009). For example, a Latino family seeking professional help in managing a loved one's psychotic illness within the home will likely find unpalatable a recommendation to place their loved one in an independent living arrangement, such as an intermediate care facility (Barrio and Yamada 2005). Given the deference afforded to professionals, such a family might not feel comfortable challenging the recommendation or pursuing a different approach with the professional, and may instead choose to discontinue treatment altogether. Despite the important role that families play in the care of Latino adults with mental illness, and their willingness to participate in treatment, these cultural incongruencies stymie their efforts and add to families' caregiving burden.

Family Involvement in Services in the Early Stages of the Illness

Families vary greatly in their initial response to the early signs of a serious psychiatric illness in a loved one. Family perceptions and responses to the illness may be culturally patterned and can affect pathways to appropriate psychiatric care. Although the research is very limited in this area, the available findings suggest a tendency for ethnic minority clients to delay seeking psychiatric treatment until the illness has progressed to an unmanageable degree (Durvasula and Sue 1996; Maynard et al. 1997; Primm et al. 1996; Snowden and Cheung 1990). In the general population, several years can pass before a serious psychiatric disorder is detected, acknowledged, and appropriately treated (Norman et al. 2004). In fact, the time between the onset of psychotic symptoms, a psychiatric diagnosis, and the initiation of formal treatment—a period of untreated psychosis—can range from one to two years (Compton et al. 2009; Johnstone et al. 1986; Loebel et al. 1992; Rabiner et al. 1986). There has been no examination of Latino populations with schizophrenia and other serious mental disorders during the early intervention period. Timely access to mental health services is critically important, as positive long-term clinical and functional outcomes for schizophrenia are associated with early intervention (Larsen et al. 2001). Treatment delay of more than one year is a strong predictor of a negative response to treatment (Loebel et al. 1992). In total, evidence suggests that our current system of care does not identify mental illnesses sufficiently early to intervene and minimize the damaging effects of psychiatric disorders, especially for young adults who are more at risk of early-onset disorders.

Family experiences during the early phase of illness have been described as an emotional "rollercoaster" (Murray-Swank et al. 2007). The months, and sometimes years, preceding appropriate psychiatric care have been characterized by misdiagnosis, misinformation, incorrect referrals, and inappropriate treatments; it is not uncommon for clients and families to experience great distress and trauma during this time. For Latino immigrant families, linguistic, cultural, and socioeconomic barriers further compound these experiences. Positive symptoms such as hallucinations, delusions, and disorganized thinking and behavior often mark the early stage of a serious mental illness. The onset of psychotic symptoms can be a very overwhelming and distressing experience for the person and the family. This is also a period of great confusion because the seriousness of the illness is often not fully grasped by the person, the family, or even professionals such as school and law enforcement personnel and, in some cases, mental health providers.

Preliminary findings from a study of the experiences of Spanish-speaking family caregivers of a loved one with schizophrenia provided further insights into how families perceive the onset of mental illness and the uneven pathway to psychiatric care (Barrio and Yamada 2010). Early symptoms were interpreted by families as social withdrawal, isolation, insomnia, laziness, aggressiveness, rebelliousness, and out-of-control behavior. For many, the illness trajectory was described as insidious, with a gradual deterioration in functioning. For others, the illness trajectory was described as sudden, leading to tumultuous crisis events. Some family members initially attributed the unusual behavior to supernatural causes, which led them to consult folk healers. Many families attributed the cause of the illness to adolescent behavior, suspicion of drug use, and bad friends. For the vast majority of caregivers, the route to treatment was circuitous and seemingly interminable, until finally they received a referral to psychiatric services by emergency room personnel, a primary care physician, a school counselor, or law enforcement. In retrospect, several families appreciated the role of law enforcement during a severe crisis that eventually served as the catalyst to obtain proper psychiatric care. Surprisingly, many clients in the study had never been hospitalized and had received primarily outpatient psychiatric services.

However, family members' experiences were marked by great distress, confusion, suffering, and great personal, social, and financial burden. Our combined research and practice experience shows that during the early phase of the illness, while families grappled with understanding the psychotic symptoms and behavioral changes in their loved one, they constantly searched for information and help both within and outside their social, spiritual, and community networks. A common scenario involved seeking advice from more acculturated persons with higher levels of education to help them acquire information and access to resources. However, often the persons consulted did not possess the requisite level of knowledge of mental illness to navigate the pathway to appropriate care. Thus, in many cases seeking assistance within the family's own social support network did not produce the desired result.

Similarly, in another qualitative examination of Latino family experiences with a loved one with schizophrenia, we found support for the notion that the early stage of the illness was characterized by great ambivalence and confusion (Barragán et al. 2010). When family members attributed behavioral changes in their loved one to a situational crisis or event (e.g., death in a family, incarcerations, divorce), such changes were recognized as a significant concern and brought stress for the family. Frequently, at the initial stage family members viewed behavioral changes as manageable and only sought assistance from within their social network. As the symptoms worsened, family caregivers sought outside help, which came in a variety of forms: first responders from a psychiatric emergency team, police intervention leading to incarceration, hospital emergency room and/or a psychiatric hospitalization. The onset of mental illness brings severe stress and burden for the person and the family, ultimately resulting in crisis-driven interventions that involve more restrictive and intense treatments (Barragán et al. 2010). Innovative outreach and program strategies are needed to provide Latino families with information and referral services that expedite entry into appropriate psychiatric care for their loved ones and essential psychoeducational and support services for the entire family.

Psychoeducational Approaches with Latino Families

Unquestionably, timely intervention for schizophrenia and other serious mental disorders results in better outcomes (Larsen et al. 2001). It is reasonable to expect that increasing knowledge about mental illness and the importance of early intervention at the family and community levels would decrease the delay between illness onset and treatment. Psychoeducational approaches geared specifically toward clients with a serious mental illness and their families already in the treatment system have formed a central part of the standard of care for several decades. Extensive research supports the use of family psychoeducation as an evidence-based practice, particularly for schizophrenia spectrum disorders (Dixon et al. 2001; McFarlane et al. 2003; Mueser et al. 2003). Increasing family members' knowledge of mental illness, and providing them with the support and tools to deal with a difficult illness, has proven effective in reducing relapse rates, facilitating recovery, improving family well-being, alleviating family burden, and increasing the quality of family relationships (Dixon et al. 2001; McFarlane et al. 2003; Mueser et al. 2003). The principles that underlie effective psychoeducational models attend to the sociocultural needs of the family and include an assessment of strengths and limitations of the family in supporting their loved one (Dixon et al. 2001). Such practical and comprehensive models combine both educational and therapeutic services. They promote an emotionally supportive environment for the person living with mental illness and foster collaborative relationships among providers, clients, and their families. Studies have shown the usefulness of adapting a psychoeducational framework of interventions to the needs of ethnic minority groups (Jordan et al. 1995; Lefley 1990; Lefley and Bestman 1991; Rivera 1988; Rodriguez 1986). For example, multiple-family psychoeducational groups conducted by professional staff, in particular, have been used with Mexican immigrant families and appear to be well received and effective in community-based mental health settings (Vega et al. 2007).

La CLAve: Promoting Early Entry into Mental Health Treatment

There is one innovative psychoeducational program, currently in the pilot stages of development, that is focused on increasing an understanding of psychosis among Spanish-speaking people within community settings (López et al. 2009). This program uses popular cultural icons derived from Latino art and music videos, as well as a mnemonic device—La CLAve (The Clue)—to deliver culturally relevant psychoeducation that will promote early entry into mental health treatment. Psychoeducational content targets four domains: (a) knowledge of psychosis, (b) efficacy beliefs that one can identify psychosis in others, (c) attributions to mental illness, and (d) professional help-seeking. La CLAve is organized as a set of 42 PowerPoint slides with 5 audio clips, 3 video clips, and 4 paintings/drawings. Symptoms are described in clear, everyday language to facilitate participants' recall of the symptoms of psychosis and to enhance their belief that they can identify psychosis in others. The program consists of a one-time educational meeting administered by a mental health professional. In the pilot phase, audiences ranged in size from 14 to 30 persons per educational session (60 to 75 minutes in duration).

The La CLAve program has been pilot-tested with community residents and family caregivers of persons with schizophrenia, and there is persuasive pre- and post-test evidence showing increases in the tested domains. For community residents, the authors observed increased ability in four domains: symptom knowledge, efficacy beliefs, illness attributions, and recommended help-seeking behaviors. For caregivers, increased ability was observed in symptom knowledge and efficacy beliefs—the belief that one can accurately identify psychiatric symptoms (López et al. 2009). A promising program like La CLAve, with its developing empirical base, could be used to implement effective and simple psychoeducation practices that are culturally tailored and would benefit the general Latino community. Ultimately, the widespread use of such educational campaigns could contribute to the early recognition and treatment of mental illness and an improvement in the quality of care for Latino clients and their families (see López et al. 2009).

CFIMA: A Manualized, Multifamily Intervention for Latino Families

Family psychoeducational models—like most psychosocial rehabilitative approaches—are based on Western notions of mental health and illness. Often, though, these approaches do not consider the role of culture in service delivery. Given the cultural issues previously discussed, we were prompted to consider intervention approaches that prioritize the cultural context and that use cultural strengths and resources to help families cope with caring for a family member who has serious mental illness. We embarked on a process to develop an intervention informed by our extensive clinical experience with Latinos, evidence-based practices, the literature on protective factors, and findings from an ethnographic study with Spanish-speaking Latinos. Given the strong research support for family psychoeducation models and their relevance to working with Latino families, we retained evidence-based elements of multifamily psychoeducation groups and added new components for use with Spanish-speaking families. We titled the intervention "A Culturally based Family Intervention for Mexican Americans" (CFIMA).

In our prior work, we explored the perspectives of Spanish-speaking Mexican American clients with schizophrenia, their families, and mental health service providers to examine the cultural fit between Latino families and the provider system. Our ethnographic study comprised a series of focus groups, in-depth interviews with participants from each stakeholder group, and an overt participant observation component in community mental health settings. The results from our ethnographic work drove the development of CFIMA. We uncovered five salient cultural domains that acted as protective factors against family burden and interpersonal problems: (a) the centrality of familism, (b) the role of spirituality and religiousness, (c) nonjudgmental cultural attributions that convey interpersonal warmth, (d) biculturalism, and (e) cross-border resources (Barrio and Yamada 2010). We found that these five domains represented valuable family sociocultural resources—and that they were largely untapped by community-based service providers. We also learned that a culturally based intervention must include a proactive and planned approach to involvement of family members, to ensure their inclusion in the treatment process.

The process of cultural adaptation can include a surface-structure or a deeper-structure approach (Kumpfer et al. 2002). *Surface-structure strategies* refer to outward modifications that may include gaining general knowledge about ethnocultural factors and sociostructural needs of the families' culture and incorporating these into service system modifications. Surface-structure modifications may include bilingual/bicultural staffing, using Latino interpersonal cultural style (*personalismo*), and community outreach to increase cultural responsiveness and access to program. Typically, community mental health treatment programs that serve large numbers of Latinos utilize a basic surface-structure approach to the cultural adaptation of their services. *Deeper-structure strategies* go further by incorporating values, traditions, and practices consistent with the worldview and help-seeking patterns of the cultural group (Kumpfer et al. 2002). Guided by the literature on the cultural adaptation of interventions (Bernal et al. 2009; Kumpfer et al. 2002; López et al. 2002), we applied a deeper-structure approach and in addition incorporated the cultural findings from basic and cross-cultural research to inform intervention strategies: a method delineated by López et al. (2002). For example, cross-cultural research on expressed emotion and protective factors (e.g., family warmth, a prosocial orientation) (López et al. 2004) was used in a central component of the model, intended to help families conserve and cultivate positive family characteristics that value interdependent functioning and family warmth.

We used a theory-driven, culturally centered approach guided by our cultural exchange framework and the tenets of strengths-oriented approaches (Rapp 1998). The intervention process focused on the transactional exchange of knowledge, attitudes, and practices that occurs between Latino families and service providers. The CFIMA includes three stages of cultural exchange in the intervention process: (a) cultural assessment, (b) cultural accommodation, and (c) cultural integration of strengths and resources. At each stage, CFIMA facilitators assess family strengths, learn from families, and impart culturally relevant information to enhance the cultural fit between the families and the mental health provider system. For example, families' notions and explanations about mental illness were explored and taken into account before they were provided with information on the biological perspective of the illness. The content of sessions focused not only on psychoeducational information, but also on raising awareness about the culturally mediated coping resources embedded in Latino family culture (such as the salience of spirituality/religiousness in coping with the illness in their lives).

We pilot-tested this model in actual practice settings. The CFIMA facilitators were master's level Latino bilingual social workers trained in the manualized intervention. CFIMA uses a 16-week multifamily group format that meets in two-hour sessions. Group sessions were held within typical mental health service settings, but during the early evening to accommodate work schedules. The format and structure of the CFIMA was based on ethnographic study findings, which indicated a strong preference by family participants for family-specific services centered on psychoeducation and support. Hence, the CFIMA groups were for family members only—clients were excluded—and each group included 10 to 15 family members.

The CFIMA was pilot-tested with 59 Spanish-speaking Latino families in a randomized control trial comparing the CFIMA with usual care (see Barrio and Yamada 2010). We collected data on family- and client-level outcomes and conducted post-study focus groups with intervention participants. Preliminary evidence from the quantitative assessments indicates that the intervention effectively increased illness knowledge and reduced the experience of burden in caring for a family member with a serious mental illness. In the following paragraphs, we highlight some key experiences and lessons learned in conducting this study. Regarding the five cultural domains from our earlier ethnographic study, we learned that familism and spirituality/religiousness were the most salient, receiving greater emphasis within each of the three stages of the cultural exchange process. This was not surprising given the attention these two domains have received in the Latino mental health literature. The other three domains appeared to have different but important roles in the process. For example, cultural attributions—conveying acceptance and affection for their loved one—were salient in typical communication and biculturation; references to cross-border living were present but appeared to be more in the background. As to the last three domains, it was helpful for the interventionists to have an awareness of them and to competently highlight them in the group process.

The strength of CFIMA's culturally relevant approach became evident throughout the intervention. Family participants reported perceived changes in knowledge, attitudes, and practices related to the mental illness. They expressed gratitude for the cultural exchange framework, which emphasized knowing about mental illness, learning from different points of view, providing mutual support, and fostering hope in each other. Whereas the participants valued the professional expertise of the group facilitators, they also benefited from sharing "testimonials" about cultural resources, especially those practices that reflected their spiritual and religious beliefs. Family members frequently indicated their desire that the group continue to meet, even though they were well aware that they were participating in a time-limited group. They expressed appreciation for the respect and warmth shown by those who recruited and enrolled them in the study and by the group facilitators who conducted the intervention. Successful recruitment was facilitated by established collaborations with administrators and clinical staff from two community mental health centers in predominantly Latino communities in Los Angeles. Potential participants were recruited and enrolled by bilingual, bicultural bachelor's level research staff trained in culturally and clinically competent recruitment and engagement strategies.

Positive comments about the group's structure were a reoccurring theme. The fact that the groups were well organized and informative conveyed to the participants that their time and involvement were both valued and respected. They liked the psychoeducational and cross-cultural curricula, the use of an agenda for each session, and the process of summarizing cultural strengths and lessons learned at the end of each session and then reviewing those summaries at beginning of the next session. They appreciated the accessibility of the group—the convenient location and the early evening schedule—that made their attendance possible. Whereas most multiple-family groups include the relative affected by the illness, the CFIMA families unanimously agreed that the group should remain for family members only. The group provided them a space of their own and some respite from the many responsibilities associated with their caregiving role. They also shared that their loved ones conveyed their appreciation of family members' prioritizing a time for a group that centered on their illness.

Frequently and spontaneously, participants shared how much they had learned, and how much they were applying what they had learned at home. They greatly appreciated learning about the illness from the provider perspective and also liked the group's emphasis on validating their Latino family cultural context. Many family members enjoyed learning about the recovery orientation to mental illness, which comes from a strengths-based approach and supports achievement of the person's full human potential. Such discussions seemed to inspire verbalizations of hope and faith in a promising future both for loved ones living with mental illness and for themselves. We found that CFIMA's emphasis on using language and terms that are person-centered and respectful to be a powerful therapeutic tool. We also found that our explanations for using person-first language helped patients and family participants focus on the person and to prioritize human potential over pejorative terms related to the psychiatric diagnosis that perpetuate stigma of the mental illness.

Families also reported increased self-knowledge and cultural knowledge. They often remarked that their "eyes had been opened" and their increased self-knowledge helped them become a better person, parent, and friend. Increased cultural knowledge was attributed to a culturally supportive environment with other Latino families dealing with similar challenges and to the empowerment they felt in helping the group facilitators learn about their own family's cultural approaches in dealing with their loved one's mental illness. Families readily shared stories filled with warmth, unity, and unconditional acceptance. They shared rituals for prayer and discussed how their spiritual faith helped them to deal with the illness. They expressed a renewed pride in their Mexican heritage, which they identified as helping them deal with the challenges of mental illness. The participants reflected on their immigrant experience and commented on insights gained in persevering, overcoming hardships, and finding meaning in the protective qualities of Mexican culture.

Many participants indicated that the group experience helped them reframe their view of their loved ones and enhanced their understanding that certain behaviors were due to the illness. Family members reflected on the shift in their attitudes and many attributed their new outlook to an increased knowledge of mental illness and a decreased sense of burden in caring for their loved one. At the beginning of the intervention, participants, like many Latino families, demonstrated a lack of awareness of their potential to assume advocacy and activism roles through organizations such as NAMI. However, over the course of the CFIMA, family members expressed a growing sense of empowerment to become more assertive about seeking treatment. They made statements such as "knowledge is power," and recognized that their newly acquired understanding of mental illness and their renewed pride in their Mexican heritage had compelled them to become more active in the treatment process. There were many examples of how the cultural exchange process extended beyond the group setting. Families shared day-to-day examples of how they found themselves teaching other family members, friends, neighbors, and co-workers about mental illness and the importance of culture. Moreover, many reported improved coping skills and an improved relationship with their affected relative, and noted that their home environment seemed more peaceful. Our experience in developing and implementing the CFIMA shows that it has promise, warranting a larger trial of this culturally based approach.

Conclusion

The cultural strengths and resources provided by Latino families are an underutilized resource within existing mental health services. The caregiving ideology that characterizes the Latino family provides strong evidence for the critical and valuable role these families play in the lives of their loved ones and in compensating for service disparities in systems of care. We encountered numerous examples indicating that families were both eager for psychoeducational information and in need of supportive services. They were open to learning about current research on the illness—biological and genetic information as well as facts about the course of the illness, pharmacotherapy, and psychosocial treatments—and were motivated to partner with providers throughout the treatment process. Unfortunately, the current public mental health system, driven by client-centered financial reimbursement, does not promote, and in fact often discourages, family-centered approaches. Given the strong role played by families in the care of Latinos with serious mental disorders, billing mechanisms that fail to reimburse family services harm Latino families that need support to cope with caring for a loved one with an episodic, and often persistent, mental illness.

With regard to intervention services during the early stages of the illness, we found no published research documenting the pathways to care for Latinos with schizophrenia and other serious disorders. What literature does exist suggests that Latinos experience serious delays in accessing treatment and that these service delays could be contributing to disparities in Latino mental health use (Barragán et al. 2010). As shown by the preliminary evidence on La CLAve, culturally tailored psychoeducational programs may be a viable avenue to reach families in immigrant communities and equip them with tools for avoiding service delays and reducing the illness burden for the individual and the family.

In several sections of this chapter, we delineated various cultural strengths and resources that characterize the Latino family, and that are often ignored or untapped by existing interventions. We also recognized that certain concepts may be experienced as culturally foreign by Latino families, such as the expectation to assume an advocacy role on behalf of their loved one. Culturally relevant programs for Latinos must be able to address how culture intersects with service provision, and train service providers to attend to cultural dynamics to better align their expectations with those of Latino clients and their families. The excellent participation in the CFIMA demonstrates that psychoeducation and support services prioritizing cultural values can be very gratifying for both families and providers, and can translate to positive outcomes at both the client and family levels. Through our work, we recognized that Latino families preferred support groups led by professional staff. They often indicated great satisfaction from the cultural exchange process with mental health professionals.

In sum, helping Latino families deal with serious mental illness in a loved one requires careful consideration of multiple cultural issues. Most importantly, family members must be included using a planned and purposeful approach, not just as an afterthought. There is strong empirical support for engaging families in the treatment of mental illness, and such approaches are now being adapted to include more culturally congruent interventions with Latino families. With the increase in the Latino population, we are witnessing a concomitant increase in the number of Latinos with serious mental disorders. In light of this fact, we should not ignore the numerous Latino family caregivers providing essential care to their loved ones, often with minimal support from formal mental health services. Perhaps it is now time that, as researchers and practitioners, we not only continue to advance the field with more culturally relevant, evidence-based family interventions, but also begin to more strongly challenge current organizational service structures to better accommodate and prioritize the services needs of Latino and other underserved families.

References

Barragán, A., López, S., & Lorenzo-Blanco, E. (2011). *Pathways to mental health treatment among Mexican Americans with schizophrenia*. Unpublished manuscript.

Barrio, C. (2000). The cultural relevance of community support programs. *Psychiatric Services, 51*(7), 879–884.

Barrio, C., & Dixon, L. (in press). Clinician interactions with patients and families. In J. Lieberman & R. M. Murray (Eds.), *Comprehensive care of schizophrenia: A textbook of clinical management* (2nd ed.). New York, NY: Oxford University Press.

Barrio, C., & Hughes, M. (2000). Kinship care: A cultural resource of African-American and Latino families coping with parental substance abuse. *Journal of Family Social Work, 4*(4), 15–31.

Barrio, C., & Yamada, A.-M. (2005). Serious mental illness among Mexican immigrants: Implications for culturally relevant practice. *Journal of Immigrant & Refugee Services, 3*(1/2), 87–106.

Barrio, C., & Yamada, A.-M. (2010). Culturally-based intervention development: The case of Latino families dealing with schizophrenia. *Research on Social Work Practice, 20,* 483–492.

Barrio, C., García, P., & Atuel, H. (2000). *Ethnic minority participation in support and self-help groups for families of the mentally ill*. Paper presented at the annual meeting of the National Alliance for the Mentally Ill, San Diego, CA.

Barrio, C., Yamada, A.-M., Atuel, H., Hough, R., Yee, S., Berthot, B., et al. (2003a). A tri-ethnic examination of symptom expression on the positive and negative syndrome scale in schizophrenia spectrum disorders. *Schizophrenia Research, 60*(2–3), 259–269.

Barrio, C., Yamada, A., Hough, R., Hawthorne, W., García, P., & Jeste, D. (2003b). Ethnic disparities in use of public mental health case management services among patients with schizophrenia. *Psychiatry Services, 54*(9), 1264–1270.

Behnke, A., MacDermid, S., Coltrane, S., Parke, R., Duffy, S., & Widaman, K. (2008). Family cohesion in the lives of Mexican American and European American parents. *Journal of Marriage & Family, 70,* 1045–1059.

Bernal, G., Jiménez-Chafey, M., & Domenech Rodríguez, M. (2009). Cultural adaptation of treatments: A resource for considering culture in evidence-based practice. *Professional Psychology: Research & Practice, 40*(4), 361–368.

Biegel, D., Sales, E., & Schulz, R. (1991). *Family caregiving in chronic illness: Alzheimer's disease, cancer, heart disease, mental illness, and stroke* (Family Caregiver Applications Series, Vol. 1). Newbury Park, CA: Sage Publications.

Brekke, J., & Barrio, C. (1997). Cross-ethnic symptom differences in schizophrenia: The influence of culture and minority status. *Schizophrenia Bulletin, 23*(2), 305–316.

Compton, M., Goulding, S., Gordon, T., Weiss, P., & Kaslow, N. (2009). Family-level predictors and correlates of the duration of untreated psychosis in African American first-episode patients. *Schizophrenia Research, 115*(2), 338–345.

Cook, J., & Knox, J. (1993). NAMI outreach strategies to African American and Hispanic families: Results of a national telephone survey. *Innovations & Research, 2,* 35–42.

Dixon, L., McFarlane, W., Lefley, H., Lucksted, A., Cohen, M., Falloon, I., et al. (2001). Evidence-based practices for services to families of people with psychiatric disabilities. *Psychiatric Services, 52*(7), 903–910.

Durvasula, R., & Sue, S. (1996). Severity of disturbance among Asian American outpatients. *Cultural Diversity & Mental Health, 2,* 43–52.

Guarnaccia, P. J. (1998). Multicultural experiences of family caregiving: A study of African American, European American, and Hispanic American families. *New Directions for Mental Health Services, 77,* 45–61.

Guarnaccia, P., & Parra, P. (1996). Ethnicity, social status, and families' experiences of caring for a mentally ill family member. *Community Mental Health Journal, 32,* 243–260.

Hall, G. (2001). Psychotherapy research with ethnic minorities: Empirical, ethical, and conceptual issues. *Journal of Consulting & Clinical Psychology, 69,* 502–510.

Hooper, K. (2004). Interrogating the meaning of "culture" in the WHO international studies of schizophrenia. In J. H. Jenkins & R. J. Barrett (Eds.), *Schizophrenia, culture, and subjectivity* (pp. 62–86). New York, NY: Cambridge University Press.

Jablensky, A., Sartorius, N., & Ernberg, G. (1992). Chapter 2: Sociodemographic, clinical and diagnostic description of the study population. *Psychological Medicine, 20* (Suppl.), 18–42.

Johnstone, E., Crow, T., Johnson, A., & MacMillan, J. (1986). The Northwick Park Study of first episodes of schizophrenia. I. Presentation of the illness and problems relating to admission. *British Journal of Psychiatry, 148*(2), 115–120.

Jordan, C., Lewellen, A., & Vandiver, V. (1995). Psychoeducation for minority families: A social work perspective. *International Journal of Mental Health, 23,* 27–43.

Kopelowicz, A. (1998). Adapting social skills training for Latinos with schizophrenia. *International Review of Psychiatry, 10,* 47–50.

Kumpfer, K., Alvarado, R., Smith, P., & Bellamy, N. (2002). Cultural sensitivity and adaptation in family-based prevention interventions. *Prevention Science, 3*(3), 241–246.

Larsen, T., McGlashan, T., & Johannessen, J. (2001). Shortened duration of untreated first episodes of psychosis: Changes in client characteristics at treatment. *American Journal of Psychiatry, 158,* 1917–1919.

Lefley, H. (1990). Culture and chronic mental illness. *Hospital & Community Psychiatry, 41,* 277–286.

Lefley, H., & Bestman, E. (1991). Public-academic linkages for culturally sensitive community mental health. *Community Mental Health Journal, 27,* 473–488.

Loebel, A., Lieberman, J., Alvir, J., Mayerhoff, D., Geisler, S., & Szymanski, S. (1992). Duration of psychosis and outcome in first-episode schizophrenia. *American Journal of Psychiatry, 149*(9), 1183–1188.

López, S., Hipke, K., Polo, A., Jenkins, J., Karno, M., Vaughn, C., et al. (2004). Ethnicity, expressed emotion, attributions, and course of schizophrenia: Family warmth matters. *Journal of Abnormal Psychology, 113*(3), 428–439.

López, S., Kopelowicz, A., & Cañive, J. (2002). Strategies in developing culturally congruent family interventions for schizophrenia: The case of Hispanics. In H. Lefley & D. Johnson (Eds.),

Family interventions in mental illness: International perspectives (pp. 61–90). Westport, CT: Praeger.

López, S., Lara, M., Kopelowicz, A., Solano, S., Foncerrada, H., & Aguilera, A. (2009). La CLAve to increase psychosis literacy of Spanish-speaking community residents and family caregivers. *Journal of Consulting & Clinical Psychology, 77,* 763–774.

Magaña, S., Ramirez, J., Hernández, M., & Cortez, R. (2007). Psychological distress among Latino family caregivers of adults with schizophrenia: The roles of burden and stigma in the stress-process model. *Psychiatric Services, 58,* 378–384.

Maynard, C., Ehreth, J., Cox, G., Peterson, P., & McGann, M. (1997). Racial differences in the utilization of public mental health services in Washington state. *Administration & Policy in Mental Health & Mental Health Services Research, 24*(5), 411–424.

McFarlane, W., Dixon, L., Lukens, E., & Lucksted, A. (2003). Family psychoeducation and schizophrenia: A review of the literature. *Journal of Marital & Family Therapy, 29,* 223–245.

Medvene, L., Mendoza, R., Lin, K., Harris, N., & Miller, M. (1995). Increasing Mexican American attendance in support groups for parents of the mentally ill: Organizational and psychological factors. *Journal of Community Psychology, 23,* 307–325.

Mueser, K., Torrey, W., Lynde, D., Singer, P., & Drake, R. (2003). Implementing evidence-based practices for people with severe mental illness. *Behavior Modification, 27,* 387–411.

Murray-Swank, A., & Dixon, L. (2004). Family psychoeducation as an evidence-based practice. *CNS Spectrums, 9,* 905–912.

Murray-Swank, A., Dixon, L., & Stewart, B. (2007). Practical interview strategies for building an alliance with the families of patients who have severe mental illness. *Psychiatric Clinics of North America, 30,* 167–180.

NAMI. (2008). *NAMI multicultural planning guide.* Retrieved from http://www.nami.org/template.cfm?section=Resources

Norman, R., Malla, A., Verdi, M., Has Sall, L., & Fazekas, C. (2004). Understanding delay in treatment for first-episode psychosis. *Psychological Medicine, 34,* 255–266.

Pickett, S., Cook, J., & Heller, T. (1998). Support group satisfaction: A comparison of minority and White families. *New Directions of Mental Health Services, 77,* 63–73.

Primm, A., Lima, B., & Rowe, C. (1996). Cultural and ethnic sensitivity. In W. Breakey (Ed.), *Integrated mental health services: Modern community psychiatry* (pp. 145–159). New York, NY: Oxford University Press.

Rabiner, C., Wegner, J., & Kane, J. (1986). Outcome study of first-episode psychosis. I: Relapse rates after 1 year. *American Journal of Psychiatry, 143*(9), 1155–1158.

Ramirez García, J., Hernández, B., & Dorian, M. (2009). Mexican American caregivers' coping efficacy. *Social Psychiatry & Psychiatric Epidemiology, 44,* 162–170.

Rapp, C. (1998). *The strengths model: Case management with people suffering from severe and persistent mental illness.* New York, NY: Oxford University Press.

Rivera, C. (1988). Culturally sensitive aftercare services for chronically mentally ill Hispanics: The case of the psychoeducational treatment model. *Fordham University Hispanic Research Center Research Bulletin, 11.*

Rodriguez, O. (1986). Overcoming barriers to clinical services among chronically mentally ill Hispanics: Lessons from the evaluation of Project COPA. *Fordham University Hispanic Research Center Research Bulletin, 9.*

Snowden, L., & Cheung, F. (1990). Use of in-client mental health services by members of ethnic minority groups. *American Psychologist, 45,* 347–355.

Solomon, P. (1998). The cultural context of interventions for family members with a seriously mentally ill relative. In H. P. Lefley (Ed.), *New directions for mental health services, families coping with mental illness: The cultural context* (pp. 5–16). San Francisco, CA: Jossey-Bass.

Stroul, B. (1989). Community support systems for persons with long-term mental illness: A conceptual framework. *Psychosocial Rehabilitation Journal, 12,* 11–26.

Sue, S., Zane, N., Nagayama Hall, G. C., & Berger, L. K. (2009). The case for cultural competency in psychotherapeutic interventions. *Annual Review of Psychology, 60,* 10.11–10.24.

United States Department of Health and Human Services [USDHHS]. (2001). *U.S. Surgeon General & Substance Abuse and Mental Health Services Administration Center for Mental Health Services. Mental Health: Culture, Race, and Ethnicity: A Supplement to Mental Health: A Report of the Surgeon General.* Rockville, MD: U.S. Department of Health and Human Services (USDHHS).

Vega, W. (1995). Theoretical and conceptual overview: A point of departure. In R. E. Zambrana (Ed.), *Latino families: Developing a paradigm for practice, research and policy.* Newbury Park, CA: Sage Publications.

Vega, W., Karno, M., Alegría, M., Alvidrez, J., Bernal, G., Escamilla, M., et al. (2007). Research issues for improving treatment of U.S. Hispanics with persistent mental disorders. *Psychiatric Services, 58*(3), 385–394..

Chapter 9
The Plight of Latino Youth in the Juvenile Justice System: Considerations for Mental Health Treatment

Michelle M. Weemhoff and Francisco A. Villarruel

Abstract Latino youth are disproportionately represented at each point in the juvenile justice system, and receive harsher treatment than non-Latino White youth, even when charged with the same offenses. This chapter explores how mental health and trauma contribute to the overrepresentation of Latino youth in the juvenile justice system, and analyzes the infrastructure in which mental health services are delivered to this population. Recommended solutions point to the need for courts, facilities, and service providers to use culturally and linguistically competent approaches when serving Latino youth and their families.

The juvenile justice system was established in the late 1800s, upon the premise that incorrigible youth who were in conflict with the law should be rehabilitated rather than punished. An alternative juvenile court allowed an individualized approach to each case, while still affording youth the right to due process and other legal protections (*In re* Gault 387 U.S. 1 (1967). Throughout the twentieth century, however, policies began to shift toward punitive sanctions that favored incarcerating youth for extended periods of time (Bishop 2000; Scott and Steinberg 2003). The Knitzer (1982) report brought public attention to abused, traumatized, and emotionally and behaviorally disordered children being warehoused in the system without receiving any form of community-based services.

In 2000, the federal Office of Juvenile Justice and Delinquency Prevention (OJJDP) funded the National Center for Mental Health and Juvenile Justice (NCMHJJ) to initiate the largest national effort ever to review mental health needs in the juvenile justice system. The study revealed that that as many as 50–75% of youth in the juvenile justice system had a diagnosable mental illness (Skowyra and Cocozza 2006). In response to these findings, the study authors developed a comprehensive framework for both the juvenile justice and mental health systems to improve ser-

M. M. Weemhoff (✉)
Michigan Council on Crime and Delinquency, Lansing MI, USA
e-mail: mweemhoff@miccd.org

vice delivery at critical intervention points, from arrest to incarceration to reentry (Skowyra and Cocozza 2006).

Multiple research studies have reported that Latino youth are disproportionately represented at each of the critical intervention points, and receive harsher treatment than non-Latino White youth, even when charged with the same offenses (Burgess-Proctor et al. 2006; Villarruel and Walker 2002, Walker et al. 2004). Despite these findings, few statistics exist to document the prevalence of mental health issues among this population. This chapter explores how mental health and trauma contribute to the overrepresentation of Latino youth in the juvenile justice system, and analyzes the infrastructure in which mental health services are delivered to this population. We provide recommendations and solutions, with the caveat that significant gaps in research prevent us from fully understanding the plight of adjudicated Latino youth.

Latino Youth in the Juvenile Justice System

Over the past three decades, Latino civil rights organizations, community practitioners, and researchers have drawn increased national attention to underserved Latino youth involved in the juvenile justice system (Ayra et al. 2009; Burgess-Proctor et al. 2006; Ramiu and Shoenberg 2009; Villarruel and Walker 2002; Walker et al. 2004). The urgency of this issue has become even more pressing since the turn of the century, when, according to the US Census Bureau, Latinos became the largest ethnic minority group in the nation. Latinos account for approximately 25% of children under the age of five (U.S. Census Bureau 2009).

Unfortunately, the growth of the Latino population has coincided with increasing overrepresentation in the juvenile and criminal justice systems. At the federal level, Latinos account for more than one-third of the incarcerated population (Walker et al. 2004). Researchers estimate that Latinos have a one-in-six chance of imprisonment during their lifetimes (Walker et al. 2004). Although most of the research focuses on adults, scholars are increasingly concerned over the increase of the Latino population in the juvenile justice system (Ayra et al. 2009; Ramiu and Shoenberg 2009).

It is estimated that on any given day, approximately 18,000 Latino youth are held within secure juvenile detention facilities and adult prisons in the United States (Ayra et al. 2009). Data compiled by Human Rights Watch (2002) indicate that incarceration rates for Latino youth are at least two to three times those of White youth (Villarruel and Walker 2002), and the average length of incarceration for every offense category is longer for Latinos than for any other racial or ethnic group (Walker et al. 2004). Moreover, scholars have found that one-in-four Latino minors are detained in adult facilities, despite the increased risks for violence, rape, and suicide in that setting (Villarruel and Walker 2002).

Disproportionate Minority Contact

The overrepresentation of youth of color at varying points in the system is referred to as "disproportionate minority contact" (DMC) (Feyerherm et al. 2009). The focus on DMC emerged as a national priority in 1992, when DMC reduction was added as a core requirement of the Juvenile Justice and Delinquency Prevention Act (JJDPA). Originally established in 1974, the JJDPA is the primary federal policy that provides funding, research, training, technical assistance, and evaluation to improve juvenile justice systems. Under the JJDPA, states are required to assess and address the disproportionate contact of youth of color at nine key contact points: arrest, referral to court, diversion, case petitioned, secure detention, delinquency finding, probation, confinement, and transfer to the adult system.

In its 2002 reauthorization of the JJDPA, the OJJDP required states to collect data to: (a) identify the extent to which DMC exists within their jurisdictions; (b) assess the reasons for DMC, if it exists; (c) develop and implement strategies to address DMC, if it exists; and (d) evaluate and monitor the effectiveness of the intervention strategies (Feyerherm et al. 2009). The OJJDP helps states to effectively assess and appropriately address DMC through use of a five-phase model (identification, assessment, intervention, evaluation, and monitoring).

Despite the national requirement to assess the extent of DMC, the ability to adequately gather data at each of these nine contact points is negated when jurisdictions do not systematically collect data on Latino youth, or alternatively, categorize Latino youth as White or African American (Villarruel and Walker 2002). In October of 2010, one of the authors of this chapter was asked to offer guidance to a state that was reviewing the nine points of contact to help identify the extent of DMC across eight jurisdictions. Disparities at each contact point are calculated based on a Relative Rate Index that compares the proportions of Latino and non-Latino White youth in the justice system to their proportions in the community. When disparities are noted, states can apply for Title II and Title V monies to introduce efforts to better respond to the needs of ethno-racial youth. In the section on the suitability of the existing data, the counties involved used three different approaches: One merged Hispanic/Latino populations into the "White" racial category; a second elevated Hispanic/Latino to a racial category in itself; the third simply did not "count" Latino populations, even though census data indicated that there was a sizable population of Latino youth in these communities. An unfortunate reality is that these practices are not unique. Until a systematic approach is employed throughout the nation, justice programs and researchers will continue to misrepresent the prevalence and incidence of Latino youth involvement with the juvenile justice system. The complexity of the issue is exacerbated by the facts that few jurisdictions disaggregate Hispanic/Latino ethnicity and that many fail to collect information related to generational status.

Many researchers have focused on systemic bias as a primary cause of DMC (Armour and Hammond 2009; Piquero 2008; Soler 2007), citing racial profiling among police, prejudice in the courtroom, or culturally insensitive policies (Villarruel and Walker 2002; Walker et al. 2004). Without adequate data, however, it is difficult, if not impossible, to distinguish the true causes of DMC and develop appropriate responses.

Mental Health and Juvenile Justice

Although systemic bias and policy reform likely contribute to Latino overrepresentation, researchers cannot discount the potentially significant ways in which mental illness and trauma might also contribute to DMC. Researchers have noted that youth with mental health diagnoses often engage in behaviors that are likely to bring them to the attention of the juvenile justice system (Grisso 2004, 2008). The NCMHJJ found conduct disorders to be prevalent among system-involved youth (46.5%), leading substance-use disorders (46.2%), anxiety disorders (34.4%), and mood disorders (18.3%) (Cocozza and Shefelt 2006; Shefelt and Cocozza 2006). Among those youth with a psychiatric diagnosis, 79% had two or more co-occurring disorders, and more than 60% also had a substance-use disorder (Shefelt and Cocozza 2006).

Although research has not yet explored the prevalence of mental health issues among Latino youth in the juvenile justice system, studies indicate that Latino populations in general, especially immigrants, are at higher risk for mental health conditions such as depression, anxiety, post-traumatic stress, and substance abuse (Miranda and Matheny 2000). Alegría and Woo (2009) noted that the prevalence of some mental health issues for Latinos in the United States is equivalent to or lower than the rate experienced by non-US Latinos (Alegría et al. 2008), but they also reported that, overall, Latinos are less likely to receive services and their treatment outcomes are less favorable. Further, scholars note significant disparities in access to and utilization of mental health services between Latinos and non-Hispanic Whites (Alegría et al. 2007; Alegría and Woo 2009). Latinos are the least likely of all groups to access specialty care (5.0%), even though Latino and Black children have the highest rates of need (10.5%) based on measures in the National Health Interview Survey (NHIS) (Ringel and Sturm 2001). For many young people, entrance into the juvenile justice system is the first time a mental health condition may be identified (Skowyra and Cocozza 2006).

Research also reveals that the neurological, psychological, and social effects of trauma may be strongly linked to involvement in the juvenile justice system (cf. Abram et al. 2004; Cauffman et al. 1998; Sprague 2008; Stouthamer-Loeber et al. 2002). Adams (2010) estimates that 75–93% of youth in the juvenile justice have experienced some level of trauma. Research suggests that trauma during critical points in development (particularly infancy and teen years) can cause emotional disregulation, high levels of stress hormones, and decreased executive functions, all potentially contributing to a lesser ability to effectively manage behaviors (Adams 2010; Giedd 2004). Not surprisingly, individuals who experienced childhood trauma are also more likely to experience lifelong mental health issues, such as personality disorders, conduct disorder, ADHD, depression, anxiety, substance abuse disorders, and post-traumatic stress disorder (PTSD) (Adams 2010).

The Impact of Acculturative Stress on Mental Health

The findings regarding the prevalence of trauma in the juvenile justice system raise questions about whether trauma experienced due to cultural misunderstanding of Latino youth and acculturative stress among immigrant youth could potentially increase the risk of delinquency. Latino youth are especially vulnerable to acculturative stress because of the pressure to rapidly adapt to the values of their new culture. Researchers have argued that the challenges of negotiating between two cultural worlds tend to reduce the social capital and benefits that can be derived from peers and adults (e.g., Barcallao and Smokowski 2009; Benet-Martínez et al. 2002; Gonzales et al. 2009). Although acculturation may affect these youths' developmental understanding of societal mores, it also places them in a position of stress when their societal context and cultural background present conflicting views of behavior. These conflicting value sets may increase the risk for mental health problems, engagement in risk behaviors (e.g., school failure or underachievement, increased likelihood of substance use and abuse, involvement in the juvenile justice system), and other negative life outcomes (Kiang et al. 2006).

In many circumstances, the acculturation process can produce significant stress for families, especially if children adapt to the host culture more quickly than their parents. Tensions are amplified when parents prefer that their children retain traditional mores, language, and behaviors. Cultural adaptation and family dissonance can be especially difficult for immigrant children and adolescents, who generally reside in what might be described as closed communities (i.e., neighborhoods with a higher concentration of immigrants) and in multifamily households (Hernandez et al. 2008). However, the support of family may ameliorate the effects of acculturative stress, particularly in the initial periods of acculturation (Miranda and Matheny 2000).

Immigrant youth who live in families that speak only Spanish are often pressed into becoming language brokers (Buriel et al. 1998), especially if they possess greater linguistic mastery than their parents (Hernandez et al. 2008). Buriel et al. (2011) hypothesize that the demands of language brokering may be a particular stressor dividing older adolescents and their parents. This type of stress is likely compounded when families enter unfamiliar systems, like juvenile justice or mental health, and rely upon their children to understand and adequately interpret directives and service plans.

Barriers to Access and Utilization of Services

To best understand the connection between Latino mental health and juvenile justice, one must recognize how these findings are inextricably linked to the lived realities that Latinos face, such as poverty, discrimination, and lack of access to services. Before Latino youth ever enter the justice system, social and economic disparities already put them at a disadvantage. Although Latino children account for nearly 20% of the current youth population, they represent nearly 35% of the youth living in poverty (Hernandez et al. 2008). The 2007 economic recession was particularly hard on Latinos, who experienced the greatest decline in household median income across all groups (DeNavas-Walt et al. 2009). Tienda and Mitchell (2006) reported that foreign-born Latinos are more likely than native-born Latinos to live in conditions of economic hardship and poverty. In 2006, 37% of Latino children lived in a family in which neither parent had full-time, year-round employment, compared to only 25% of White children living in a similar situation (Annie E. Casey Foundation 2008a). Researchers have noted that families living in the lowest socioeconomic status are two to three times more likely than those in higher strata to have mental health issues (Vega et al. 1998).

Barriers to accessing and utilizing mental health services are closely tied to economic disparities, including lack of health insurance and prohibitive cost (Vega and Alegría 2001). According to the National Health Interview Survey, approximately 7% of families with a child with need (based on NHIS measures) claimed financial barriers as the reason for not getting any mental health care (Ringel and Sturm 2001). Unfortunately, youth with untreated mental health needs are at far greater risk for entering the juvenile justice system (Skowyra and Cocozza 2006).

Health care, education, and social service systems are often viewed as the first lines of defense to prevent delinquency. However, these systems do not always recognize the social stigma and cultural and linguistic barriers that may prevent Latino clients from fully benefiting from their services. Researchers note that lack of awareness of cultural issues, bias, inability to speak the client's language, and the client's own fear or mistrust of treatment can be huge barriers to service delivery (Adler et al. 2000; Vega and Alegría 2001).

Many of the same cultural and linguistic barriers encountered with community-based services are experienced at the various decision points in the juvenile justice system. Non-English-speaking youth may have difficulties understanding what is being requested of them by juvenile justice professionals or respond in a way that is viewed as disrespectful or noncompliant (such as avoiding eye contact or remaining silent). Likewise, parents' limited English proficiency may be a barrier for youth who need to comply with court-mandated directives or are required to participate in intervention programs (Vera Institute of Justice 2010). When immigrant youth and their families are unable to understand the process, they are likely to feel that the system is not sympathetic to their challenges or even unsupportive of them (Ramiu and Shoenberg 2009).

Juvenile Justice Involvement

Although Latino youth are disproportionately affected at all contact points in the juvenile justice system, little empirical research has been conducted to document how considerations of mental health or trauma are linked to this overrepresentation. Likewise, cultural influences on behavior are often disregarded by systemic approaches that address mental health needs as a cause or outcome of involvement with the justice system. The following section explores how Latino youth fare at various contact points in juvenile justice (arrest, petition, court process, probation, and secure confinement); how mental health or trauma may play a role; and systemic approaches to addressing these issues.

Arrest and Intake

Due to difficulties in data collection (noted previously), arrest information about Latinos is imprecise and inconsistent. Analyses from California and Arizona indicate that Latino youth make up a large proportion of the youth who are arrested in each state (51% in California, 38% in Arizona) (Ayra et al. 2009), despite representing less than 10% of the total arrests in each state. An analysis of arrest data reveals little individual differences in factors that tend to produce crime. The majority of Latino arrests are for nonviolent offenses, including curfew violations, loitering, theft, and liquor-law violations (Ayra et al. 2009). However, Latino youth arrested for nonviolent offenses are 28% more likely to be detained than White youth (Ayra et al. 2009).

Contact with police is only one way a youth may be referred to the juvenile justice system. Schools are providing a greater number of referrals, consistent with an increased presence of officers in the schools and the enactment of zero-tolerance policies (Losen and Skiba 2010). Even parents may press charges against their own children, particularly for status offenses (e.g., illegal behavior for youth which would not be considered criminal behavior for adults, such as running away, truancy, or smoking).

It is important to note that a youth's disruptive or inappropriate behavior is often the result or a symptom of undiagnosed or untreated mental health issues (Skowyra and Cocozza 2006). Although delinquent behaviors may initially be identified by or referred to law enforcement, an early assessment of a child's needs may reveal that mental health services are more appropriate. Unfortunately, studies suggest that many jurisdictions do not systematically screen for mental health or trauma-related symptoms at the point of entry into the system (Adams 2010).

There is, however, a growing trend toward utilizing the juvenile justice system as a means of accessing mental health services that are otherwise unavailable or inaccessible in the community (Skowyra and Cocozza 2006). According to the General Accounting Office and Congress, parents placed more than 12,700 children into child welfare or juvenile justice systems in fiscal year 2001 solely to gain access to mental health care (General Accounting Office 2003). The report further speculates that this figure is a significant underestimate.

Petitions

After arrest, the prosecutor's office reviews the case and weighs numerous factors, such as age, history of delinquency, severity of offense, and threat to public safety, to determine whether the case should be (a) dismissed, (b) handled informally, or

(c) processed formally through the court. Prosecutors may dismiss a case if they feel the youth does not pose a risk or if there is not sufficient evidence to warrant further processing. A case may be handled informally, through a process called *diversion*, if the youth agrees to informal supervision or to participation in a community-based service or sanction in lieu of court involvement. If the prosecutor feels that court involvement is necessary to address the charges, a formal delinquency petition is filed and a court date is set.

The National Center on Juvenile Justice analyzed data from the National Juvenile Justice Court Data Archive and found that nearly 150,000 cases involving Latino youth were handled formally by filing a delinquency petition in the juvenile courts in 2005 (Ayra et al. 2009). Given inconsistencies in data collection, it is suspected that these numbers are actually much higher. Latino youth were 4% more likely than White youth to be formally petitioned (Ayra et al. 2009).

Many youth and families are unfamiliar with the expectations, roles, and processes in the juvenile justice system. Language barriers and economic concerns further compound their confusion. Many youth and their families may not fully understand their rights, such as the right to due process, the right to avoid self-incrimination, the right to remain silent, or even the right to counsel.

If a family cannot afford an attorney, a public defense attorney is appointed to help the youth navigate the court process. The National Juvenile Defender Center (2008) recommends that public defenders play an active role in identifying mental illness and developmental impairments, legally addressing these needs, and making appropriate referrals for these clients as an essential component of quality legal representation. Without further research, it is unclear how many public defender offices actively engage in partnerships with mental health professionals to screen for referrals, and whether making mental health referrals at this point in the process has an effect on reducing DMC.

Court Process/Adjudication

The court process involves a hearing in which the judge may or may not find the youth responsible ("guilty") for the offense with which he or she is charged. This process is referred to as *adjudication*. Not surprisingly, Latino youth are 16% more likely than non-Hispanic White youth to be adjudicated delinquent (Ayra et al. 2009). Although not a criminal conviction, adjudication in the juvenile justice system may have lifelong consequences. Despite popular belief, most juvenile records are public and can be accessed by potential employers and colleges as part of a criminal background check. Certain offenses can bar a youth from receiving a driver's license, living in public housing, owning a firearm, or serving in the military. Adjudication can also affect one's immigration status, occasionally resulting in deportation (MacArthur Foundation 2010). Depending on state law and sentencing guidelines, a juvenile adjudication often results in sentencing enhancements if the person is later convicted in the criminal justice system as an adult.

Once a youth has been adjudicated, the judge can choose from an array of "sentencing" options, referred to as *dispositions*, which include, but are not limited to, probation, community-based treatment programs, nonsecure residential placement, and secure confinement. As mental health awareness increases, many jurisdictions are developing partnerships with their local community mental health agencies or creating their own court-operated mental health treatment services (Skowyra and Cocozza 2006). Still, despite research on the prevalence of mental health concerns, Adams (2010) noted that more than 50% of juvenile and family court judges had not received training on the assessment or treatment of childhood trauma, nor were they aware of the psychological impact of trauma exposure. Adams further noted that when judges were made aware of trauma-related issues, they felt overwhelmed by the degree of trauma exposure among children in their courtrooms and frustrated with the lack of evidence-based treatments available. The question remains as to whether juvenile and family court judges would make different decisions about dispositions if they had a greater understanding of mental health and trauma needs and if evidence-based programs were available to meet those needs.

Probation

Juvenile probation may be imposed to provide community supervision for court-involved youth. Considerations for probation can occur at multiple contact points. For example, a judge may suspend the formal filing of a petition if the juvenile participates in a community-based treatment program. If a formal petition is filed, the adjudication hearing may also result in a judicial decision that includes mandatory completion of a program or programs, as well as conditions of post-release treatment. Many times, decisions about conditions of probation are negotiated by legal advocates, counsel, or families that know there are alternatives to secure confinement.

Research demonstrates that community-based programs contribute to lower levels of recidivism and subsequent re-arrest than incarceration, especially for youth on probation (Lyons and Walsh 2010). Children with post-traumatic stress disorder who are diverted to mental health treatment have higher recovery rates and lower recidivism rates than youth sent to secure placement (Adams 2010; Lyons and Walsh 2010).

In recent years, the use of electronic monitoring has increased the ability of nonviolent offenders to remain in their homes while remaining under supervision. Research involving the use of electronic monitoring devices is mixed (Bonta et al. 2000), citing benefits of decreased recidivism and also keeping youth at home with their families. However, there is a dearth of information about the impact that this may have on Latino youth and families, and more specifically, on the social and psychological impact of stigma. Researchers need to better understand if the use of electronic monitoring adversely affects stress levels and mental health of Latino youth on probation. Research should also focus on culturally sensitive approaches to community-based probation services, to address the experiences of Latino youth.

Secure Confinement

Latino youth are 40% more likely than White youth to be removed from their homes and placed in some type of secure confinement (Sickmund 2005). Secure confinement can be a group home, a treatment facility, or a training school. Researchers note that the majority of youth who spend time in secure confinement are rearrested within three years, and that more than half of those released are reincarcerated as adults (Nellis and Hooks Wayman 2009).

Although each facility must be evaluated on its own merit, research suggests that, in general, confinement may exacerbate the symptoms of certain mental disorders, including PTSD (Adams 2010). Additionally, processing a youth through intake at a facility often involves the use of handcuffs, searches, isolation, and restraints, and may trigger a catastrophic reaction in a youth who has experienced traumatic life events. Highly publicized incidents of verbal, physical, and sexual victimization in juvenile facilities, between staff and youth and among youth themselves (Beck et al. 2010) raise concerns about the safety and well-being of incarcerated youth nationwide.

The average length of secure confinement is longer for Latino/a youth than for any other racial or ethnic group, in every offense category (Villarruel and Walker 2002). Limited information is available to document the use of culturally competent and evidence-based interventions in confinement settings. Although more than 50% of states report some form of evidence-based treatment for youth with mental health needs, many of these programs do not include culturally competent or trauma-informed services (Adams 2010).

Any length of stay away from one's family and the comforts of home can be traumatic for youth. Depending on the conditions of confinement, youth may have few personal belongings or reminders of home life. Contact with family may be extremely limited, due to the distance of the facility or strict visitation policies. Likewise, both conversations and physical contact between a youth and family members may be closely monitored or restricted. Families in which one or more members are undocumented immigrants may feel particularly uncomfortable about visiting an incarcerated youth, for fear of discovery of or retribution against their own legal status; this creates further family disconnection.

Solutions and Recommendations

The heterogeneity of the Latino population in the United States makes it incredibly difficult to prescribe a one-size-fits-all solution to some of the barriers found in the juvenile justice system. Despite significant gaps in research, a number of options are emerging to address the mental health needs of Latino youth in the juvenile justice system. The most promising solutions have focused on building structures to reduce DMC, increasing coordination and collaboration across systems, and developing culturally competent interventions within community-based agencies and in secure confinement settings.

Jurisdictions must prioritize early identification of mental health needs by increasing access to and utilization of preventative systems and using culturally appropriate screening and assessment to inform court decisions. It is critical to address the underlying causes of discrimination and economic, social, and political disparities to ensure that Latino children are given equal access to education, human services, and mental health services. Of particular importance is increasing the availability of culturally specific programs that support adjustment of Latino immigrants (Alegría and Woo 2009) and providing adequate mental health services to Latino populations. A strategic and planned increase in the identification of children with mental health issues and referral to appropriate services may help reduce the number of Latino youth processed within the juvenile justice system. Because most assessments are normed on non-Latino White males, it is imperative that additional research be conducted to design culturally appropriate screening and assessment instruments based on Latino youth (Ramiu and Shoenberg 2009).

Increase research aimed at understanding the prevalence and causes of disproportionate minority contact, as well as the responses most effective in reducing DMC. The JJDPA core requirement to reduce DMC has been a significant step forward in encouraging states to identify and address racial and ethnic overrepresentation in their jurisdictions. Although the JJDPA does not establish numerical quotas, many states are proactively pursuing strategies for better data collection and analysis, and subsequent use of that data to develop appropriate interventions. In 2007, the MacArthur Foundation DMC Action Network, managed by the Center for Children's Law and Policy, brought together state and local leaders from 17 select jurisdictions to expose them to the latest tools and ideas to effectively and sustainably reduce the disproportionate contact of youth of color within the juvenile justice system. Some of the interventions include tools to promote objective decision making, improve language and cultural competency, and build cultural competencies in detention alternatives, community services, education, and workforce development. Ultimately, the goal of the DMC Action Network is to replicate effective strategies throughout the country.

Courts must recognize the importance of culturally and linguistically competent practices and train juvenile justice stakeholders at every level to utilize these practices effectively. Police, court workers, and residential treatment staff who come into contact with youth at all decision points must be trained in cultural sensitivity and cross-cultural communication. Intake and clinical staff must learn to identify mental health needs through use of culturally appropriate, standardized assessment instruments and be aware of the range of referral options available in the community to address these issues. Likewise, residential treatment staff must be trained to employ a range of evidence-based practices designed to meet the needs of Latino youth, especially those with mental health issues. Jurisdictions must enhance their capacity regarding linguistic competency to ensure that court, secure confinement, and community-based services have Spanish-speaking staff who can effectively communicate with Latino youth and families. One strategy that has been recommended is the increased use of translated materials and interpreters (Ramiu and Shoenberg 2009), which would help dispel fears and misunderstandings among non-English-speaking families. Training on adolescent development may also help staff understand the impact of trauma, mental health, and incarceration at key developmental phases of adolescence (Bullis et al. 2002). Jurisdictions can ensure continued commitment to culturally based practices and ongoing training by incorporating this information into policies and procedures.

All child-serving systems should be involved in developing a coordinated plan to ensure that children are being referred to the correct system for services and to address the multiple needs of youth in a coordinated way. The coordination of key systems (e.g., juvenile justice, mental health, child welfare, education) is critical to ensure that children do not slip through the cracks. Systems of Care, promoted by the federal Substance Abuse and Mental Health Services Administration, is recognized as the leading approach to improving access to and the quality of mental health services for youth. Impact System of Care, an initiative in Ingham County, Michigan, is one example of successful collaboration among multiple agencies that results in improved outcomes for youth and families. Impact System of Care, which is facilitated by the local community mental health agency, provides services to youth with severe emotional disturbance and their families; the majority of referrals come from the juvenile court. Their family-driven and youth-guided approaches are built upon values that embrace accessible and effective services, coordinated and collaborative care, and culturally and linguistically competent services. Through a range of family-focused interventions, including home-based therapy, wraparound approaches, and family advocates, Ingham County has witnessed increased levels of functioning among youth as well as increased family participation. As of November 2008, 69% of the 181 youth referred had not had new delinquency petitions filed since receiving services through Impact System of Care (Impact System of Care 2009).

Culturally competent diversion and community-based programs must be increased in an effort to prevent out-of-home placement but still address behavioral issues effectively. The Alternatives to Detention Initiative in Santa Cruz, California, for example, has established an important framework for engaging community members, service providers, and youth to reduce DMC across multiple contact points. In particular, the Santa Cruz DMC Taskforce implemented a series of strategies to reduce the number of Latino youth in detention through the increased use of diversion (Annie E. Casey Foundation 2008b). Through implementation of standardized assessments and an increase of community-based programs, the proportion of Latinos in detention fell by 50% in 2001 (Ayra et al. 2009).

Juvenile facilities should employ evidence-based programs that are individualized, family centered, strength based, gender responsive, and culturally competent. The Missouri Model is nationally recognized for its developmentally appropriate approach to treating youth in residential placement (Mendel 2010). The most important element of the Missouri Model is its focus on building relationships, rather than only managing behavior. Treatment-oriented services are delivered in group homes rather than large institutions, and staff are trained to provide eyes-on supervision over isolation. Through effective programming and supportive after-care, the Missouri Model produces positive outcomes for youth, results in lower recidivism (reoffending) rates than other states, and remains more cost-effective than many residential programs across the country (Mendel 2010).

When youth are placed in secure confinement, it is imperative that facilities offer culturally competent programs as well as quality mental health services. Research-ers advocate for case plans that focus on successful reintegration and family reuni-fication from the first day in the facility, rather than shortly before release from con-finement (Griffin et al. 2007). The Youth Reentry Task Force of the Juvenile Justice and Delinquency Coalition emphasizes the need for individualized and culturally competent residential services aimed at improving thinking and behavior, such as educational tutoring, job skills training, cognitive behavioral therapy, and family and individual counseling (Nellis and Hooks Wayman 2009).

Conclusion

The face of juvenile justice continues to change, with more Latino youth experienc-ing contact across the system. This chapter has attempted to introduce the mental health needs and the infrastructure for providing mental health services to Latino youth in the juvenile justice system, but there are still multiple unresolved issues that merit further research. Empirical studies are needed to determine why Latino youth are disproportionately represented at each of the nine contact points identi-fied by the OJJDP and if overrepresentation in juvenile justice is related to Latinos' lesser access to other human service and mental health delivery systems. Research is also needed to identify the most effective interventions for reducing recidivism and increasing positive outcomes for adjudicated Latino youth, especially in view of the unique impact that immigration, acculturation issues, and lived realities may have on this population. A critical direction within that avenue of research is under-standing the impact that surveillance techniques (i.e., electronic monitoring) and secure confinement have on the mental health of Latino youth and their families.

Most importantly, empirical research, and subsequent evidence-based interven-tions, may help reduce the number of Latino youth who eventually become in-volved in the adult criminal justice system. Without attention to the critical needs of this vulnerable population, there is a great concern that the current approaches may strip youth of important developmental building blocks that foster their successful transition to adulthood (Butts et al. 2010) and perpetuate a cycle of crime. Profes-sionals at all points of contact who understand cultural differences and recognize mental health needs can enhance the outcomes of Latino youth who encounter the juvenile justice system. Of paramount importance is creating an infrastructure with juvenile justice and mental health systems that addresses the cultural, linguistic, and developmental needs of Latino youth and their families, making this a priority rather than an afterthought.

References

Abram, K. M., Teplin, L. A., Charles, D. R., Longworth, S. L., McClelland, G. M., & Dulcan, M. K. (2004). Posttraumatic stress disorder and trauma in youth in juvenile detention. *Archives of General Psychiatry, 61,* 403–410.

Adams, E. (2010). *Healing invisible wounds: Why investing in trauma-informed care for children makes sense.* Washington, DC: Justice Policy Institute.

Adler, N., Epel, E., Castellazzo, G., & Ickovics, J. (2000). Relationship of subjective and objective social status with psychological and physiological functioning: Preliminary data in healthy white women. *Health Psychology, 19*(6), 586-592.

Alegría, M., & Woo, M. (2009). Conceptual issues in Latino mental health. In F. A. Villarruel, G. Carlo, J. M. Grau, M. Azmitia, N. J. Cabrarra, & T. J. Chahin, (Eds), *The U.S. handbook of Latino research: Developmental and community-based perspectives* (pp. 15–30). Thousand Oaks, CA: Sage.

Alegría, M., Mulvaney-Day, N., Torres, M., Polo, A., Cao, Z., & Canino, G. (2007). Prevalence of psychiatric disorders across Latino subgroups in the United States. *Journal of Public Health, 97,* 68–75.

Alegría, M., Canino, G., Shrout, P. E., Woo, M., Duan, N., Vila, D., et al. (2008). Prevalence of mental illness in immigrant and non-immigrant U.S. Latino groups. *American Journal of Psychiatry, 165,* 359–369.

Annie E. Casey Foundation. (2008a). *Kids Count data center.* Baltimore, MD: Author. Retrieved from http://www.kidscount.org/datacenter

Annie E. Casey Foundation. (2008b). *Juvenile detention alternatives initiative.* Baltimore, MD: Author. Available at http://www.jdaihelpdesk.org/pages/SantaCruzCountyCA.aspx

Armour, J., & Hammond, S. (2009). *Minority youth in the juvenile justice system: Disproportionate minority contact.* Washington, DC: National Conference of State Legislators. Retrieved from http://www.modelsforchange.net/publications/183

Ayra, N., Villarruel, F. A., Villanueva, C., & Augartan, I. (2009). *America's invisible children: Latino youth and the failure of justice.* Washington, DC: Campaign for Youth Justice. Available at http://www.campaign4youthjustice.org

Barcallao, M. L., & Smokowski, P. R. (2009). *Entre dos mundos*/Between two worlds: Bicultural development in context. *Journal of Primary Prevention, 30,* 421–451.

Beck, A., Harrison, P., & Guerino, P. (2010). Sexual Victimization in Juvenile Facilities Reported by Youth, 2008-2009. Washington, DC: Bureau of Justice Statistics.

Benet-Martínez, V., Leu, J., Lee, F., & Morris, M. W. (2002). Negotiating biculturalism: Cultural frame switching in biculturals with oppositional versus compatible cultural identities. *Journal of Cross-Cultural Psychology, 33,* 492–516.

Bishop, D. (2000). Juvenile offenders in the adult criminal system. *Crime & Justice, 27,* 81–167.

Bonta, J., Wallace-Capretta, S., & Rooney, J. (2000). Can electronic monitoring make a difference? An evaluation of three Canadian programs. *Crime & Delinquency, 46*(1), 61–75.

Bullis, M., Yovanoff, P., Mueller, G., & Havel, E. (2002). Life on the "outs": Examination of the family-to-community transition of incarcerated youth. *Exceptional Children, 69,* 7–22.

Burgess-Proctor, A., Holtrop, K., & Villarruel, F. A. (2006). *Youth transferred to adult court: Racial disparities.* Washington, DC: Campaign for Youth Justice. Available at http://www.campaign4youthjustice.org/news.htm

Buriel, R. Love, J. A. & Villanueva, C. M. (2011). Language brokering in Latino immigrant families: Developmental challenges, stressors, familial supports, and adjustment. In N. Cabrera, F. Villarruel, & H. E. Fitzgerald (Eds.), *Latina and Latino child mental health: Volume 1 Development and context* (pp. 91-116). Santa Barbara, CA: Prager.

Buriel, R., Perez, W., De Ment, T., Chavez, D. V., & Moran, V. R. (1998). The relationship of language brokering to academic performance, biculturalism and self-efficacy among Latino adolescents. *Hispanic Journal of Behavioral Sciences, 20,* 283–297.

Butts, J. A., Bazemore, G., & Meroe, A. S. (2010). Positive youth justice: Framing justice interventions using the concepts of positive youth development. Washington, DC: Coalition for Juvenile Justice. Available at http://juvjustice.org/media/resources/public/resource_390.pdf

Cauffman, E., Feldman, S. S., Waterman, J., & Steiner, H. (1998). Posttraumatic stress disorder among incarcerated females. *Journal of the American Academy of Child & Adolescent Psychiatry, 37,* 1209–1216.

Cocozza, J. J., & Shefelt, J. L. (2006). *Juvenile mental health courts: An emerging strategy.* Retrieved from National Center for Mental Health and Juvenile Justice website: http://www.ncmhjj.com/pdfs/publications/JuvenileMentalHealthCourts.pdf

DeNavas-Walt, C., Proctor, B. D., & Smith, J. C. (2009). *Income, poverty, and health insurance coverage in the United States: 2008* (Current Population Reports, P60-236). Washington, DC: U.S. Census Bureau.

Feyerherm, W., Snyder, H. N., & Villarruel, F. A. (2009). Chapter 1: Identification and monitoring. In *Disproportionate minority contact technical assistance manual* (4th ed.). Washington, DC: Office of Juvenile Justice and Delinquency Prevention. Available at http://www.ncjrs.gov/html/ojjdp/dmc_ta_manual/dmcch1.pdf

General Accounting Office. (2003). *Child welfare and juvenile justice: Federal agencies could play a stronger role in helping states reduce the number of children placed solely to obtain mental health services.* Washington, DC: Author. Retrieved from: http://www.gao.gov/new.items/d03397.pdf

Giedd, J. N. (2004). Structural magnetic resonance imaging of the adolescent brain. *Annals of the New York Academy of Sciences, 1021,* 77–85.

Gonzales, N. A., Fabrett, F. C., & Knight, G. P. (2009). Acculturation, enculturation, and the psychosocial adaptation of Latino youth. In F. A. Villarruel, G. Carlo, J. M. Grau, M. Azmitia, N. J. Cabrarra, & T. J. Chahin, (Eds), *The U.S. handbook of Latino research: Developmental and community-based perspectives* (pp. 115–134). Thousand Oaks, CA: Sage.

Griffin, P., Steele, R., & Franklin, K. (2007). *Aftercare reality and reform. Pennsylvania progress.* Pittsburgh, PA: National Center for Juvenile Justice.

Grisso, T. (2004). *Double jeopardy: Adolescent offenders with mental disorders.* Chicago: University of Chicago Press.

Grisso, T. (2008). Adolescent offenders with mental disorders. *The Future of Children, 18,* 143–164.

Hernandez, D. J., Denton, N. A., & Macartney, S. E. (2008). Children in immigrant families: Looking to America's future. *Social Policy Report* (Society for Research in Child Development), *22*(3), 1–24.

Human Rights Watch. (2002). *Race and incarceration in the United States.* Washington, DC: Author. Available at http://www.hrw.org/en/reports/2002/02/27/race-and-incarceration-united-states

Impact System of Care. (2009). *Annual report to the community.* Lansing, MI: Author. Available at http://www.impactsystemofcare.org/images/pubs/09-IMP-168-annualreport.pdf

Kiang, L., Yip, T., Gonzales-Backen, M., Witkow, M., & Fuligni, A. J. (2006). Ethnic identity and the daily psychological well-being of adolescents from Mexican and Chinese backgrounds. *Child Development, 77,* 1338–1350.

Knitzer, J. (1982). *Unclaimed children: The failure of public responsibility to children and adolescents in need of mental health services.* Washington, DC: Children's Defense Fund.

Losen, D. J., & Skiba, R. J. (2010). *Suspended Education - Urban middle schools in crisis.* Montgomery, AL: Southern Poverty Law Center.

Lyons, S., & Walsh, N. (2010). *Money well spent: How positive social investments will reduce incarceration rates, improve public safety, and promote the well-being of communities.* Washington, DC: Justice Policy Institute. Available at http://www.justicepolicy.org/images/upload/10-09_REP_MoneyWellSpent_PS-DC-AC-JJ.pdf

MacArthur Foundation. (2010). *Understanding the long-term consequences of juvenile adjudication: Models for change.* Available at http://www.modelsforchange.net/newsroom/163

Mendel, R. (2010). The Missouri Model: Reinventing the practice of rehabilitating youthful of-fenders. Baltimore, MD: Annie E. Casey Foundation.

Miranda, A. O., & Matheny, K. B. (2000). Socio-psychological predictors of acculturative stress among Latino adults. *Journal of Mental Health Counseling, 22,* 306–317.

National Juvenile Defender Center. (2008). *Ten core principles for providing quality delinquency representation through public defense delivery systems.* Washington, DC: Author. Available at http://www.njdc.info/pdf/10_Core_Principles_2008.pdf

Nellis, A., & Hooks Wayman, R. H. (2009). *Back on track: Supporting youth reentry from out-of-home placement to the community.* Washington, DC: Youth Reentry Task Force of the Juvenile Justice and Delinquency Prevention Coalition. Available at http://www.sentencingproject.org/doc/publications/CC_youthreentryfall09report.pdf

Piquero, A. R. (2008). Disproportionate minority contact. *The Future of Children, 18,* 59–80.

Ramiu, M. F., & Shoenberg, D. (2009). Chapter 7: Strategies for serving Hispanic youth. In *Disproportionate minority contact technical assistance manual* (4th ed.). Washington, DC: Office of Juvenile Justice and Delinquency Prevention. Available at http://www.ncjrs.gov/html/ojjdp/dmc_ta_manual/dmcch1.pdf

Ringel, J. S., & Sturm, R. (2001). National estimates on mental health utilization for children in 1998. *Journal of Behavioral Health Services & Research, 28,* 319–333.

Scott, E. S., & Steinberg, L. (2003). Blaming youth. *Texas Law Review, 81,* 799–840.

Shefelt, J. L., & Cocozza, J. J. (2006). Youth with mental health disorders in the juvenile jus-tice system: Results from a multi-state prevalence study. Retrieved from National Center for Mental Health and Juvenile Justice website: http://www.ncmhjj.com/pdfs/publications/Preva-lenceRPB.pdf

Sickmund, M. (2005). New survey provides a glimpse of the youth reentry population. *Corrections Today, 30–31.*

Skowyra, K. R., & Cocozza, J. J. (2006). *Blueprint for change: A comprehensive model for the identification and treatment of youth with mental health needs in contact with the juvenile justice system.* Delmar, NY: The National Center for Mental Health and Juvenile Justice [NC-MHJJ] and Policy Research Associates, Inc.

Soler, M. (2007). *Disproportionate minority contact: Practical applications and implications.* Washington, DC: Center for Children's Law and Policy. Available at http://cclp.org/media/documents/doc_40.pdf

Sprague, C. (2008, August). *Informing judges about child trauma.* NCTSN Service System Briefs, 2(2). Retrieved from www.NCTSN.org

Stouthamer-Loeber, M., Wei, E. H., Homish, D. L., & Loeber, R. (2002). Which family and demo-graphic factors are related to both maltreatment and persistent serious juvenile delinquency? *Children's Services: Social Policy, Research, & Practice, 5,* 261–272.

Tienda, M., & Mitchell, F. (Eds.). (2006). *Multiple origins, uncertain destinies: Hispanics and the American future.* Washington, DC: National Academies Press.

U.S. Census Bureau. (2009). Census Bureau estimates nearly half of children under age 5 are mi-norities. *U.S. Census Bureau News.* Retrieved September 3, 2010 from http://www.census.gov/newsroom/releases/archives/population/cb09-75.html

Vega, W., & Alegría, M. (2001). Latino mental health and treatment in the United States. In M. Aguirre-Molina, C. Molina, & R. Zambrana (Eds.), *Health issues in the Latino community* (pp. 179–208). San Francisco, CA: Jossey-Bass.

Vega, W. A., Kolody, B., Aguilar-Gaxiola, S., Alderete, E., Catalaon, R., & Caraveo-Anduga, J. (1998). Lifetime prevalence of DSM-III-R psychiatric disorders among urban and rural Mexi-can Americans in California. *Archives of General Psychiatry, 55,* 771–778.

Vera Institute of Justice. (2010). *If parents don't speak English well, will their kids get locked up? Language barriers and disproportionate minority contact in the juvenile justice system.* Available at http://www.aecf.org/~/media/Pubs/Topics/Special%20Interest%20Areas/Immi-grants%20and%20Refugees/IfParentsDontSpeakEnglishWellWillTheirKidsGet/ifparents.pdf

Villarruel, F. A., & Walker, N. E. (2002). *¿Dónde está la justicia?: A call to action on behalf of Latino and Latina youth in the U.S. justice system.* Washington, DC: Building Blocks for Youth. Available at www.buildingblocksforyouth.org

Walker, N. E., Senger, J. M., Villarruel, F. A., Arboleda, A. (2004). *Lost opportunities: The reality of Latinos in the U.S. criminal justice system.* Washington, DC: National Council of La Raza.

Chapter 10
Promoting the Well-Being of Unaccompanied Immigrant Minors

Etiony Aldarondo and Rachel Becker

Abstract The presence of undocumented unaccompanied Latino immigrant children and youth in our communities poses a formidable challenge for this nation. This chapter highlights the plight of unaccompanied migrant minors (UIM) in the United States and around the world, what we know about their mental health and resiliency, and the government's response to this issue; it also discusses the creation and evolution of an innovative community–university partnership designed to promote the human rights and well-being of UIMs in South Florida. Throughout this discussion, the authors urge readers to consider opportunities for infrastructure building at the community level, and the important role of local and federal governmental responses in the provision of specialized services for this population.

*One of the basic American values is to be a welcoming nation
but to be a rule of law nation. The 14th Amendment was
passed in 1866 to prevent states from disenfranchising the free
slaves. The Amendment says that if you are [a] naturally born
person under the jurisdiction laws of the United States you are
automatically a citizen. That protected the freed slaves. Fast
forward 160 years, we got people selling trips across the border.
They will sneak you into America, go to American hospitals
so that you can have your baby here and that baby becomes
an American citizen. That incentivizes illegal immigration....
We just can't have people swimming across the river having
children here. That is chaos. So that is why they do it.*
Senator Lindsey Graham (Scott 2010)

AGUA CALIENTE, Guatemala—*He was warned the journey
north would be hard, so Gilmar Morales beefed up on eggs and
sausage, bought some ham sandwiches from the bodega across
the street, told his mother he loved her and set off with two
other relatives on a path well-travelled by young people here in
one of Latin America's poorest countries.*

E. Aldarondo (✉)
Dunspaugh-Dalton Community and Educational Well-Being Research Center, School of
Education, University of Miami, Miami, FL, USA
e-mail: etiony@miami.edu

> *Then, a few weeks later his mother, watching a television show,*
> *looked hard at the picture of the bodies of 72 Central and*
> *South American migrants killed last week in northeast Mexico*
> *near the Texas border. Was it Gilmar, the one with the familiar*
> *yellow-and-white striped T-shirt, his blue pants?*
>
> (Archibold 2010)

Today as in the past, political fervor and xenophobic attitudes permeate popular conversation about immigrants and their place in the United States. Hardly a day goes by without stark reminders of how affectively loaded the issue of immigration has become. Social tensions run high—from immigration raids in workplaces, to vigilante patrols in border states, to reactive legislation in Arizona and Alabama requiring legal immigrants to carry documentation at all times. The backlash is palpable, as reflected in heated discussions about "anchor babies" that question the wisdom of the 14th Amendment in protecting the birthright citizenship of the native born. These sentiments, though ill informed, affect public opinion and contribute to the creation of a hostile social context, with grave implications for the well-being of the individual and families, and for the development of community policies and programs (Aldarondo and Ameen 2010; Zayas 2010). Widespread fear of foreign people and a dislike for their customs, culture, and language thwart collective efforts to promote the well-being of society's most vulnerable members—its children. The act of questioning the citizenship of the native-born children of immigrants reflects a troublesome failure in popular imagination for creative responses to the challenges posed by immigration. Moreover, such a line of questioning creates a context that leaves immigrant children—those with the least say in their fate and the least power to alter their circumstances, those caught in a process not of their making—particularly vulnerable to exploitation and death.

In fact, the growing number of undocumented unaccompanied Latino immigrant children and youth in our communities poses a particular challenge for this nation. This chapter highlights the plight of unaccompanied immigrant minors (UIMs) in the United States and around the world, what we know about their mental health and resiliency, and the government's response to this issue; it also discusses the creation and evolution of an innovative community–university partnership designed to promote the human rights and well-being of these children in South Florida. Throughout this discussion, the authors urge readers to consider opportunities for infrastructure building at the community level, and the important role of local and federal governmental responses in the provision of specialized services for this population.

Unaccompanied Immigrant Minors and Their Journey to the United States

Unaccompanied immigrant minors are in the United States without guardians, facing arrest, detention, and removal. The professional discourse on unaccompanied minors has largely centered on their legal plight; immigration status significantly influences the degree of benefits, services, and legal rights afforded to foreign-born individuals in the United States (Pine and Drachman 2005). The Bureau of Citizenship and Immigration Services (CIS), a branch of the Department of Homeland Security (DHS), defines an *immigrant* as a non-US citizen who is lawfully admitted for permanent residence (Immigration Policy in the United States 2006). However, thinking within this legal context often causes the lived experiences of immigrants to be overlooked or disregarded. Migrating involves uprooting; losing home, parents, friends, social networks, familiar environments, customs; and much more. The disruption of social and cultural belonging may result in social isolation, the loss of self-identification, and the loss of a sense of security and well-being (Derluyn and Broekaert 2008). Thus, these minors often face a host of stressors that lead them to migrate, an arduous journey to their host destination, and a cascade of difficulties upon their arrival to the host country.

Unaccompanied children are frequently found in situations of military conflict, natural disasters, and political unrest (Ressler et al. 1988). The United Nations High Commission for Refugees defines *unaccompanied minors* as "those who are separated from both parents and are not cared for by an adult who, by law or custom, is responsible to do so" (Kohli 2007, p. 4). Unaccompanied immigrant minors, according to the Homeland Security Act (HSA) of the United States, are children who have no lawful immigration status in the United States, have not attained 18 years of age, and with respect to whom (a) there is no parent or legal guardian in the United States, or (b) no parent or legal guardian in the United States is available to provide care and physical custody (Haddal 2009).

The portions of these definitions that refer to "minors" must be considered in terms of three important caveats. First, the age limit denoting minor status (typically 18) is not a worldwide standard. Second, experiences of childhood differ significantly across cultures and contexts, such that an official age limit is not necessarily a proxy for the cultural idea of transition to adulthood. Finally, the development of a minor into an adult is an idiosyncratic process, such that minors of the same age may differ significantly in maturity level (Derluyn and Broekaert 2008).

Another challenge posed by the definition of UIMs concerns the determination of "unaccompanied." Some definitions of *unaccompanied* indicate that these children migrate without parents or a legal caregiver. Others specify that the minor has migrated in the absence of parents or a legal guardian. Strictly interpreting "unaccompanied" affords some benefits: It helps to prevent the trafficking of children and adolescents for exploitative purposes. However, a strict interpretation can also result in youth becoming separated from an adult who was previously a caregiver, but not a parent or legal guardian. The process of discerning whether an accompanying adult is an actual caregiver poses a difficult challenge to authorities, especially because documentation to verify the purported ties is often unavailable (Bhabha and Young 1999).

The motivations behind migrating as an unaccompanied minor vary. Many of these minors leave their home countries to join family already in the United States; escape abuse, persecution, or exploitation in the home country; or to seek employment or educational opportunities in the United States. At times, UIMs are sent to the United States by their families or other traffickers for labor or commercial

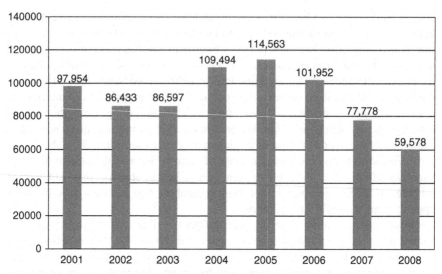

Note: These figures reflect data combined from various government agencies and should be regarded as conservative estimates of the number of youth apprehended by the government each year.

Fig. 10.1 Apprehensions of unaccompanied immigrant minors by customs and border protection, 2001–2008. (Sources: Haddal (2009) and Homeland Security, Office of Immigration Statistics (2009))

sex exploitation (Haddal 2009). Minors also become unaccompanied for a variety of reasons. Some are explicitly sent by their families to prepare the way for other family members, others find themselves separated during the migration process, and still others are left behind by parents who began the family's migration process (Derluyn and Broekaert 2008).

As shown in Fig. 10.1, over 700,000 immigrant children have been apprehended by Customs and Border Protection (CBP) since 2001. In 2006, the CBP averaged 279 undocumented juvenile apprehensions per day (Haddal 2009). Approximately four out of every five of these juveniles are Mexican citizens (Haddal 2009). Although the majority of these children were immediately repatriated, more than 8,000 were detained and placed under the guardianship of the Office of Refugee Resettlement (ORR); the ORR, in turn, houses these children in one of more than 40 detention facilities located throughout the country while their legal situation is investigated. The average amount of time a child spends in a detention facility ranges from one month to more than 1 year (Florida Immigrant Advocacy Center [FIAC] 2006).

In spite of these figures, UIMs have received minimal attention outside of the legal field, which may partially be attributed to the constricted popular conversation about immigration alluded to at the beginning of the chapter and the ensuing lack of awareness about their presence in our communities by professionals and ordinary citizens alike. Additionally, several scholars suggest that official government statistics do not provide a complete picture of the situation of UIMs. They believe that the statistics are not comprehensive because each government agency that interacts with the youth keeps its own records. More specifically, ORR's records do not include children who are apprehended by the DHS but are never placed in ORR's care (Bhabha and Schmidt 2006). Additionally, most governmental statistics do not attempt to account for unaccompanied youth who do not come into contact with governmental authorities (Mahoney 2002).

The majority of UIMs, approximately 74%, are males between the ages of 15 and 18 years. This predominance of adolescent boys is consistent with international reports documenting that the vast majority of unaccompanied children seeking asylum worldwide are males (UNHCR 2004). Girls comprise roughly 26% of the unaccompanied-child population. These children come from around the world; however, three countries in particular—Honduras, Guatemala, and El Salvador—account for approximately 85% of the unaccompanied minors held in detention in the United States (Haddal 2009).

A recent study by Scot (2009) paints a more detailed picture of these youth. Most of the 118 youth sampled had attended some school in their home countries, with the majority attending school for only 4–6 years. Two-thirds of the children worked while living at home. Of these youth, the majority worked as laborers; others sold goods or worked as housekeepers or childcare providers. Almost all children surveyed lived with their families before they journeyed to the United States. Approximately two-thirds of the youth lived with their parents, whereas the remainder resided with extended family members. The youth were also asked to reflect on their goals for their futures. Consistent with the opening statements in this chapter, the majority of the youth reported the desire to work; one-fourth said they wanted to attend school; the remainder expressed other goals (e.g., having a family of their own, reunifying with existing family, or returning to their home countries).

Unaccompanied minors' reasons for immigration vary. Some are fleeing political upheaval, extreme poverty, child labor, and abusive homes (Florida Immigrant Advocacy Center [FIAC] 2006), whereas others are attempting to reunite with family members who previously immigrated to the United States. Although a variety of sources cite abuse as a frequent determinant in the decision to migrate, one study found that 90% of all youth reported that they were not abused in their home country (Scot 2009). The most common reason given for migration was to attend school or to locate employment. One-third of children reported migrating in order to reunite with family currently residing in the United States (Scot 2009), a motivation which appears to characterize the decision to migrate for many Latino youth (Dreby 2010). Finally, these youths' journeys differ in a variety of ways: Some are transported by traffickers or by hired smugglers, others make the perilous journey alone (Florida Immigrant Advocacy Center [FIAC] 2006). It is not uncommon for a child's parent to journey to the United States to establish stable employment and housing, and then pay a smuggler ("coyote") $ 5,000–$ 10,000 to bring their children into the country (Gonzalez 2004).

The vast majority of youth from Central American countries leave on foot or by bus to travel into Mexico. While in Mexico, the children must be careful because routes to the north are well known and therefore are heavily monitored by authorities and criminals. Once the UIMs reach the northern part of the country, they must jump on a train that will take them across the border. This part of journey is one of the most perilous; many have been injured or killed during their attempts. After the UIMs arrive at the border, they can pay a coyote to transport them across the Rio Grande or lead them into the Arizona desert where they can enter the United States (Scot 2009).

Unlike the anticipation experienced by many documented immigrant children as they journey to the United States, undocumented children tend to characterize the journey as stressful and traumatic (Suarez-Orozco and Suarez-Orozco 2002). Unaccompanied immigrant minors risk becoming victims of a variety of crimes before or during their journey. These children are often vulnerable to smugglers and child traffickers. Girls may be smuggled for domestic servitude or sex work (Gonzalez 2004). When reflecting on their journey, one-fifth of all youth indicated that they were abused either by a stranger, by a smuggler who was hired to take them across the border, or by Mexican or US Border Patrol (Scot 2009). Immigration and Naturalization Service (INS) operations attempted to restrict immigration during the mid 1990s; however, these measures contributed to an increase in the number of deaths, rapes, and accidents at the US borders (Eschbach et al. 1997; Suarez-Orozco and Suarez-Orozco 2002).

Unaccompanied Immigrant Minors Around the World

Given the current anti-immigrant fervor, we run the risk of assuming that the increase in UIMs is unique to the United States. A closer look at international reports on UIMs around the world, however, reveals a profile similar to that seen in the United States. In 2003, asylum requests for UIMs were filled in 28 industrialized countries (UNHCR 2009). The ubiquitous spread of poverty, global capitalism, political unrest, and war has led to increasing rates of immigration worldwide (Cemlyn and Briskman 2003). The United States, the United Kingdom, Australia, Canada, Sweden, the Netherlands, and Finland have all received unaccompanied youth in the past few years, and have all noted an increase in the number of immigrants (Bean et al. 2007; Bhabha and Schmidt 2006; Bhabha and Young 1999; Ferenci 2000; Kohli and Mather 2003; Rousseau et al. 2001; Russell 1999; Sourander 1998).

The experience of unaccompanied immigrant youth in Mexico provides a rich example of UIMs' journeys outside the United States. In 2009, the International Organization for Migration reported that as many as 20,000 unaccompanied immigrant youth may be migrating through Mexico each year. Of these, the Mexican government repatriated 4,555 unaccompanied Central American children in 2008. In a recent study conducted by Catholic Relief Services (2010), researchers documented the conditions of unaccompanied immigrant migrants from Honduras, El Salvador, and Guatemala who were en route to Mexico and beyond. Though the overall rate of Central American migration has decreased since 2006, a larger number of those who do migrate now are children. For example, the Mexican government reported in 2008 that unaccompanied migrants made up 72% of all children migrants in detention. Seventy-five percent of the 12- to 15-year-old youths were male; however, females tended to migrate at younger ages than males. Prior to migration, the girls in this study were less likely to live with both parents and more likely to live with neither parent than were boys. Guatemalan youth were more likely to live with both parents and, on average, had the greatest number of siblings (i.e., 41% reported six or more siblings). Overall, migrants from El Salvador were much younger than those in Honduras and Guatemala.

The profile of youth who spoke an indigenous language (17% of those interviewed) had a slightly different profile from the majority. These youth were more likely to live with both parents, have more siblings, and have less formal education than nonindigenous migrant youth. More specifically, 90% of indigenous-speaking youth had a primary education or less, whereas this number was only 70% in nonindigenous-speaking youth. These indigenous-speaking youths were also more likely to report having worked to aid their family in their home country (Catholic Relief Services 2010).

The majority of minors in this Catholic Relief Services study (59%) reported migrating for the primary reason of obtaining employment, even though many had already been working in their home countries. This motivation was more prevalent in youth who had a pre-primary level of education. Twenty-one percent of youth migrated primarily to reunite with their family. These numbers were higher for Salvadorans and younger children. Most youth reported that this was their first time attempting to migrate. More than half stated that they had left their home countries with $100 or less for the journey.

The Mental Health of Unaccompanied Immigrant Minors

During migration, youth may experience of variety of stressors that negatively affect their long-term health and well-being. Youth who migrate alone frequently experience physical and emotional abuse during their journey. Those migrant children who reach their families in a host country often face difficulties reintegrating and adapting to shifts in family structure, language, and culture (Catholic Relief Services 2010). The complex circumstances surrounding UIMs provide fertile soil for psychological distress. Because war and political violence have often accounted for forced migration, the majority of previous research has centered on the psychological impact of war-related violence exposure and parent–child separations, chiefly during the migratory and resettlement phases of refugees' experiences. For example, Kinzie et al. (1986) interviewed 46 Cambodian refugees aged 14–20 years and found that 90% of these youth were sent to age-segregated concentration camps when they were 8–12 years old. Almost half of the subjects met the diagnostic criteria for either post-traumatic stress disorder, major depressive disorder, or both.

More recently, Jaycox et al. (2002) investigated newly arrived immigrant children's risk for violence exposure and related psychological distress resulting from experiences before, during, and after immigration. One thousand and four recent immigrant children, aged 8–15 years, from Spanish, Korean, West Armenian, and Russian regions, were interviewed. The study participants reported high levels of violence exposure, both personal victimization and witnessing violence. The researchers found that 32% of these children reported post-traumatic stress symptoms and 16% reported depressive symptoms within the clinical range. The post-traumatic stress symptoms were predictive of recent and lifetime violence exposure, whereas depressive symptoms were predictive of recent violence exposure.

There is a paucity of literature examining the impact of unaccompanied migration on youths' mental health. The few extant studies consistently argue that unaccompanied youth are at greater risk for mental health problems than accompanied youth (Thomas and Lau 2002). By the sheer process of immigrating alone, these children and adolescents become more susceptible to victimization. This negatively affects their developmental and emotional self-regulatory capacities. Sourander (1998) studied premigratory trauma exposure and emotional and behavioral symptoms of 46 unaccompanied refugee children held in an asylum center in Pernio, Finland. The results indicated that UIMs endure a significant number of separations, losses, and violence exposure and that younger UIMs showed more vulnerability to clinical levels of psychological distress than the older children. In addition, several studies have highlighted age at separation from parental figures as an important factor in children's subsequent adaptation. For example, a study of unaccompanied Cambodian children in the Khao Dang Holding Center in Thailand found that children who were younger than age 5 when they experienced the loss of their parents demonstrated greater psychological disturbances (Ressler et al. 1988). Studies from a variety of different countries support these findings (i.e., an increase in vulnerability is associated with earlier age at separation) (Ajdukovic and Ajdukovic 1998; Almqvist and Broberg 1999; Garmezy and Rutter 1983; Lustig et al. 2004; Rousseau 1995; Sourander 1998). However, there is also evidence suggesting that that older unaccompanied minors may experience more psychological trauma than their younger counterparts (Bean et al. 2007). The Derluyn and Broekaert (2008) study of UIMs in Belgium found that age made little difference to the level of emotional distress experienced by unaccompanied children. The lack of clear findings highlights the complicated relationship between human development and adaptation, as youth are adapting to their environmental situations while experiencing biological and cognitive developmental changes (Berry et al. 2006).

Research suggests that migration is associated with the disruption of mental health, the ultimate manifestation of which may be a severe psychopathology (Ponizovsky et al. 1999; Short and Johnston 1997). There is evidence suggesting that this situation may be more pronounced for unaccompanied youth. Derluyn et al. (2008) found that unaccompanied refugee youth are five times more likely than accompanied refugee youth to report very severe symptoms of anxiety, depression, and post-traumatic stress. A large body of literature delineates the stressful nature of transitions and their ability to trigger a variety of reactions, both adaptive and maladaptive. These circumstances become particularly stressful when one is unable to call upon a traditional support network and employ past successful coping techniques (Suarez-Orozco and Suarez-Orozco 2002). Successful coping mechanisms can be further compromised for the unaccompanied immigrant child when removed from family and predictable contextual factors.

A study by Bean et al. (2007) further explored the relationship between psychological distress and a variety of factors in the lives of the unaccompanied minors. The authors found higher severity levels of internalizing complaints and traumatic stress reactions in unaccompanied youth as compared to refugee minors and Dutch adolescents. A one-year follow-up study demonstrated that the strongest predictor of psychological distress was the baseline psychopathology at the first measurement (Bean et al. 2007). Additionally, the traumatic stress reactions and internalization of distress in this population converge with previous research on other populations, where traumatization was strongly associated with high levels of psychological distress. After controlling for initial severity level, the total number of self-reported stressful life events remained a significant predictor of self-reported traumatic stress reactions, emotional distress, and behavioral problems. Other significant predictors of psychological functioning included age, residence in shelter, time of stay in shelter, gender, and absence of local family members. Not surprisingly, unaccompanied immigrant children in this study reported elevated levels of traumatic stress reactions as compared with normative populations.

We are aware of only one published study evaluating an intervention designed to assist UIMs reduce the impact of traumatic stress. Descilio et al. (2010) conducted a field-based open trial to examine the effectiveness of a trauma resolution method, "traumatic incident reduction," in 40 unaccompanied minor refugees with significant histories of "troubling trauma/loss events" in their histories. They found a significant reduction in post-traumatic symptoms following treatment. The effects were most pronounced in youth with recorded "clinical level trauma scores" prior to treatment. They also found a significant post-intervention reduction in depression symptoms. In terms of gender differences, unaccompanied immigrant young women reported greater reduction in depression symptoms and higher happiness ratings scores following treatment than their male counterparts.

Resiliency in Unaccompanied Immigrant Minors

Although there is clearly good reason to be concerned about the impact of separation, loss, and trauma on the mental health of UIMs, perhaps the most remarkable characteristic of this group is their resilience and drive to move forward in life. Loughry and Flouri (2001) explored the well-being of unaccompanied Vietnamese refugee children several years after their return to Vietnam. The study revealed that unaccompanied minors reported levels of social support and coping ability comparable to those of minors who had never left Vietnam. Similarly, Kohli and Mather (2003) found that unaccompanied children in the United Kingdom demonstrated the ability to successfully manage day-to-day stressors. In another study, Wolff et al. (1995) compared the social–emotional state and cognitive development of 4- to 7-year-old Eritrean children orphaned during war with those of refugee children residing with families. Although both groups had the same exposure to the traumatic stresses of war and drought, the authors discovered that the unaccompanied children outperformed accompanied children on measures of cognition and language. A handful of qualitative studies have also underscored the existence of positive adaptation and a need to explore the presence of resilience in unaccompanied children (German 2004; Kohli and Mather 2003; Maegusuku-Hewett et al. 2007; Rousseau et al. 1998). These studies suggest that UIMs have the capacity to recover from early psychological traumas and that interventions have the potential to protect children against the adverse effects of loss (Wolff et al. 1995). Moreover, the mere fact that many UIMs exhibit symptoms of emotional distress need not lead to the conclusion that as a group they require extensive psychological or therapeutic interventions (Derluyn and Broekaert 2008). Ressler et al. (1988, p. 165) highlight the complex relationship between trauma response and resilience:

> While recollections of family separation and loss have been the primary source of … older children's persisting grief, and underlying depression, they also have been at the heart of their continuing personal stamina and resiliency. Through the process of idealization and identification, memories of better times along with previously acquired parental and cultural values have continued to guide the older children; informing their effort in school, helping them determine right from wrong and encouraging them toward more hopeful futures.

Other qualitative research has fleshed out the nature of resilience in this population. Goodman (2004) explored coping skills employed by unaccompanied refugees from Sudan. Qualitative narratives revealed four themes of how the participants coped with trauma and life stressors: collectivity and the communal self, suppression and distraction, making meaning, and emerging from hopelessness to hope. Grant-Knight et al. (2009) conducted national surveys of Sudanese UIMs. Their results were encouraging, as they suggested positive outcomes despite years of deprivation, trauma, and separation from families during childhood.

In a recent study, Scot (2009) explored resilience and protective factors in UIMs in the United States. She found that children who were raised by their parents in their country of origin valued school more than children who were raised by extended family members. Interestingly, the data revealed that children who reported being treated poorly on their journey to the United States placed greater value on attending school than those who did not report being abused. Children whose main goal was to have a family of their own, reunite with family, or return to their home countries scored higher on personal competence than those with other goals. Moreover, the UIMs in this study scored in the moderate range on three important dimensions of resilience: social bonding, social competence, and personal competence. Thus, as a whole, studies of resilience in UIMs suggest that although these youths have encountered a host of life difficulties, they demonstrate individual abilities to deal effectively with adversity and thrive in safe and supportive environments.

Government Responses to the Needs of Unaccompanied Immigrant Minors

Government responses to UIMs vary significantly around the world. Unfortunately, no international body, UN department, institute, or treaty body is specifically charged with the responsibility of caring for migrant children. The lack of a unified approach has resulted in such youth tending to fall through the cracks of safety nets developed to protect them; however, international awareness has begun to grow. The 1989 Convention on the Rights of the Child is the most widely ratified and signed human rights instrument (the United States and Somalia are the only members of the UN who have not become full parties). This Convention unifies all of the protections related to the "best interests of the child," which in turn stipulates protective measures and addresses issues of process. More specifically, the Convention requires states to pay attention to the youth's views and attend to them when possible. Additionally, the UN Committee on the Rights of the Child recently issued a General Comment on the treatment of UIMs, stating:

> This comment calls on states to take seriously their obligations not to discriminate against these children because of their alien status but to make available to them the full range of protective services offered to vulnerable domestic children, including education, shelter, and health provision. The General Comment also urges states to balance the requirements of best interest, through appointment of a guardian for each separated or unaccompanied child, with the complementary need to accord careful attention to the expressed wishes and views of the children themselves (Committee on the Rights of the Child 2005).

A report produced by the Harvard University Committee on Human Rights Studies (2006) offers a comparative analysis of the implementation of international law concerning UIMs. Overall, the study concluded that at the time neither the United States, the United Kingdom, nor Australia had a unified, coherent legal framework that specifically targets the international welfare of youth immigrating alone. Since then, all three countries have started to carve out specific legal procedures for this population (Australian Government 2007; Bhabha and Schmidt 2006).

The United Kingdom has made considerable gains in recognizing the special status of unaccompanied youth. Its system establishes procedures for the protection of youth traveling without a responsible adult. The Immigration and Nationality Directorate of the Home Office determines whether to grant asylum to a youth. Eligibility for asylum depends on the youth's ability to meet the definition of *refugee* in the 1951 Refugee Convention. Additionally, the Immigration Rule explicitly states that priority should be given to the cases of unaccompanied minors, and official proceedings reflect this: Child asylum seekers are not interviewed directly after the initial screening, they are given longer application deadlines than adults, and officials perform special screenings to identify at-risk youth. This stance can also be seen in a European directive stating that the best interest of the child should be the guiding consideration for all matters related to children. Additionally, the UK asylum system allows for the right to appeal in most cases. Finally, the UK's Children Act (1989) dictates that the government is responsible to support, accommodate, and protect all children, regardless of nationality or immigration status. This provides unaccompanied youth with the same rights to state protection as domestic children.

Over the past several years, Australia has adopted the most progressive policy toward UIMs. Australia's Unaccompanied Humanitarian Minor Program coordinates the efforts of the Commonwealth and state governments to provide settlement services to these minors (Australian Government 2007). This program provides protection to all UIMs, regardless of whether they arrive legally or illegally. The program aims to guarantee that the minors receive welfare supervision and settlement support while residing in Australia. After arriving in Australia, unaccompanied minors can apply for protection. If this protection is granted, they receive permanent protection visas which provide them access to the full range of government benefits and services and enable them to live in Australia permanently. The Department of Immigration and Citizenship (DIAC) assists in visa determinations and employs psychologists and state welfare authorities to guide the department's response to the youths' educational, social, and medical needs.

Australia's current procedures under the Unaccompanied Humanitarian Minor Program differ significantly from other countries' approaches to UIMs. After DIAC requests that the department's Director General accept a UIM, the Senior Advisors of Cultural Diversity are notified and assign a liaison to the child (Department for Child Protection 2010). For children who arrive with an adult nonrelative caregiver, DIAC conducts an assessment of the caregiver and provides that person with a "foster carer subsidy." In addition, both the child and the caregiver can receive services from the Integrated Humanitarian Settlement Strategy. Therefore, Australia's procedures provide an integrated care system for all UIMs, incorporating knowledge of psychological needs (e.g., attachment to a caregiver or liaison) with a dedication to serve the best interests of the child.

US Government's Response

During the 1980s, there was a sharp rise in the number of UIMs arriving in the United States, as many fled civil wars in Central America and the resulting hardships. At that time, UIMs were placed under the legal custody of the INS. The Community Relations Service (CRS), a separate agency and part of the Department of Justice, was responsible for the daily care of unaccompanied youth until 1987, when the two agencies joined resources to provide care and child welfare services. Less than a decade later, complete responsibility was shifted to the DHS—some argue as a result of budget cuts (Bhabha and Schmidt 2006).

Following the terrorist attacks of September 11th, Congress passed the HSA, which had implications for the care of unaccompanied youth. The act created the DHS and eliminated the INS. The DHS is comprised of three divisions: US CIS, US Immigration and Customs Enforcement (ICE), and US CBP. After the INS closed, care of unaccompanied children was placed with the ORR, a division of the Department of Health and Human Services.

Once a child is apprehended by federal immigration authorities (e.g., one of the subsidiary agencies of DHS), the child is placed in ORR custody. The youth who is assumed to be an unaccompanied immigrant is then taken to a detention facility, where DHS begins a process to determine whether the individual is unaccompanied and younger than 18 years old. If the individual does not meet both of these requirements, he or she remains in DHS custody. DHS determines an individual's age through the use of forensic evidence, such as dental exams and bone x-rays, even if birth certificates are available. Critics have noted that these methods are outdated, and may lead to instances of wrongful identification, such that a minor is misidentified as an adult (Smythe 2004). The implications of this are significant: Children have sometimes erroneously been placed in adult detention facilities (Nugent 2006). Age determinations also consume a substantial portion of governmental resources—and resources of lawyers contesting wrongful age determinations. Therefore, some critics recommend that DHS adopt more accurate methodology for assessing age (Smythe 2004).

To determine whether a minor is unaccompanied, DHS uses the HSA's criteria: "a child who has no lawful immigration status in the United States, has not attained 18 years of age, and with respect to whom there is no parent or legal guardian in the United States, or no parent or legal guardian in the United States is available to provide care and physical custody." In addition, if DHS determines that a parent or legal guardian was not present with the child or "within a geographical proximity" when the minor was apprehended, then the child is deemed "unaccompanied" (Haddal 2009). Although these procedures appear straightforward, several critics say that their application is inconsistent (Bhabha and Schmidt 2006; Nugent 2006). After transfer to ORR custody, DHS is no longer involved in a minor's custody. However, if the minor faces removal proceedings in front of an immigration judge, ICE (a branch of DHS) prosecutes the case for the government. If these proceedings lead to the youth's removal, then DHS becomes responsible for returning the minor to his or her home country (Nugent 2006).

These proceedings and the conditions in which the unaccompanied minors are held have been criticized over the past three decades. In the late 1980s, the CRS was responsible for the care of unaccompanied minors and housed these youth in facilities that were a mix between a detention center and a shelter. When these housing responsibilities were transferred to INS, the agency attempted to balance its roles of being responsible for caring for the youth with being the law-enforcing body. A comparison of the United States at this time to other countries housing significant numbers of unaccompanied minors showed that the United States frequently detained youth for longer periods of time and under harsher conditions (Bhabha and Schmidt 2006). The INS sent one-third of unaccompanied youth to secure detention centers, where some were subjected to shackling or handcuffing during court appearances and while being transported (Human Rights Watch 1998).

A class action lawsuit, *Flores v. Reno*, was filed against the INS in 1985. This suit challenged the agency's arrest, processing, detention, and release of minors in its custody (Unaccompanied Minors Project [UMP] 2009). In 1993, the Supreme Court ruled in favor of the INS on many issues, but the parties were able to negotiate a settlement on other key issues, including the detention, release, and treatment of minors in INS custody (Unaccompanied Minors Project [UMP] 2009). These compromises were termed the Flores agreement:

> The Flores agreement recognizes two fundamental principles: (1) minors should be treated with dignity, respect, and special concern for their particular vulnerability; and (2) children should be held in the least restrictive setting possible or, when appropriate, released from detention to an individual or entity willing to ensure the child's safety and timely appearance in immigration court.

When the *Flores v. Reno* settlement agreement was reached in 1997, it established the first consistent standards for the care and treatment of immigrant and refugee minors in INS custody. Many observers noted that the INS continually violated this agreement by failing to follow the settlement's guidelines. When ORR assumed the INS's role in caring for UIMs, it also fell short of meeting the *Flores v. Reno* standards (Taverna 2004). A common violation was excessive use of confinement, handcuffs, and restraints; other violations included placing children in secure facilities when they were not escape risks or delinquents, commingling nondelinquent children with juvenile delinquents, denying minors adequate education, denying children psychological services, failing to explain legal proceedings to youth, failing to provide medium-security facilities for nondelinquent children with special needs, failing to provide adequate access to telephones, and refusing to release children unless the children's undocumented parents and relatives surrendered themselves for removal (Unaccompanied Minors Project [UMP] 2009).

The ORR website clearly delineates its role in being responsible for unaccompanied youth. It notes that the "Division of Unaccompanied Children's Services (DUCS) program recognizes the importance of providing a safe and appropriate environment for UAC from the time they are placed into ORR custody and are reunified with family members or sponsors in the United States or until they are removed to their country of origin by the DHS immigration officials. DUCS takes into consideration the unique nature of each UAC's situation and incorporates child welfare principles when making placement, clinical, case management, and release decisions that are in the best interest of the child" (Unaccompanied Minors Project [UMP] 2009).

The ORR has made many improvements over the INS system: Most detention facilities are nonsecure shelters, foster care is provided in some cases, the overall amount of time spent in the detention facilities has been reduced, and county lock-down facilities are no longer in use (Nugent 2006). To date, there are more than 40 DUCS detention facilities across the nation. These facilities endeavor to ensure that all youth have medical, dental, psychological, and religious needs met within 90 days of placement. In addition, they aim to provide youth with English as a Second Language programs, life skills, tutorials, and social activities. Advocates for UIMs note, however, that the standards outlined by ORR are not always met, and that the detention facilities run by nonprofit agencies under contract with ORR at times fail to commit the resources necessary to keep pace with the increasing number of unaccompanied youth (Unaccompanied Minors Project [UMP] 2009).

Building Infrastructure to Promote the Well-being of Unaccompanied Immigrant Minors: The Immigrant Children Legal and Service Partnership

Despite advances in the US response to the needs of UIMs, ambivalence with regard to the protection of the rights of children has contributed to the slow development of more comprehensive systems of protections and services. This ambivalence is evidenced by the US failure to ratify the Convention on the Rights of the Child, Congress's inability to move forward a discussion about the "H.R. 1172 [109th]: Unaccompanied Alien Child Protection Act of 2005," and the lack of agreement between DHS and ORR on issues such as information sharing, location of facilities, age determination, and provision of services. Ambivalence also fuels a polarized debate on how best to approach the needs of these youth. Should UIMs be treated as humanitarian refugees and victims of hardship circumstances? Should these children be treated as unauthorized immigrants, a cost burden to US citizens, and a potential security threat? Human right advocates view these children as victims of abuse and economic necessity and argue that the government has the responsibility to safeguard their rights and promote their well-being. In contrast, immigration and national security officials link the presence of undocumented immigrants in our communities to increases in illegal activities and argue for stricter enforcement of the law. Not surprisingly, the lack of a clearly articulated commitment from the top to promote the welfare of these youths translates into lack of material and human resources at the community level to attend to multiple legal, health, and social needs of this population. Therefore, a special legal category is required to address the needs of children who enter the United States without documentation, whether accompanied or unaccompanied.

In 2006, a group of citizens concerned over the condition of UIMs in South Florida and the lack of appropriate resources to respond to their needs formed a human services, legal, education, and policy advocacy network dedicated to safeguarding the best interest, welfare, and rights of UIMs in our communities. The Immigrant Children and Legal Services Partnership (ICLASP), as this group is called, is guided by a vision of society in which UIMs are welcome to remain in the United States and have access to human services, legal representation, medical and mental health services, housing, and education that will promote their healthy development and well-being. ICLASP aims to achieve this vision through the creation and dissemination of an integrated, child-centered model of expert legal counsel and advocacy, trauma-oriented mental health services, resilience-building youth development programming, and professional development of staff caring for UIMs in local detention facilities. The ICLASP members include the FIAC, the Clinical Program at Florida University College of Law, the University of Miami Law School Children and Youth Clinic, Victim Services Center, Sisters of the Humility of Mary, and the University of Miami School of Education.

Rather than substituting for existing programs and services provided to UIMs by local detention facilities, ICLASP is designed to strengthen and enhance the ability of these facilities to care for UIMs and help catalyze other community resources to promote the well-being of these children. ICLASP aims to address a core set of needs not met by the facilities by:

1. Providing legal counsel not afforded to UIMs by immigration law.
2. Conducting language-specific and culturally appropriate assessments of children from diverse cultural backgrounds and with limited English proficiency.
3. Providing UIMs with knowledge of the US legal system and the immigration processes, because many such youths have little or no understanding of the system in which crucial decisions about their immigration status are being made.
4. Harnessing expert knowledge of trauma resolution to better respond to the needs of children with histories of victimization and loss.
5. Utilizing expert knowledge of positive youth development strategies and programs to build and sustain UIMs' resilience and sense of hope while waiting through uncertainty for the resolution of their situation.
6. Providing detention facility staff with education in child development and best practices for well-being promotion.

In accordance with this aim, our team of approximately 15 lawyers, law students, psychologists, psychology graduate students, and trauma response professionals provides UIMs with "Know Your Rights" training, individual legal assessment and court representation, culturally and linguistically appropriate mental health services by trained professionals, and participation in a positive youth development program specifically designed for this population (i.e., The Immigrant Children Affirmative Network Program (Aldarondo et al. 2010)). In addition, we provide the administration and staff of the facilities with professional development opportunities in areas of interest to them (i.e., bullying, well-being, sexual development in youth, multicultural communication skills, and problem solving) and serve as community liaison with other community organizations and individual patrons with expert knowledge or material resources that can contribute to the well-being of the youth in the facilities. Within this context, we offer trainings for juvenile and family court judges about immigration requirements for UIMs and interpreter services when needed.

With the financial support of the Children's Trust of Miami, over the past 4 years ICLASP has served more than 1,500 UIMs; created and implemented the only youth development program in the nation specifically designed for this population of youth; and offered trainings and professional development activities to more than

200 judges, lawyers, mental health professionals, community leaders, and care staff at the detention facilities for UIMs. We have made presentations at local and national professional meetings about the plight of UIMs and about how networks of professionals like ICLASP can help strengthen communities' ability to address UIMs' multiple legal, health, and social needs. Moreover, we have cultivated a respectful and collaborative relationship with the ORR even while continuing to advocate for a more comprehensive response from the government.

During this time, we have witnessed with pleasure ORR's growing responsiveness to the mental health needs of this population, and coordinated efforts to assist with its care of UIMs while they remain in the custody of the US government. Local detention facilities now see us a resource for both the children and their organizations and often request our input to address special needs of particular children as they arise. The UIM facilities in our area now resemble social services shelters more than correctional facilities for youth. Although we do not claim credit for the progress made in the care of UIMs in our region, we do believe we have been an important catalytic agent in this process.

Conclusion

Despite all the hardships and perils that stand before them—a raging drug war in Mexico, walls, border agents, National Guard troops, anti-immigrant fervor, and a fragile economy if they even make it—they still come. And they still die, often in the deserts of the Southwest, sometimes at the hands of thieves and kidnappers and now, in a startling twist, at the hands of a drug gang seeking money or possibly recruits.... (Archibold 2010, p. 4).

The presence of unaccompanied immigrant Latino minors in our communities is a reality that must be addressed with policies and programs that go beyond stricter immigration enforcement laws to intentionally and proactively address the needs of these youth. We would do well to emulate recent developments in Australia to protect all UIMs regardless of their legal status: to offer them supervision and settlement support while living among us, provide them access to the full range of government benefits and services available to other children and youth in our communities, and employ expert knowledge to make determinations on how to best respond to their specific educational, social, and medical needs. Our experience with ICLASP makes it abundantly clear that, given the current state of affairs, university–community partnerships can play an important role in advocating for these youths' rights and improving the quality of services and care they receive. Clearly, much more than a local community partnership is needed to successfully address the needs of UIMs in this country and to make significant gains in curtailing the growth of this population. Until such time as our child immigration laws and policies align with the Convention on the Rights of the Child, we are confident that the ICLASP model can help other communities protect and promote the rights and well-being of unaccompanied immigrant youth.

References

Ajdukovic, M., & Ajdukovic, D. (1998). Impact of displacement on the psychological well-being of refugee children. *International Review of Psychiatry, 10*(3), 186–195.

Aldarondo, E., & Ameen, E. (2010). The immigration kaleidoscope: Knowing the immigrant family next door. In B. Risman (Ed.), *Families as they are* (pp. 231–245). New York, NY: Norton.

Aldarondo, E., Ameen, E., Fernandez, M., Virginia, A., Gomez, J., Becker, R., Dulen, S., Weyler, A., Villamar, J., Paula, T., & Diem, J. (2010). *Immigrant Children Affirmative Network (ICAN) program: A practical manual for group facilitation, interprofessional collaboration and training purposes.* Unpublished document. Available from the first author cew@miami.edu.

Almqvist, K., & Broberg, A. (1999). Mental health and social adjustment in young refugee children 3-1/2 years after their arrival in Sweden. *Journal of the American Academy of Child & Adolescent Psychiatry, 38*(6), 723–730.

Archibold, R. (2010, September 1). Grief across Latin America for migrant killings. *The New York Times.* Retrieved from http://www.nytimes.com/2010/09/02/world/americas/02migrants.html

Australian Government. (2007). *Caring for unaccompanied minors.* Retrieved from http://www.immi.gov.au/media/fact-sheets/69unaccompanied.htm

Bean, T., Eurlings-Bontekoe, E., & Spinhoven, P. (2007). Course and predictors of mental health of unaccompanied refugee minors in the Netherlands: One year follow-up. *Social Science & Medicine, 64,* 1204–1215.

Berry, J., Phinney, J., Sam, D., & Vedder, P. (Eds.). (2006). *Immigrant youth in cultural transition: Acculturation, identity and adaptation across national contexts.* Mahwah, NJ: Lawrence Erlbaum Associates.

Bhabha, J., & Schmidt, S. (2006). *Seeking asylum alone: Unaccompanied and separated children and refugee protection in the U.S.* Cambridge, MA: Harvard University Committee on Human Rights Studies.

Bhabha, J., & Young, W. (1999). Through a child's eyes: Protecting the most vulnerable asylum seekers. *Interpreter Releases, 75*(21), 757–791.

Catholic Relief Services. (2010). *Child migration: The detention and repatriation of unaccompanied Central American Youth.* Retrieved from http://www.ccadm.org/ourministries/ump

Cemlyn, S., & Briskman, L. (2003). Asylum, children's rights and social work. *Child & Family Social Work, 8,* 163–178.

Committee on the Rights of the Child. (2005). *General comment no. 6: Treatment of separated and unaccompanied children outside their country of origin.* Geneva, Switzerland: United Nations. (CRC/GC/2005/6)

Department for Child Protection. (2010). *Unaccompanied humanitarian minors.* Retrieved from http://manuals.dcp.wa.gov.au/manuals/cpm/Pages/05UnaccompaniedHumanitarianMinors.aspx

Derluyn, I., & Broekaert, E. (2008). Unaccompanied refugee children and adolescents: The glaring contrast between a legal and a psychological perspective. *International Journal of Law & Psychiatry, 31,* 319–330.

Derluyn, I., Broekaert, E., & Schuyten, G. (2008). Emotional and behavioral problems in migrant adolescents in Belgium. *European Child & Adolescent Psychiatry, 17,* 54–62.

Descilio, T., Greenwald, R., Schmitt, T. A., & Reslan, S. (2010). Traumatic incident reduction for urban at-risk youth and unaccompanied minor refugees: Two open trials. *Journal of Child & Adolescent Trauma, 3*(3), 181–191.

Dreby, J. (2010). *Divided by borders.* Berkeley, CA: University of California Press.

Eschbach, K., Hagan, J., & Rodriguez, N. (1997). *Death at the border.* Houston, TX: Center for Immigration Research.

Ferenci, B. (2000). Separated refugee children in Australia. *International Journal of Refugee Law, 12,* 525–547.

Florida Immigrant Advocacy Center (FIAC). (2006, September). *Unaccompanied immigrant children: Nuts & bolts.* Meeting conducted at FIAC headquarters, Miami, FL.

Garmezy, N., & Rutter, M. (Eds.). (1983). *Stress, coping and development in children.* Baltimore, MD: The John Hopkins University Press.

German, M. (2004). Enabling reconnection: Educational psychologist supporting unaccompanied, separated, asylum-seeker/refugee children. *Educational & Child Psychology, 21*(3), 6–29.

Gonzalez, D. (2004, May 23). Growing number of migrant kids held in U.S. shelters. *The Arizona Republic.* Retrieved from www.azcentral.com.

Goodman, J. H. (2004). Coping with trauma and hardship among unaccompanied refugee youths from Sudan. *Qualitative Health Research, 14*(9), 1177–1196.

Grant-Knight, W., Geltman, P., & Ellis, B. H. (2009). Physical and mental health functioning in Sudanese unaccompanied minors. In D. Brom, R. Pat-Horeczyk, & J. D. Ford (Eds.), *Treating traumatized children* (pp. 102–116). New York, NY: Routledge.

Haddal, C. C. (2009, March). *Unaccompanied alien children: Policies and issues.* (CRS Report for Congress [RL 33896, pp. 1–34]). Washington, DC: Congressional Research Service, Domestic Social Policy Division.

Harvard University Committee on Human Rights Studies. (2006). *Seeking asylum alone.* Retrieved from http://www.humanrights.harvard.edu/images/pdf_files/SAA_Comparative_Report.pdf

Human Rights Watch (1998). *Detained and deprived of rights: children in the custody of the U.S. Immigration and Naturalization Service.* Retrieved from http://www.hrw.org/reports98/ins2/berks98d.htm#P61_1500

Immigration Policy in the United States. (2006, February). *A CBO paper: A series on immigration* (pp. 1–19). Washington, DC: Congress of the United States, Congressional Budget Office.

Jaycox, L., Stein, B., Kataoka, S., Wong, M., Fink, A., Escudero, P., et al. (2002, September). Violence exposure, posttraumatic stress disorder, and depressive symptoms among recent immigrant schoolchildren. *Journal of the American Academy of Child & Adolescent Psychiatry, 41*(9), 1104–1110.

Kinzie, J. D., Sack, W., Angell, R., Manson, S., & Ben, R. (1986). The psychiatric effects of massive trauma on Cambodian children, I: The children. *Journal of American Academy of Child & Adolescent Psychiatry, 23,* 370–376.

Kohli, R. (2007). *Social work with unaccompanied asylum seeking children.* New York, NY: Palgrave Macmillan.

Kohli, R., & Mather, R. (2003). Promoting psychosocial well-being in unaccompanied asylum seeking young people in the United Kingdom. *Child & Family Social Work, 8*(3), 201–212.

Loughry, M., & Flouri, E. (2001). The behavioral and emotional problems of former unaccompanied refugee children 3–4 years after their return to Vietnam. *Child Abuse & Neglect, 25,* 249–263.

Lustig, S., Kia-Keating, M., Knight, G., Geltman, P., Ellis, H., Kinzie, D., et al. (2004, January). Review of child and adolescent refugee mental health. *American Academy of Child & Adolescent Psychiatry, 43*(1), 24–36.

Maegusuku-Hewett, T., Dunkerley, D., Scourfield, J., & Smalley, N. (2007). Refugee children in Wales: Coping and adaptation in the face of adversity. *Children & Society, 21,* 309–321.

Mahoney, S. (2002).TransAtlantic workshop on unaccompanied/separated children: Comparative policies and practices in North America and Europe. *Journal of Refugee Studies, 15,* 102–119.

Nugent, C. (2006, Spring). Whose children are these? Towards ensuring the best interests and empowerment of unaccompanied alien children. *Boston University Public Interest Law Journal, 15,* 219–235.

Pine, B. A., & Drachman, D. (2005). Effective child welfare practice with immigrant and refugee children and their families. *Child Welfare, 84,* 537–562.

Ponizovsky, A., Ritsner, M., & Modai, I. (1999). Suicidal ideation and suicide attempts among immigrant adolescents from the former Soviet Union in Israel. *Journal of the American Academy of Child & Adolescent Psychiatry, 38,* 1433–1441.

Ressler, E. M., Boothby, N. & Stienbock, D. J. (1988). *Unaccompanied children: Care and protection in wars, natural disasters, and refugee movements.* Oxford, UK: Oxford University Press.

Rousseau, D. M. (1995). *Psychological contracts in organizations: Understanding written and unwritten agreements.* Thousand Oaks, CA: Sage Publications.

Rousseau, C., Mekki-Berranda, A., & Moreau, S. (2001, Spring). Trauma and extended separation from family among Latin American and African refugees in Montreal. *Psychiatry, 64*(1), 40–59.

Rousseau, C., Said, T., Gagne, M., & Bibeau, G. (1998). Resilience in unaccompanied minors from the north of Somalia. *Psychoanalytic Review, 85,* 615–637.

Russell, S. (1999). Unaccompanied refugee children in the United Kingdom. *International Journal of Refugee Law, 11,* 126-154.

Scot, S. (2009). *Resilience in undocumented unaccompanied children: Perceptions of the past and future outlook.* Unpublished doctoral dissertation, The Catholic University of American, Washington, DC.

Scott, J. (Producer). (2010, August 4). *Happening now* [Television broadcast]. New York, NY: Fox Broadcasting.

Short, K. H., & Johnston, G. (1997). Stress, maternal distress, and children's adjustment following immigration: The buffering role of social support. *Journal of Counseling & Clinical Psychology, 65,* 494–503.

Smythe, J. (2004). Age determination authority of unaccompanied alien children and demand for legislative reform. *Interpreter Releases,* 81(23), 753–762.

Sourander, A. (1998). Behavior problems and traumatic events of unaccompanied refugee minors. *Child Abuse & Neglect, 23,* 719–727.

Suarez-Orozco, C., & Suarez-Orozco, M. (2002). *Children of immigration* (pp. 16–165) [The Developing Child Series]. Cambridge, MA: Harvard University Press.

Taverna, J. (2004). Did the government finally get it right? An analysis of the former INS, the Office of Refugee Resettlement, and unaccompanied minor aliens' due process rights. *William and Mary Bill of Rights Journal, 12,* 939-977.

Thomas, T., & Lau, W. (2002, June). Psychological well being of child and adolescent refugee and asylum seekers: Overview of major research findings of the past ten years. *National inquiry into Children in Immigration Detention* (pp. 1–24). Australia: Human Rights and Equal Opportunity Commission.

Unaccompanied Minors Project (UMP). (2009). Center for Human Rights and Constitutional Law. Retrieved from http://74.125.47.132/search?q=cache:jwoVLruWDfsJ:immigrantchildren.org/mission/+flores+v.+reno+settlement+agreement+%22mission+and+services%22&cd=1&hl=en&ct=clnk&gl=us&client=firefox-a

UNHCR. (2004, July). *Trends in unaccompanied and separated children seeking asylum in industrialized countries, 2001–2003* (pp. 1–14). Geneva, Switzerland: United Nations High Commissioner for Refugees.

UNHCR. (2009, December). *Guidelines on international protection: Child asylum claims related to the status of refugees* (pp. 1–28). Geneva, Switzerland: United Nations High Commissioner for Refugees.

Wolff, P., Bereket, T., Egasso, H., & Tesfay, A. (1995). The orphans of Eritrea: A comparison study. *Journal of Child Psychology & Psychiatry, 36*(4), 633–644.

Zayas, L. (2010). Protecting citizen-children safeguards our common future. *Journal of Health Care for the Poor & Underserved, 21*(3), 809–814.

Chapter 11
Latinos in Rural Areas: Addressing Mental Health Disparities in New Growth Communities

Sergio Cristancho, Karen E. Peters and D. Marcela Garcés

Abstract Although many communities fail to provide adequate mental health support for immigrants, the problem is particularly evident in rural areas. In these areas, access barriers—geographic isolation, the lack of public transportation systems, and the shortage of health care providers—are particularly acute. In this chapter, we draw on our research and outreach experience with Latino immigrants in the Midwest to illustrate the gaps between this population's needs and the available resources. We also provide some possible strategies for bridging those gaps and make recommendations regarding much needed changes to augment the technical capacity to serve Latinos in rural areas.

While significant progress has been made to respond to the mental health service needs of the Hispanic population in general, relatively little attention has been directed to identifying, understanding and addressing the mental health service problems, concerns and needs of Hispanics/Latinos residing in rural America.

—Soto 2000

Any program focused on building mental health infrastructure for Latinos must address the needs of the growing population of rural immigrants throughout the United States (U.S. Senate 2007). Although Latino immigrants face many mental health threats associated with the migration and acculturation process, overwhelming evidence exists that current mental health infrastructures are both insufficient and inadequate to meet their needs (Atdjian and Vega 2005; Lopez 2002; Sentell et al. 2007; Stroul and Blau 2008; Vega and Lopez 2001; U.S. Department of Health and Human Services [DHHS] 2001, 2003). The implications of these structural shortcomings are serious. Often, the system remains unresponsive until the situation has escalated to violence, substance abuse, or other serious family disruption (Klostermann and Kelley 2009).

S. Cristancho (✉)
College of Medicine, University of Illinois, Rockford, IL, USA

Facultad Nacional de Salud Pública, Universidad de Antioquia, Medellín, Colombia
e-mail: scrista@uic.edu

Although many communities fail to provide adequate mental health support for immigrants, the problem is particularly evident in rural areas. In these areas, access barriers—geographic isolation, the lack of public transportation systems, and the shortage of health care providers—are particularly acute (U.S. Department of Health and Human Services [DHHS] 1999, 2001; Gamm et al. 2003; Mueller et al. 1999; Murray and Keller 1991; Ricketts 1999). In this chapter, we draw on our research and outreach experience with Latino immigrants in the Midwest to illustrate the gaps between this population's needs and the available resources. We also provide some possible strategies for bridging those gaps, and make recommendations regarding much needed changes to augment the technical capacity to serve Latinos in rural areas.

The chapter is organized as follows. First, we review the experiences of immigrant Latinos who have settled in rural areas, and give an overview of the health care service provision landscape in these areas. We follow this discussion with an overview of the mental health needs of newly arrived Latino immigrants in the upper Midwest, and the challenges associated with meeting their needs. Next, we discuss our research program with the rural Latino population and present some key findings from that research. Finally, we provide recommendations for ways to overcome these gaps and ultimately improve the health and well-being of the rural Latino population.

Challenges in Meeting the Mental Health Needs of Latino Immigrants in the Rural United States

The growing Latino migration to rural areas of the United States (Kandel and Cromartie 2004) challenges both immigrants and their host communities (Fry 2008; Kochhar et al. 2005). For immigrants, the migration process itself can be challenging both physically and psychologically. Many are separated from their families and encounter stressful events on their journey to the United States. For some, traumatic experiences include enduring life-threatening conditions when crossing the border, being physically or sexually victimized, being financially exploited, or witnessing the injury or death of others. These experiences can be so devastating that post-traumatic stress disorder (PTSD), depression, substance abuse, and anxiety disorders may develop in this population (Hitchen 2009).

Although the promise of employment opportunities draws immigrants to rural communities, finding decent work can be extremely challenging for newcomers. Available work is often physically demanding, low paying, uncertain, and sometimes dangerous. Laborers work nights, double shifts, and weekends, experiencing high pressure for increased productivity. They suffer mistreatment from supervisors or other co-workers, and are frequently uncertain as to how long the job will last (Gouveia and Stull 1995). In rural Illinois, immigrants work long hours in the service sector or in industries such as food processing, meat packing, and car assembly, in plants where the risk of injury from occupational hazards is high and little compensation is available for work-related injuries (Blewett et al. 2003).

Immigrants also face significant family and adjustment pressures (Berry and Ataca 2000; Berry and Sam 1997). Many send significant portions of their salary to their families back home. When they are not working, they encounter a society with a very different language and culture than their native culture (U.S. Department of Agriculture [USDA] 2005). Cultural differences have health behavior and health status implications (Betancourt and Fuentes 2001). The geographic dispersion of the rural population and the individualistic culture of the United States (Triandis 1994) contribute to social isolation and loneliness. The long work hours, lack of public transportation options, and limited English proficiency make it particularly difficult for newcomers to establish new friendships.

Recently arrived immigrants in the upper Midwest, most of whom arrive from rural areas of Mexico, confront simple logistical challenges as well. Many arrive during the winter months when they encounter climates that they are neither accustomed to nor prepared for. The winter months in northern rural areas of the United States require additional—and often expensive—protective clothing such as coats and boots. Snow equipment such as shovels, salt, blowers, and plows are unknown in their native countries. Moreover, because of the lack of public transportation, many newcomers without access to a car must depend on others for their transportation needs.

For the host communities, the influx of new immigrants raises several challenges. Immigrants may be perceived as a threat because they are sometimes seen as "taking away" limited employment opportunities from native-born residents. Community members may conflate negative stereotypes such as low levels of education with criminality, and thus perceive new immigrants as a threat to local security. In addition, questions of whether to share public resources and increase linguistic access often mask larger questions of social inclusion and community belonging (Engstrom 2006; Piedra 2006). Questions we have heard from non-Latino rural residents during our field research include: "Why should these Latinos benefit from my tax contributions by using our public library, driving on our streets, or using our local school system?" or "Why do they speak Spanish in public places if the official language in the US is English?" These comments reflect a subtle form of discrimination that, when experienced by Latinos on a daily basis, may be psychologically damaging (Pérez et al. 2008; Sanchez and Brock 1996).

Within this context, rural Latinos with mental health needs find a lean service environment composed of service providers who, until recently, did not need to consider linguistic and cultural differences in their client population. The current state of rural health and mental health services, therefore, calls for the creation of new health and mental health infrastructures to serve the population at large and, more specifically, to provide services tailored to the Latino population. The delivery of such infrastructure requires creativity in how current structures are used and in the development of new ones. It also requires an understanding of the current infrastructure, a topic we take up next.

Rural Health Care Landscape

For most of its history, the United States has been an agricultural nation with the majority of its population residing in rural areas. The period between 1850 to1910, however, was one of great industrial growth that fueled increased urbanization. The 1920 census marked the first time that the urban population exceeded the rural population. Since then, urban areas have continued to drive most of the nation's growth (Glasgow et al. 2004). In comparison, the rural population growth rate of the United States has remained fairly stable, with rural residents currently representing approximately 20% of the total US population, or a total of 55 million (U.S. Census Bureau 2008). Specifically, of the 55 million, about 46 million (84%) are non-Latino White, 4.5 million (8%) are Black, 2.6 million (5%) are Latino, 870,000 are American Indian/Alaska Native, and 745,000 are Asian/Pacific Islanders (U.S. Census Bureau 2005).

The rural health infrastructure is plagued with challenges. It has inadequate transportation systems for emergency response, as well as a shortage of personnel and funds (Peters and Gupta 2009c). Hospital closures in recent years have left many without a source of care within a reasonable driving distance (Peters and Gupta 2009c). The lack of public transportation options and lower levels of employer-based health insurance, prescription drug coverage, and Medicaid further compound the problem, resulting in rural populations having lower access to both primary and specialty care than urban residents (Gamm et al. 2003; Mueller et al. 1999; National Rural Health Association [NRHA] 2010; Starfield and Fryer 2007). The health of rural individuals is further compromised by fewer opportunities for economic advancement, fewer or no educational opportunities, and a weak political power base at the policy-making level (Geyman 2000). Disadvantages in economic, educational, and political capital translate into higher rates of chronic illness and disability and poorer overall health status. Reflecting these factors, recent federal data (Centers for Disease Control and Prevention [CDC] 2010) indicate that rates of heart disease, cancer, and diabetes are higher in rural areas, and that the rural population is less likely to use preventive screening services and engage in regular physical activity than the urban population.

Differences in health care service delivery are also striking. Although 20% of the US population lives in rural areas, only about 10% of physicians practice there, a factor that significantly limits access to general primary care (Rabinowitz et al. 2005). Similarly, sizeable disparities exist in the distribution of specialists. In rural areas, there are 40.1 specialists per 100,000 residents, compared to 134.1 in urban areas (NRHA 2010). Rural hospitals, a critical organization in the health care system, receive considerably less Medicare reimbursement than urban hospitals (90% vs. 100% payment-to-cost ratio), and Medicare spends 15% less per capita on rural patients compared to urban patients (NRHA 2010). The closing of more than 470 rural hospitals over the past 25 years highlights the negative impact of Medicare reimbursement policy on rural health care infrastructure (Ricketts 1999).

Funding for health care services in rural areas is closely related, in fact, to policy decisions. Definitions of *rural* at the federal and state levels dictate the allocation of funds and determine which rules and regulations apply to health and mental health programs serving these communities. Nevertheless, this term remains subject to conceptual difficulties due to a lack of consensus on how to define it. For example, the US Census Bureau defines *rural* as 2,500 persons living in an incorporated place (U.S. Census Bureau 2005), whereas the Office of Management and Budget defines *rural* at the county level, using terminology such as "metropolitan," "micropolitan," or "non-metropolitan" in designating counties (Cromartie and Bucholtz 2008). The USDA, in turn, has created several classifications within the non-metropolitan county designation and uses a scaled approach to classify the degree of "rurality" of an area (NRHA 2010).

To promote the development of health infrastructure for underserved communities, the federal government designates counties or parts of counties as health professional shortage areas (HPSAs), mental health HPSAs (MH-HPSAs) or medically underserved areas (MUAs). These area designations create eligibility for federal and state grant programs for clinic construction, practitioner recruitment and placement programs, and increased Medicare and Medicaid reimbursement payments. The majority of HPSAs ($n = 2,157$) and MH-HPSAs ($n = 910$) are in rural areas. Strikingly, 79% of non-metropolitan counties are MH-HPSAs. This designation reflects the fact that 20% of non-metropolitan counties do not have mental health services, compared with 5% in metropolitan counties. Moreover, more than half of the nation's rural counties do not have a licensed psychologist or psychiatrist (Rabinowitz et al. 2005). The lack of mental health service providers in rural areas—a key component of any mental health infrastructure—has a profoundly detrimental effect on the mental health status of rural residents, particularly Latinos who may require specialized or tailored services due to language barriers and immigration status concerns.

Federally Qualified Healthcare Centers (FQHCs) and local public health agencies are two health care system infrastructure components that play a critical role in rural health. Often the provider of last resort, FQHCs and public health agencies may be the only sources of care available in rural areas. Compared to their urban counterparts, these health care organizations are generally smaller, have less staff, and fewer staff with mental health training. Smaller operating budgets and limited technical capacity constrain their ability to provide mental health services (Primm et al. 2010). Thus, these agencies are often unprepared to address those who present service delivery challenges.

To gain an understanding of rural Latinos' mental health service needs, we designed a research program that we implemented in the upper Midwest. In the next section, we present our research model and discuss some key findings that provide a context for the infrastructure gaps and recommendations we identify in a subsequent section of this chapter.

Research Model and Key Findings with Mental Health Infrastructure Implications

Our team has devoted several years to the identification of health and mental health disparity issues for rural Latinos, and has identified effective ways to bridge some of the identified gaps. During the past decade, we have undertaken 3 large investigations with 10 rural communities throughout the state of Illinois. One of them was part of the Project EXPORT Center for Excellence in Rural Health Disparities Research funded by NIH/NCMHD, which focused on identifying major health concerns and barriers to health care for rural Latinos. Another one was the "*Mentes Sanas, Cuerpos Sanos*" Project on mental health, chronic disease, and acculturation among Latino immigrants, funded by the CDC through the National Association for Chronic Disease Directors (NACDD). Finally, we undertook the "Acculturation and Cardiovascular Disease" study among rural Latino immigrants, funded by the University of Illinois Excellence in Academic Medicine Program. Products from this work include published articles, reports, and unpublished manuscripts (Cristancho et al. 2010; Cristancho et al. 2009; Cristancho et al. 2008; Peters et al. 2009a, 2010). We begin the section with a conceptual overview of our work, including our conceptual model and choice of research methodology. This will provide a useful context for the findings and implications presented in the remainder of the chapter.

According to Lopez (2002), investigations that have the greatest capacity to transform existing community-based infrastructures and services are those that draw on multidisciplinary perspectives and are informed by multiple stakeholders (e.g., service providers, consumers, policymakers). Thus, in our work we used participatory and community-based approaches, which allowed communities to be actively involved in identifying and addressing priority mental health concerns, and empowered community leaders and organizations throughout the research process (Casey et al. 2004). Specifically, we developed an approach we term Community-Based Participatory Action Research (CBPAR). CBPAR borrows from participatory action research through its commitment to social transformation using research, community engagement, and communicative action (Fals-Borda 1987; Habermas 1984; Lewin 1946). It also draws on community-based participatory research, given that the investigation is grounded in a social justice agenda, exhibits scientific rigor, involves diverse partnerships, and focuses on an ecological model of health (Israel et al. 2005; Israel et al. 2003).

Broadly, CBPAR begins by forming or strengthening existing partnerships with community members. A community-based needs assessment occurs concurrently with relationship building. Next, with a complete assessment and established relationships, the partners devise and carry out an implementation plan to address priority issues, followed by an evaluation. Finally, the partners develop a plan to disseminate the results of the project to relevant audiences, such as other communities, organizations, providers, policymakers, and academics. These various phases are iterative, suggesting that several cycles are needed to build community capacity around a certain issue. We have found that, within each of these large phases, it is important to: (a) explore all the available options in order to make an informed decision; (b) select the best approach; (c) reflect individually and collectively about each decision made and the role of each participant; and (d) maintain permanent communication within the partnership and to external actors. In our work in the upper Midwest, we used CBPAR in partnership with several rural Latino immigrant communities to understand their mental health status and infrastructure needs. Consistent with our model, here we present findings from our assessment phase, as well as a description of several approaches we discovered during the implementation phase to address mental health disparities.

Assessment Phase: Key Findings

The CBPAR assessment phase uncovered a troubling picture, in which residents have great mental health service needs, yet have little access to services in a context ill prepared to meet their needs. The key findings associated with the need for mental health services infrastructure are:

- The majority (52%) of immigrant Latinos surveyed did not have health insurance. Those who had been in the United States for less than five years represented a high proportion of the uninsured (72%). Longer residency in the United States increased the likelihood that individuals would have some type of health insurance more than twofold (Amezola et al. 2006).
- Qualitative data showed that there is a severe shortage of Spanish-speaking health and mental health providers. Furthermore, those who do serve Latinos have limited capacity to understand their cultural beliefs and backgrounds. Moreover, there is an alarming lack of interpreters to facilitate patients' communication with English-speaking monolingual providers (Cristancho et al. 2008).
- There is a high prevalence of self-reported mental health conditions. Participants reported greater concern about problems with depression (26%), stress (17%), and anxiety (9%) than with physical conditions such as obesity (8%), diabetes (6%), and cancer (5%). Similarly, they reported suffering from mental problems more often than from physical problems (Peters et al. 2009a).
- The majority of participants (55%) reported experiencing depression or another emotional problem during the past 30 days. This proportion differed as a function of time in the United States, with the highest prevalence among those who had been US residents for less than 5 years (76%), followed by those who had lived in the United States between 5 and 10 years (51%), and more than 10 years (50%) (Cristancho et al. 2009).
- Compared to men, women reported a lower quality of life, more days with mental and physical health problems, and more sleepless nights (Peters et al. 2009a).
- As length of US residence increased, so did perceptions of social support from trusted others, close friends, and relatives in the community (Peters et al. 2009a).
- To obtain health information, rural Latinos reported a preference for workshops in Spanish in community settings. A preference for mailed printed materials increased in the second generation (Cristancho et al. 2010).

Based on our findings from the assessment phase, we worked with communities to develop action plans and strategies to address their top mental health needs. Thus, during the implementation phase we addressed a number of key infrastructure needs.

Table 11.1 Community assessment findings and corresponding implementation strategies

Community	Assessment Findings	Implementation Strategies
Community A	• High levels of stress, anxiety, depression, and loneliness • Difficulties in family life in United States and distance from social support in home country • Economic pressures due to job loss	• Created speaker series on depression and stress • Sponsored sports leagues • Offered social support groups (gender specific) • Developed health resource directory/newsletter • Offered social activities promoting physical activity through walking clubs
Community B	• Feelings of isolation due to legal status issues and family separation • Language barriers between Latinos and mental health care providers • Lack of health knowledge	• Offered social/recreational activities • Offered classes at the multicultural center (language, cooking, computers) • Offered health fair
Community C	• Concern with mental health issues, obesity, and dental problems • Legal issues • Limited or inadequate medical interpretation • Lack of support groups	• Established social clubs • Sponsored community workshops
Community D	• High levels of stress, loneliness, insomnia, depression, and domestic violence • Discrimination and lack of self-esteem • Lack of community resources	• Provided bilingual counseling services • Sponsored workshops on depression, stress, and anxiety
Community E	• High levels of depression, stress, loneliness, and fear • Concern about substance abuse and violence • Lack of location for activities	• Organized Family Nights at local community center • Sponsored workshops • Sponsored sports leagues

Implementation Phase

During the implementation stage, community groups developed several different approaches to address their mental health services infrastructure needs (see Table 11.1), which they subsequently implemented with our professional and monetary support. Given the stipulations of a small grant we had obtained from the CDC/NACDD, the budget for each of the five communities was US $5,000, with a one-year implementation period.

As indicated in Table 11.1, there are similarities and differences in the way communities addressed their needs. The strategies addressed a wide range of issues depending on the community's needs. For example, some communities created a speaker series where Latino health professionals addressed mental health topics and provided the community with a forum to ask questions. Other counties established social clubs based on age groupings to increase the community's involvement in activities that promote mental health and well-being, provided vouchers for exercise and fitness facilities, sponsored "family nights" with movies and family-friendly activities in a local community center, and provided bilingual mental health counseling services at a local community facility free of charge. Mental health topics prioritized by rural Latino communities for educational workshops included parenting advice (e.g., cultural norms, substance abuse, cultural identity, academic performance, adolescent sexuality), cultural adaptation, adult sexuality, stress, anxiety (e.g., PTSD as a result of traumatic events in the home country or of the immigration process), and depression (seasonal depression was particularly relevant in the winter months).

In our research, we noted that mental health promoters helped serve as liaisons between the partnerships and community members, and also acted as mental health educators. To avoid the negative stereotyping associated with the concept of mental health, we suggest calling these persons *"promotores de bienestar"* (which literally translates to "promoters of well-being"). Moreover, our research communities succeeded in developing community-based mental health infrastructure and created a coalition known as the *Alianza*. Members of the *Alianza*, in collaboration with the research team, shared their experiences with federal government agencies and other local and state venues, and they advocated for the local development of infrastructure to facilitate the delivery of services (Peters et al. 2009a). The lack of an existing transportation infrastructure generates particular concern among the *Alianza*. The resolution of transportation barriers remains critical in the development of infrastructures that address mental health and health care needs of rural populations.

Taken together, the assessment data and implementation experiences of the five communities underscore the need to conceptualize rural Latino mental health as a complex and multifaceted construct: (a) encompassing both positive and negative dimensions, (b) having various social determinants (Adler Institute on Social Exclusion 2010), (c) involving not only individuals but also their unique social environment (e.g., family, community), (d) being context-dependent, and (e) being inclusive of acculturation processes. For example, Community B (see Table 11.1) prioritized services to address social isolation because many of its members suffered from family separation, language barriers, and legal status issues. They also prioritized lifestyle issues, including diet, exercise, and sleep. Based on this prioritization, they proposed an action plan that included social/recreational activities, classes in the multicultural center (cooking, swimming, martial arts, nutrition, legal issues, etc.), and a community health fair. They used mini-grant resources to provide incentives to community members to attend the activities (e.g., monthly gift cards) and to pay for two *promotores de bienestar* who helped recruit community participants and implement the exercise component. As a result, 20 people (10 adults and 10 children) are exercising regularly at local recreation facilities. They also paid for 200 copies of an exercise brochure and a community newsletter. Finally, they paid for health education activities, including workshops on depression and immigrant legal issues. The variety of actions implemented by this community highlight the importance of developing mental health infrastructure for rural Latinos based on a multifaceted definition of mental health.

Our evaluation showed that the programming implemented in the five participating communities was very effective in addressing basic mental health infrastructure needs among local Latino community members, despite the limited budget we had at our disposal. For example, these are qualitative quotes from committee members in response to our request to summarize the main benefits this program has had for the community (Peters et al. 2009b):

- "We can provide services to the community and the opportunity to receive professional help with mental health problems."
- "Latinos are exercising. They are less isolated and their health is improving. Others see, hear and read about Latinos exercising. This affects their attitudes, knowledge and eventually, their behaviors. Latinos learn about health and legal issues. Leadership development and mentoring."
- "Youth leaders participated freely and with great enthusiasm, kids, teens and elderly participants."

Recommendations for Infrastructure Improvements

Given the complex and multifaceted nature of mental health and the many mental health issues faced by rural Latino communities, we advocate for infrastructure development that strengthens the provision of services along a prevention-oriented continuum. Consistent with the Institute of Medicine (IOM), we conceptualize prevention for the mental health field in terms of three core activities: prevention, treatment, and maintenance (IOM 1994). Broadly, *prevention* is aimed at avoiding the onset of mental health problems, whereas treatment and maintenance are aimed at minimizing their impact at the individual, family, and community levels. As a result, *prevention* should encompass mental health promotion and education, patient navigation services, and effective patient–provider communication strategies. *Treatment* and *maintenance* should include a focus on inpatient and outpatient treatment services and the coordination of mental health care plans and systems for follow-up. In addition, part of the infrastructure to support the provision of these activities requires attention to *program administrative* elements, including ongoing service evaluation, dissemination of program or treatment options, advocacy for mental health awareness raising, and access to treatment and competent care. In the remainder of this section, we provide recommendations organized by levels of prevention.

Prevention Activities

We urge the development of new programs and the tailoring of existing programs to reflect the priorities of the particular community, as indicated by

community-focused assessments. Current mental health promotion and patient education efforts assume that Latinos have high levels of health literacy and reflect a preference for printed materials and other impersonal strategies. In most cases, these printed materials are just a literal translation of those available to the majority population, and thus fail to influence Latinos. The absence of basic prevention-oriented services through community-level mental health promotion and educational outreach warrants attention. However, offering these services requires access to bilingual and bicultural mental health professionals, or at least to qualified interpreters, as well as extensive outreach efforts. To implement these services, we recommend hiring a coordinator (to handle recruitment, logistics, etc.) and Spanish-speaking (and ideally also bicultural) mental health professionals (e.g., psychologists, counselors, social workers, nurses, educators). The sites where these activities are held should be Latino-friendly, with culturally sensitive staff; ideally, the physical environment would recreate Latinos' favorite decoration patterns, music, videos, and other elements, thus developing a sense of identity and ownership. For example, there should always be Spanish-speaking staff available to Latino patients in the reception area. Bilingual signage would help guide the rural Latino consumer within the facility. Institutional waiting rooms may have available mental health promotion materials in Spanish other than printed materials; these might include videos or other interactive strategies to present mental health promotion information. Offering a means for transportation to community activities is highly desirable, as distance from the workplace or home to community sites may be a barrier to accessing these services in rural contexts.

Facilities within the existing infrastructure (e.g., clinics, schools) should broaden their activities and collaborate with other organizations to meet mutually compatible goals. For example, health care clinics could meet the interests of schools by promoting early childhood literacy and giving parents and children books (Butera et al. 2000; Willis et al. 2007). Likewise, schools could offer physical space for satellite clinics for health screenings for parents and tailor health promotion materials for both children and their parents. By sharing resources across physical spaces and coordinating services through enhanced communication systems (Leisey 2009), a rural infrastructure could be developed to better serve the community. Because of language barriers and the shortage of bilingual providers, such coordination is essential in assisting Latino immigrants who live in rural parts of the country (Partida 2007).

Treatment and Maintenance Activities

Health care organizations should supplement their current outreach strategies by recruiting, hiring, and training *promotores* or community liaisons who could assist rural Latinos to access the local resources that are available to them and help them navigate the US mental health care system. Such a remedy would go far in helping rural Latinos acquire a basic understanding of the health and mental health care system, especially given the alarming scarcity of bilingual health and mental personnel. Therefore, infrastructure-building efforts must prioritize making navigation services more readily available to rural Latinos.

We propose the name of *"promotores de bienestar"* (well-being promoters) for peer community workers (Arcury and Quandt 2007; Rhodes et al. 2007; Swider 2002). *Promotores* can go door-to-door in Latino neighborhoods to assess each household's specific needs and offer resources to address their needs. They can also offer advice to community members on issues such as basic health rights, transportation, insurance, access to psychotherapy and medications, support groups, and referral and translation services. Based on their knowledge of the mental health care system and of the local social service institutions, *promotores* can advocate for patients who have had difficulties accessing mental health care or promotion services. They can also develop access plans, disseminate maps to the local mental health care facilities, and deliver educational workshops to community members regarding how to access these resources. Finally, a strategy that we think might help with the navigation component is to provide Hispanic community-based organizations (HCBOs) and mental health care providers with support through small mini-grants to develop these access and navigation plans and their related resources, as we have done in the upper Midwest.

Program Administration

Engage in advocacy at the policy level to increase funding for, and awareness of, mental health risks of and treatment options for rural Latinos. Policy advocacy is essential for mental health infrastructure development in rural areas. Community organizations should engage in advocacy at local, state, and national levels to promote a healthy infrastructure. For example, advocating for linkages that bridge service sectors is essential to building an infrastructure that will improve the delivery of health and mental health services (Probst et al. 2004). Among these linkages, we recommend the creation of satellite clinics in schools and churches and the use of mobile units, to increase the number of service entry points and facilitate triage of less serious problems.

In addition, community members themselves can have a powerful voice in advocacy at the policy level. For example, through the *Alianza* coalition, community members have advocated at the local, state, and federal levels for actions such as the creation of public transportation systems and the recruitment of bilingual mental health care providers. They have also applied for larger funding opportunities and exchange experiences and resources to improve and enhance the impact of their local action plans.

Conclusions

Rural communities are underresourced, and experience a myriad of economic and social pressures just to survive. The influx of new Latino immigrants to rural areas presents both additional challenges to and exciting possibilities for rural America today. We contend that a healthy rural Latino population is critical to the survival and rebuilding of the rural United States.

An effective mental health infrastructure must include a continuum of services for promoting well-being and prevention, and should allow patients to access treatment at multiple sites in the community. Traditionally, mental health service treatment has focused on the individual, without regard for the social determinants that may cause or exacerbate the individual's condition. Creation of an effective mental health infrastructure for Latino immigrants in rural communities must take into account the social and environmental life circumstances that impinge upon individuals' lives. Through our experiences, we found that the CBPAR approach, which allows the community to be proactive and participate in social change, can effectively diminish the health disparities experienced by rural immigrant Latinos. The availability of high-quality services for all community members, including those who are newly arrived, is a social justice priority and will be a critical and necessary contribution to the restoration and well-being of rural communities.

Acknowledgment We acknowledge the contributions to this chapter made by Latinos living in several rural communities of Illinois that have participated in our projects (Beardstown, Belvidere, Carbondale, Cobden, DeKalb, Effingham, Galesburg, Monmouth, Rochelle, Rockford), and to the Hispanic Health Advisory Committees in those communities. We are specially indebted to community leaders Benito Luna, Evaristo Rodriguez, José Acosta (Beardstown), Earl Mainland (Belvidere), Cathy Bless, Flora Chacón (Carbondale), Aurelia Zargoza (Cobden), Gilda Madrid, Tricia Wagner, Carla Raynor (DeKalb), Rosie Gibbons (Effingham), Tony Franklin (Galesburg), Al Kulczewski (Monmouth), Vicky Bross (Rochelle), and Pat Gomez and Ed Flores (Rockford).

Projects that informed portions of this chapter were funded by National Institutes of Health/National Center on Minority Health and Health Disparities (NIH/NCMHD) (Grant No. P20 MD0000524), Centers for Disease Control and Prevention (CDC) (Grant No. CDC U48/CDC U509661), National Association of Chronic Disease Directors (NACDD), and Excellence in Academic Medicine at the University of Illinois College of Medicine at Rockford (Grant No. G7111). We also acknowledge the support we received at various stages of our community work from Ben Mueller, Michael Glasser, and Carlos Aguero, as well as the valuable comments on earlier drafts of this manuscript provided by the editors (Drs. Buki and Piedra). Research assistance was provided by Emilio Araujo, Adriana Bautista, Isidro Gallegos, Sunanda Gupta, Brittney Lilly, Cindy Harper, Lora Oswald, Gloria Rincón, María Silva, Ellen Smith-Blokus, and Alejandra Valencia.

References

Adler Institute on Social Exclusion. (2010). *Social determinants of mental health definition.* Chicago, IL: Adler School of Professional Psychology. Retrieved June 30, 2010, from http://www.adler.edu/about/SocialDeterminantsofMentalHealthDefinition.asp

Amezola, C., Mueller, B., & Peters, K. (2006, March 29). *Association between length of residence and Hispanic healthcare access in rural Illinois.* Poster presentation at the University of Illinois College of Medicine at Rockford Research Day, Rockford, IL.

Arcury, T. A., & Quandt, S. A. (2007). Delivery of health services to migrants and seasonal farmworkers. *Annual Review of Public Health, 28,* 345–363.

Atdjian, S., & Vega, W. A. (2005). Disparities in mental health treatment in U.S. racial and ethnic minority groups: Implications for psychiatrists. *Psychiatric Services 56,* 1600–1602.

Berry, J. W., & Ataca, B. (2000). Cultural factors in stress. In G. Fink (Ed.), *Encyclopedia of stress* (Vol. I, pp. 604–611). San Diego, CA: Academic Press.

Berry, J. W., & Sam, D. (1997). Acculturation and adaptation. In J. W. Berry, M. H. Segall, & C. Kağitçibaşi (Eds.), *Handbook of cross-cultural psychology: Vol. 3. Social behavior and applications* (2nd ed., pp. 291–326). Boston, MA: Allyn & Bacon.

Betancourt, H., & Fuentes, J. L. (2001). Culture and Latino issues in health psychology. In S. S. Kazarian & D. R. Evans (Eds.), *Handbook of cultural health psychology* (pp. 306–323). San Diego, CA: Academic Press.

Blewett, L. A., Smaida, S. A., Fuentes, C., & Zuehlke, E. U. (2003). Health care needs of the growing Latino population in rural America: Focus group findings in one Midwestern state. *Rural Health Policy, 19,* 33–41.

Butera, G., McMullen, L., & Phillips, R. (2000). Energy express: Connecting communities and intervention on behalf of schoolchildren in West Virginia. *Journal of Research in Rural Education, 16*(1), 30–39.

Casey, M. M., Blewett, L. A., & Call K. T. (2004). Providing health care to Latino immigrants: Community-based efforts in the rural Midwest. *American Journal of Public Health, 94*(10), 1709-1711.

Centers for Disease Control and Prevention. (2010). *Behavioral risk factor surveillance system survey data.* Retrieved August 1, 2010, from http://apps.nccd.cdc.gov/BRFSSBib/SearchV. asp?type=0&Search=rural

Cromartie, J., & Bucholtz, S. (2008). Defining the "rural" in rural America. *Amber Waves 6*(3), 28–35.

Cristancho, S., Garcés, M., & Peters, K. (2010). *Health information preferences among rural Hispanic immigrants in the Midwest: Length of residence and socio-demographic variations.* Manuscript submitted for publication.

Cristancho, S., Garcés, M., Peters, K., & Aguero, C. (2009). *Identification of key acculturation dimensions associated with cardiovascular health behavior change and maintenance in Hispanic immigrants* (Final report, Grant No. G7111). University of Illinois College of Medicine at Rockford, Excellence in Academic Medicine Program.

Cristancho, S., Garcés, D. M., Peters, K., & Mueller, B. (2008). Listening to rural Hispanic immigrants in the Midwest: A community-based participatory assessment of major barriers to health care access and use. *Qualitative Health Research, 18*(5), 633–646.

Engstrom, D. W. (2006). Outsiders and exclusion: Immigrants in the United States. In D. W. Engstrom & L. M. Piedra (Eds.), *Our diverse society: Race and ethnicity—Implications for 21st century American society* (pp. 19–36). Washington, DC: Routledge.

Fals-Borda, O. (1987). The application of participatory action-research in Latin America. *International Sociology, 2*(4), 329–347.

Fry, R. (2008). Latino settlement in the new century. Retrieved June 1, 2010, from Pew Hispanic Center at http://pewhispanic.org/files/reports/96.pdf

Gamm, L. D., Hutchinson, L. L., Dabney, B. J., & Dorsey, A. M. (2003). *Rural health people 2010: A companion document to Healthy People 2010* (Vols. 1–3). College Station, TX: The Texas A&M University System Health Science Center, School of Rural Public Health, Southwest, Rural Health Research Center.

Geyman, J. (2000). *The handbook of rural medicine.* New York, NY: Wiley.

Glasgow, N., Morton, L., & Johnson, N. E. (2004). *Critical issues in rural health.* Ames, IA: Blackwell.

Gouveia, L., & Stull, D. D. (1995). Dances with cows: Beefpacking's impact on Garden City, Kansas and Lexington, Nebraska. In D. D. Stull, M. J. Broadway, & D. Griffith (Eds.), *Any way you cut it. Meat processing and small-town America* (pp. 85–108). Lawrence: University of Kansas Press.

Habermas, J. (1984). *The theory of communicative action: Vol 1.Reason and the rationalization of society.* Boston, MA: Beacon Press.

Hitchen, A. R. (2009). *A systematic utilization review of a community mental health program for Latinos* (School of Professional Psychology Paper 67). Retrieved December 3, 2010, from http://commons.pacificu.edu/spp/67

Institute of Medicine. (1994). *Reducing risks for mental disorders: Frontiers for preventive intervention research.* Washington, DC: National Academy Press.

Israel, B. A., Eng, E., Schulz, A. J., & Parker, E. A. (2005). *Methods in community-based participatory research for health.* San Francisco, CA: Jossey-Bass.

Israel, B. A., Schulz, A. J., Parker, E. A., Becker, A. B., Allen, A., & Guzman, J. R. (2003). Critical issues in developing and following community-based participatory research principles. In M. Minkler & N. Wallerstein (Eds.), *Community-based participatory research for health* (pp. 56–73). San Francisco, CA: Jossey-Bass.

Kandel, W., & Cromartie, J. (2004). *New patterns of Hispanic settlement in rural America* (Rural Development Research Report 99). Washington, DC: Economic Research.

Klostermann, K., & Kelley, M. L. (2009). Alcoholism and intimate partner violence: Effects on children's psychosocial adjustment. *International Journal of Environmental Research & Public Health, 6*(12), 3156–3168.

Kochhar, R., Suro, R., & Tafoya, S. (2005). *The new Latino south: The context and consequences of rapid population growth.* Retrieved June 1, 2010, from Pew Hispanic Center at http://pewhispanic.org/files/reports/50.pdf

Leisey, M. (2009). The Journey Project: A case study in providing health information to mitigate health disparities. *Journal of the Medical Library Association, 97*(1), 30–33.

Lewin, K. (1946). Action Research and minority problems. *Journal of Social Issues, 2,* 34–46.

Lopez, S. R. (2002). Mental health care for Latinos: A research agenda to improve the accessibility and quality of mental health care for Latinos. *Psychiatric Services, 53,* 1569–1573.

Mueller, K., Ortega, S., Parker, K., Patil, K., & Askenazi, A. (1999). Health status and access to care among rural minorities. *Journal of Health Care for the Poor & Underserved, 10,* 230–249.

Murray, J. D., & Keller, P. A. (1991). Psychology and rural America: Current status and future directions. *American Psychologist, 46*(3), 220–231.

National Rural Health Association. (2010). *What's different about rural health care?* Retrieved August 1, 2010, from http://www.ruralhealthweb.org/go/left/about-rural-health/what-s-different-about-rural-health-care

Partida, Y. (2007). Addressing language barriers: Building response capacity for a changing nation. *Journal of General Internal Medicine, 22*(2), 347–349.

Pérez, D. J., Fortuna, L., & Alegría, M. (2008). Prevalence and correlates of everyday discrimination among U.S. Latinos. *Community Psychology, 36*(4), 421–433.

Peters, K., Cristancho, S., & Garcés, M. (2009a). *Acculturation and mental health effects on chronic disease among Hispanic/Latino immigrant populations* (Final report for the National Association for Chronic Disease Directors and the Centers for Disease Control and Prevention, Grant No. 2008-04547).

Peters, K., Cristancho, S., Garcés, M., Bautista, A., Araujo, E., Madrid, G., et al. (2009b). *Acculturation, mental health, and chronic diseases: Findings from the Mentes Sanas, Cuerpos Sanos (healthy minds, healthy bodies) Hispanic/Latino immigrant project.* Presentation by invitation at the U.S. Centers for Disease Control and Prevention (CDC), National Center for Chronic Disease Prevention and Health Promotion, Division of Adult and Community Health, Community Health and Prevention Services Branch, Atlanta, GA.

Peters, K. E., & Gupta, S. (2009c). Geographic barriers to healthcare. In R. Mullner (Ed.), *Encyclopedia of health services research* (2009 ed., Vols. 1–2). Thousand Oaks, CA: Sage.

Peters, K., Cristancho, S., & Garcés, M. (2010, June 3–4). *Participatory approaches to community mobilization around mental health and chronic disease among rural Hispanic immigrants.* Adler Institute for Professional Psychology Annual Conference, "Social Determinants of Mental Health: From Awareness to Action," Chicago, IL.

Piedra, L. M. (2006). Revisiting the language question. In D. W. Engstrom & L. M. Piedra (Eds.), *Our diverse society: Race and ethnicity—Implications for 21st century American society* (pp. 67–87). Washington, DC: NASW Press.

Primm, A. B., Vasquez, M. J., Mays, R. A., Sammons-Posey, D., MicKnight-Elly, L. R., Presley-Cantrell, L. R., et al.(2010).The role of public health in addressing racial and ethnic disparities in mental health and mental illness. *Preventing Chronic Disease, 7*(1), 1–7.

Probst, J. C., Moore, G. C., Glover, S. H., & Samuels, M. E. (2004). Person and place: The compounding effects of race/ethnicity and rurality on health. *American Journal of Public Health, 94*(10), 1695–1703.

Rabinowitz, H. K., Diamond, J. J., Markham, F. W., & Rabinowitz, C. (2005). Long-term retention of gradates from a program to increase the supply of rural family physicians. *Academic Medicine, 80*(8), 728–732.

Rhodes, S. D., Foley, K. L., Zometa, C. S., & Bloom, F. R. (2007). Lay health advisor interventions among Hispanics/Latinos: A qualitative systematic review. *American Journal of Preventive Medicine, 33*(5), 418–427.

Ricketts, T. C. (1999). *Rural health in the United States.* New York, NY: Oxford University Press.

Sanchez, J. I., & Brock, P. (1996). Outcomes of perceived discrimination among Hispanic employees: Is diversity management a luxury or a necessity? *Academy of Management Journal, 39*(3), 704–719.

Sentell, T., Shumway, M., & Snowden, L. (2007). Access to mental health treatment by English language proficiency and race/ethnicity. *Journal of General Internal Medicine 22*(suppl. 2), 289–293.

Soto, J. J. (2000, May 30). Mental health services issues for Hispanics/Latinos in rural America. *In Motion Magazine.* Retrieved September 1, 2010, from http://www.inmotionmagazine.com/soto4.html

Starfield, B., & Fryer, G. E. (2007). The primary care physician workforce: Ethical and policy implications. *Annals of Family Medicine, 5,* 486–491.

Stroul, B. A., & Blau, G. M. (Eds.). (2008). *System of care handbook: Transforming mental health services for children, youth, and families.* Baltimore, MD: Paul H. Brookes.

Swider, S. M. (2002). Outcome effectiveness of community health workers: An integrative literature review. *Journal of Public Health Nursing, 19*(1), 11–20.

Triandis, H. C. (1994). *Culture and social behavior.* New York, NY: McGraw-Hill.

U.S. Census Bureau. (2005). *Population distribution in 2005.* Retrieved August 1, 2010, from http://www.census.gov/population/www/pop-profile/files/dynamic/PopDistribution.pdf

U.S. Census Bureau. (2008). *American community survey 1-year estimate.* Retrieved August 1, 2010, from http://factfinder.census.gov/servlet/DatasetMainPageServlet?_program=ACS&_submenuId=&_lang=en&_ts=

U.S. Department of Agriculture. (2005). Rural Hispanics at a glance. *Economic Information Bulletin, 8* (December). Retrieved August 3, 2010, from http://www.ers.usda.gov/publications/eib8/eib8.htm

U.S. Department of Health and Human Services. (1999). *Mental health: A report of the Surgeon General—Executive summary.* Rockville, MD: U.S. Department of Health and Human Services, Substance Abuse and Mental Health Services Administration, Center for Mental Health Services, National Institutes of Health, National Institute of Mental Health.

U.S. Department of Health and Human Services. (2001). *Mental health: Culture, race, and ethnicity—A supplement to Mental Health: A Report of the Surgeon General.* Rockville, MD: U.S. Department of Health and Human Services, Substance Abuse and Mental Health Services Administration, Center for Mental Health Services.

U.S. Department of Health and Human Services. (2003). *Achieving the promise: Transforming mental health care in America* (Pub. No. SMA-03-3832). Rockville, MD: President's New Freedom Commission on Mental Health.

U.S. Senate. (2007). 110th Congress, 1st Session, Amendment S. 2183 on Part H—Community-based mental health infrastructure improvements. Sec. 560, Grants for community-based mental health infrastructure improvements. Retrieved July 26, 2010, from http://frwebgate.access.gpo.gov/cgi-bin/getdoc.cgi?dbname=110_cong_bills&docid=f:s2183is.txt.pdf

Vega, W. A., & Lopez, S. R. (2001). Priority issues in Latino mental health services research. *Mental Health Services Research 3,* 189–200.

Willis, E., Kabler-Babbitt, C., & Zuckerman, B. (2007). Early literacy interventions: Reach out and read. *Pediatric Clinics of North America, 54*(3), 625–642.

Part IV
Reflections on Service Opportunities in Latino Mental Health

Chapter 12
Life During and After Breast Cancer: Providing Community-based Comprehensive Services to Latinas

Jennifer B. Mayfield and Lydia P. Buki

Abstract Breast cancer can have a significant impact on the emotional and psychological well-being of Latinas who are diagnosed with the disease. Although psychosocial interventions can alleviate the psychological distress experienced by survivors, the benefits of psychosocial support remain elusive for many Latina women due to lack of access to mental health services in their community. To meet the rising need for services among Latina breast cancer survivors, new infrastructures are needed to increase access to culturally congruent and comprehensive mental health services. Within this chapter, we propose that community-based nonprofit organizations can play a key role in the expansion of mental health services for Latina breast cancer survivors. First, we describe the range of psychological concerns of breast cancer survivors to underscore the need for mental health services. Next, we present a model of comprehensive mental health services within the nonprofit sector. The final section provides further infrastructure recommendations for narrowing this critical mental health services disparity.

Despite having a longer lifespan than other populations in the United States (Arias 2010), Latinos have more negative outcomes than non-Latino Whites across a range of health conditions, including cancer, diabetes, and HIV (Beard et al. 2009; Centers for Disease Control and Prevention 2007; Institute of Medicine 2002). Factors that influence Latinos' health outcomes include difficulty accessing quality care, lack of health insurance, linguistic barriers, low levels of health literacy and formal education, cultural health beliefs, low incomes, and institutional racism in health care (Buki and Selem 2009; Institute of Medicine 2002, 2004; Livingston et al. 2008). One area of documented health disparity influenced by these factors is breast cancer survivorship among Latinas. Breast cancer is the most common form of cancer and the leading cause of cancer deaths among Latinas; approximately 14,200 women were expected to be diagnosed with breast can-

J. B. Mayfield (✉)
University of Illinois at Urbana-Champaign, 127 Huff Hall, 1206 S. Fourth St., Champaign, IL 61820, USA
e-mail: jaymay03@gmail.com

cer in 2009 and 2,200 cancer deaths were expected to occur (American Cancer Society 2009). Although Latina women have a lower incidence of breast cancer than non-Latina White women, they are diagnosed at younger ages and at more advanced stages of the disease, and with more aggressive types of tumors than non-Latina White women (Ashing-Giwa et al. 2007; Bauer et al. 2007; Patel et al. 2010; Shavers et al. 2003). Furthermore, although breast cancer incidence has decreased among women across racial/ethnic groups, Latinas' incidence has decreased at a lower rate than that of non-Latina White women. Among breast cancer survivors, Latinas report the lowest health-related quality of life of women in all ethnic groups (Ashing-Giwa et al. 2007).

To cope with the psychological impact of breast cancer, Latinas would benefit from mental health services in conjunction with their traditional cancer treatment regimen. However, research shows that they have limited access to mental health support services (Buki and Grupski 2010; Ell et al. 2005; Nápoles-Springer et al. 2007), despite evidence that psychological interventions can be effective in enhancing the quality of life of breast cancer survivors (Ganz et al. 2004). Buki and Grupski (2010) surveyed 40 programs nationwide that provide psychosocial supports for Latina breast cancer survivors and found serious service gaps. About 80% of the program administrators reported that they were unable to meet Latina breast cancer survivors' needs adequately with current resources, a fact that is particularly troubling because they also experienced a significant increase in demand for services over the past several years—a trend that is expected to continue given demographic projections. Similarly, in a study of women with breast or gynecological cancers, the majority of whom were Latina, Ell et al. (2005) found that among participants who met criteria for moderate or severe depression, only 6% perceived having emotional support from family or friends, 4% reported seeing a social worker or mental health counselor, and 2% reported attending a support group.

Within this chapter, we assert that lack of access to mental health services hinders Latina women's ability to reap the benefits that supportive services would provide. Thus, a need exists to expand mental health services to support Latinas who have been diagnosed with breast cancer. Such an expansion requires new infrastructures that are equipped to provide comprehensive mental health services. We argue that community-based nonprofit organizations can play a key role in the expansion of mental health services for Latinas with breast cancer. Toward this end, we illustrate one comprehensive service model that has dual goals of (a) narrowing the breast cancer health disparity gaps created by socioeconomic and cultural barriers, and (b) providing culturally competent mental health services to Latina breast cancer survivors. Thus, we start with a discussion of psychological concerns of breast cancer survivors, to provide a foundation for the ensuing discussion of how these needs can be met effectively at the community level. Next, we discuss the role that nonprofit organizations can potentially play in expanding the service infrastructure for Latina women by illustrating the service model of *Nueva Vida*, a nonprofit, community-based organization dedicated to providing psychosocial support to Latina breast cancer survivors. The chapter ends with specific recommendations for continued infrastructure building.

Psychological Concerns Among Latina Breast Cancer Survivors

In this section, we focus on three areas of documented concern among breast cancer survivors: depression, body image, and social support. Although there is a growing literature on Latina breast cancer survivors, a much larger literature exists documenting the breast cancer experience for non-Latina White women. Thus, we have structured this section such that for each area, we present the broad literature first, followed by a more specific focus on the experience of Latina women.

Depression

Among breast cancer survivors, depression commonly arises with the feelings of fear, shock, sadness, disbelief, and anger associated with a serious medical condition (Ell et al. 2005; Golden-Kreutz and Andersen 2004). The emotional upheaval experienced by cancer survivors can escalate into major depression; if a breast cancer survivor develops depression soon after her initial diagnosis, it can negatively affect her psychological adjustment to the disease over time and lead to increased risk of mortality (Badger et al. 2004; Burgess et al. 2005; Dausch et al. 2004; Pinquart and Duberstein 2010). Researchers have found that depressive symptoms among breast cancer survivors can persist up to five years after the initial diagnosis (Burgess et al. 2005). Depressive symptoms can also increase according to the severity of the disease (Love et al. 2004). Women diagnosed with an advanced cancer with a poor prognosis are more likely to experience moderate levels of depression compared to women diagnosed with cancer at an earlier stage and with a more optimistic forecast (Love et al. 2004).

Research has shown that depression is a major concern for Latina breast cancer survivors (Bower 2008; Dwight-Johnson et al. 2005). In one study of 269 Latina patients diagnosed with either breast or gynecological cancer, researchers found that 25% of the women suffered from major depression or exhibited symptoms of dysthymia (Dwight-Johnson et al. 2005). In another study, researchers found that among 472 breast or gynecological cancer survivors—the majority of whom identified as Latina—24% experienced moderate to severe depression and 30% of those suffering from depression were breast cancer survivors (Ell et al. 2005).

Although fear and sadness related to the cancer diagnosis can lead to depression among Latinas, financial worries and uncertainty about the physical and psychological consequences of cancer treatment contribute to their depressive symptoms (Ashing-Giwa et al. 2006; Ashing-Giwa and Lim 2010; Buki et al. 2008; Campesino et al. 2009; Ell et al. 2005). Moreover, in comparison to non-Latina Whites, Latinas report a disproportionate burden of family stress and role strain, financial pressure, and work disruption, factors that may contribute to lower levels of psychological well-being (Ashing-Giwa and Lim 2010).

Body Image Concerns

Many breast cancer treatments cause serious physical side effects, such as weight gain, hair loss, and body disfigurement, that alter a patient's physical appearance (Avis et al. 2004). Therefore, breast cancer survivors also report body image concerns. Two common surgical interventions for removal of cancerous tissue in the breast are lumpectomies and mastectomies. *Lumpectomy* (also known as *breast conservation therapy*) involves the removal of cancerous tissue and a small amount of normal tissue surrounding the tumor (American Cancer Society 2010). This procedure can create scar tissue, which leads to swelling, redness, or hardening in the area of the lump excision. Breast cancer survivors report higher satisfaction with their outward body appearance and shape when they opt for a lumpectomy to conserve their breasts rather than a mastectomy (Metcalfe et al. 2004), a choice that is available to women in less advanced stages of the disease (Fisher et al. 2002). *Radical mastectomies* (involving the removal of the entire breast and muscle wall) can lead to disfigurement of a woman's chest. Removal of the axillary (underarm) lymph nodes through axillary dissection procedure can lead to a condition known as *lymphedema*, which causes tight, swollen, or painful arms. Lymphedema occurs in up to 42% of women treated for breast cancer (Norman et al. 2008).

Post-surgical treatments administered to prevent the recurrence of cancer (known as *adjuvant therapies*), such as chemotherapy and radiation, also have unwanted physical side effects. Such side effects include hair loss, dry or reddened skin, premature menopause, and sexual dysfunction (American Cancer Society 2010; Beckjord and Compas 2007). These side effects are particularly distressing for younger women, who often worry about how these physical changes might affect their sexual lives and their romantic relationships (Beckjord and Compas 2007). Moreover, the side effects associated with cancer treatments can severely disrupt breast cancer survivors' daily routine and their ability to maintain their roles in family or work situations (Ashing-Giwa and Lim 2010; Paskett and Stark 2000).

Latina women are more likely than non-Latina White women and African-American women to experience sexual disruption after a breast cancer diagnosis, and have reported feeling unattractive, less feminine, and having a decreased libido (Christie et al. 2009; Spencer et al. 1999). Also, Latina breast cancer survivors have reported embarrassment, feelings of inadequacy, lack of self-worth, and feelings of frustration concerning weight gain (Ashing-Giwa et al. 2004), and more physical symptoms than women of other ethnicities (Ashing-Giwa et al. 2007; Giedzinska et al. 2004). Negative physical side effects accompany increased distress, social disruption, alienation from self, and fear of future adverse outcomes, further compromising women's psychological health and well-being (Petronis et al. 2003).

Social Support

Social support represents an important coping strategy that helps women manage the distress associated with a breast cancer diagnosis (e.g., depression, anxiety, fear of recurrence; Alfano and Rowland 2006; Ashing-Giwa et al. 2004). In general, people with dependable and intimate social support networks are least likely to seek professional help for their personal problems and report fewer mental health effects such as depression, anxiety, or decreased quality of life (Parker et al. 2003; Taylor and Stanton 2007). Social support networks offer women the opportunity to express their emotions, vent about their problems, and either decrease the perceived importance of the problem (e.g., breast cancer diagnosis) in their lives or serve as a distraction from the problem (Cohen 2004). In a review of the cancer support literature, Alfano and Rowland (2006) concluded that patients who receive psychosocial support services fare better than those who do not, and that areas of functioning positively influenced by intervention include stress, mood, physical functioning, health-related quality of life, and self-efficacy, among others.

Thus, as would be expected, perceived social support among Latina breast cancer survivors is associated with lower distress levels (Alferi et al. 2001; Ashing-Giwa et al. 2006). Support networks help Latinas cope with the feelings of fear, worry, denial, and concern that arise as a result of disruption of their caregiver role in their family systems (Ashing-Giwa et al. 2004; Galván et al. 2009). Family, close family friends, other survivors, and health care providers are essential sources of social support for Latina breast cancer survivors (Ashing-Giwa et al. 2004; Galván et al. 2009). However, when Latinas experience emotional distress for prolonged periods, the emotional burden can erode the social support they receive from family and friends (Alferi et al. 2001).

Inadequate social support networks place breast cancer survivors at risk for more severe psychological problems, such as higher levels of distress, lower emotional well-being, social disruption, and avoidance of cancer-related thoughts and stimuli (Figueiredo et al. 2004; Zakowski et al. 2004). Consistent with these findings, Latina breast cancer survivors, in comparison with women of other ethnicities, have reported lower levels of support, higher levels of distress and uncertainty, lower quality of life, and poorer mental health (Ashing-Giwa et al. 2007; Carver et al. 2006; Sammarco and Konecny 2010). Women who are least acculturated, speak Spanish only, and have financial problems appear to be at greatest risk for low social support, in part because they have significant barriers to obtaining support from health care professionals (Ashing-Giwa et al. 2006; Janz et al. 2009). Unfortunately, these are often the women most in need of professional supports.

However, negative psychological outcomes can be buffered with greater provision of social support. Research shows that Latinas who access support groups reap psychological benefits from the experience (Ashing-Giwa et al. 2006; Galván et al. 2009; Nápoles-Springer et al. 2007), such as (a) emotional support, validation, and reassurance; (b) help with learning how to express their feelings; (c) instillation of hope and the belief that they can survive; (d) information related to survivorship;

(e) empowerment and greater self-efficacy; and (f) ability to communicate freely in Spanish about their condition (Galván et al. 2009; Nápoles-Springer et al. 2007). In fact, support groups are an especially appropriate intervention for Latina breast cancer survivors, as they have reported feeling more comfortable speaking with their peers than with family members (who may believe that cancer is fatal or may not fully understand the women's experience; Ashing-Giwa et al. 2006). Arguably, support groups may provide a way to preserve existing family supports, which women perceive as critically important to their well-being (Ashing-Giwa et al. 2004; Galván et al. 2009), because their assistance means the woman need not overtax the family system and erode this critical source of support (Alferi et al. 2001).

Mental Health Service Gap

Given the risk for mental health sequelae that include depression, body image concerns, and need for social support among Latina breast cancer survivors, there exists a need for psychosocial interventions to help women gain the information and support they need to cope with a breast cancer diagnosis (Alfano and Rowland 2006; Institute of Medicine 2005). Unfortunately, the majority of medical hospitals do not integrate psychosocial interventions with their traditional cancer treatment regimens, and women's mental health needs are left largely unmet by the health care system (Institute of Medicine 2005). When support services exist at all, they are in English, are expensive, and require private health insurance, creating virtually insurmountable barriers for Latinas who need these services (Institute of Medicine 2005). Thus, support networks provided by community organizations, and accessing affordable mental health services through such agencies, may be the best option for Latinas without health insurance or with limited English proficiency to receive additional care outside of their informal social support networks.

The Role of Nonprofits in Provision of Breast Cancer Psychosocial Services

Many breast cancer survivors turn to community-based nonprofit organizations to receive support for issues that extend beyond their clinical and pharmacological needs, such as educational or financial aid programs, child care and transportation, and mental health counseling (Grieve 2003; Shelby et al. 2002). A number of nonprofit organizations have emerged in response to both the absence of government-based services and the lack of public support for breast cancer research (Altman 1996; Grieve 2003). These organizations advocate for the creation of public policy related to breast cancer issues and for increased psychosocial support for breast cancer survivors (Altman 1996; Grieve 2003).

Some pioneering women set up their own grassroots organizations in response to the absence of reliable breast cancer information from doctors and the government. For instance, in 1975 Rose Kushner campaigned to increase women's knowledge of breast cancer and treatment options with her book, *Breast Cancer: A Personal History and Investigative Report*. She subsequently established the Women's Breast Cancer Advisory Center (later renamed the Rose Kushner Breast Cancer Advisory Center) (Altman 1996). Since then, additional nonprofit organizations have emerged, such as The Sister Network (n.d.), Y-Me (currently known as the Breast Cancer Network of Strength; Altman 1996), and Living Beyond Breast Cancer (n.d.). These organizations created a space for women to share their experiences related to the breast cancer diagnosis, to inform them of their rights as patients, to encourage open communication between patients and their physicians, and to provide information about the disease and treatment options (Altman 1996). In the 1990s, the National Breast Cancer Coalition (NBCC) gained much clout through its advocacy for critical public policy initiatives (e.g., increased NIH funding for breast cancer research) and for the education and treatment rights of underserved and uninsured breast cancer survivors (National Breast Cancer Coalition 2006). Founded by Fran Visco, a lawyer who left her law-firm position after her own breast cancer diagnosis, the organization's efforts have led to major accomplishments, including an 800% increase in breast cancer research funding (from $ 90 million in 1991 to $ 800 million in 2003) (National Breast Cancer Coalition 2006).

As the number of breast cancer support organizations has grown, so have the number of ethnic minority women diagnosed with the disease. Many community-based nonprofit breast cancer organizations have recognized that women's knowledge and perceptions of breast cancer may differ by their racial, ethnic, or cultural background, and thus they must tailor outreach initiatives to address the needs of specific populations. However, such a call to service is not without its challenges. The complexities involved in recruiting culturally competent staff and board members, overcoming language barriers, and maintaining culturally appropriate program objectives threatens the sustainability of the organizations and their programs (Ramakrishnan and Viramontes 2006). Culturally, many nonprofit organizations that focus on a particular racial or ethnic population have few precedents upon which to model their services, because so few mainstream organizations tailor their services to meet the needs of racial and ethnic minority groups (Ramakrishnan and Viramontes 2006). Therefore, it is not surprising that despite the positive impact that nonprofit organizations have on the lives and treatment options of breast cancer survivors, little can be found in the research literature concerning how nonprofit organizations serving Latina breast cancer survivors face these cultural and economic challenges while meeting the needs of their community stakeholders and continuing to thrive. Given the purposes of this chapter in illustrating infrastructure building for Latinas with breast cancer, we expand current discourse in this area by highlighting the work of an organization, *Nueva Vida*, that was established in response to the unmet need for culturally tailored mental health services in Spanish for this population.

Meeting the Psychosocial Needs of Latina Breast Cancer Survivors: *Nueva Vida*

Nueva Vida is a Washington, DC-based nonprofit organization incorporated in 1999 in response to the need for psychosocial services for Latina breast cancer survivors. Its goals include (a) increasing knowledge and awareness about breast cancer in terms of early detection and treatment in the Latina community, and (b) providing support services to Latina women who have been diagnosed with breast cancer. The development of *Nueva Vida* merits attention. In January 1994, a group of mental health professionals working in a public health clinic that served Latinos noticed an increase in referrals for cancer survivors. Because the primary care providers observed that patients diagnosed with cancer were also reporting symptoms of anxiety and depression, they simultaneously referred the patients for mental health services. As the demand for mental health services grew, mental health providers supplemented individual therapy and psychiatric services by establishing a formal support group for patients diagnosed with cancer. Over time, this group became overwhelmingly attended by women.

As services expanded, it became increasingly clear to the staff that the clinic was an unsuitable place for hosting the groups. The building had an inadequate heating and cooling system and a faulty electrical system. Additionally, the support group members were required to climb three flights of stairs to attend the meetings. Because the building posed potential health hazards to cancer survivors, the staff tried to host the group meetings in an alternate location. Unfortunately, insurance liabilities stymied their efforts. Thus, with little recourse, the staff began to draft a plan to provide supportive group services independent of the clinic. In 1995, they received a grant from the Susan G. Komen Breast Cancer Foundation, a nonprofit organization that provides funding to decrease breast cancer health disparities, to support the cancer survivor support group. Subsequently, the group was moved to a local hospital in Washington, DC, where the meeting space was comfortable, accessible through public transportation, and met requirements for insurance liability. However, as a result of the stipulations of the grant, the group developed a focus on breast cancer and became less diverse in terms of cancer types and gender.

In 1997, the breast cancer support group was developed into a more formal psychoeducational program named *Nueva Vida* (which means "New Life" in Spanish). As time passed, the founders began to realize the potential of *Nueva Vida* to become a formal organization. In collaboration with several professional volunteers, such as psychologists, lawyers, and accountants, *Nueva Vida* became incorporated as an independent nonprofit organization in 1999 and eventually grew to become the first and largest dedicated provider of psychosocial support services to Latina breast cancer survivors in the nation. The organization's mission is to develop a collaboration of health care professionals, members of the Latino community, and Latina breast cancer survivors to provide culturally appropriate support services to Latina cancer survivors (*Nueva Vida* (n.d.), "Who We Are" section). It strives to serve every client who enters its doors with a cancer diagnosis by facilitating access to medical treatment and providing psychosocial support and psychotherapy services. The majority of the organization's clients are Latina breast cancer survivors who are recent immigrants, have low socioeconomic status, and have limited English language proficiency.

Structure of Nueva Vida

The founders of *Nueva Vida* conceptualized the psychosocial needs of Latina breast cancer survivors from a holistic perspective, recognizing that an interplay of biological, psychological, and social factors have a significant effect on breast cancer survivors' mental health. Therefore, the founders strove to provide an array of mental health services to address the complex needs of their clients, and the following three programs emerged: the Mental Health Support Program, the Access Program, and the Navigation Support Program. The Mental Health Support Program represents the evolution of *Nueva Vida,* from consisting of only one general social support group for cancer survivors to providing more extensive therapeutic services designed to assist Latina breast cancer survivors as they cope with the psychological and emotional toll of cancer. The need for an even broader range of support services led to the implementation of the Access Program and the Navigation Support Program, to ensure that survivors were receiving appropriate medical treatment for their cancer as well as to decrease social, economic, and political barriers to their access to medical and mental health services. The purpose of the Access Program is to link Latina women to available diagnosis and treatment services in local clinics, hospitals, and research institutions, regardless of their health insurance or immigration status. For example, the staff may refer clients to a free mammogram program offered by a local hospital or to a clinical trial that offers free diagnosis or treatment services. The Navigation Support Program provides assistance to Latina breast cancer survivors in their interactions with the medical system and in their communication with health care providers. Latinas with limited English proficiency are often referred to bilingual Spanish/English physicians or are provided with an interpreter. Furthermore, the Access Program and the Navigation Support Program work in tandem to connect Latina breast cancer survivors with various types of social services, including transportation, child care, food service (e.g., Meals on Wheels), and assistance with applications for Medicaid and cancer screening and treatment programs.

Each of the three programs has a coordinator who oversees the function of the individual program and the work of additional staff and volunteers within the program. The Mental Health Program has additional staff, consisting of a small team of female licensed professional counselors who work with the organization part-time and provide individual counseling services. The organization also relies on a group of volunteers to provide additional support services when needed for the Access, Navigation Support, and Mental Health Programs. All of the staff members are bilingual in Spanish and English; thus, they are able to reach and serve women who are limited English proficient in addition to those who are English monolingual. Given the focus of this chapter, we focus the remainder of the discussion on the structure and activities associated with the Mental Health Program.

Structure of the Mental Health Support Program

Nueva Vida's Mental Health Support Program is organized to provide Latina breast cancer survivors convenient access to mental health services such as individual and group therapy and peer support. When a new client contacts the organization to receive services, the Mental Health coordinator asks questions regarding the client's personal background and cancer diagnosis in order to triage and refer her for appropriate services. If the client's needs can be adequately met by the services provided by *Nueva Vida*, then she is referred to a support group and given the option of receiving individual therapy as well. If the client does not have metastatic cancer (i.e., cancer that has spread to other regions of the body, which leads to increased risk of mortality), then the client is assigned a community peer counselor for an additional source of support. Clients with metastatic cancer are always connected with a professional counselor who is trained to deal with end-of-life issues.

The Mental Health Support program offers one hour of individual therapy on a weekly basis, either within *Nueva Vida*'s offices or at the client's home, depending upon the client's preference. The weekly therapy sessions also include one to two follow-up phone conversations each week. Therefore, counselors involved in individual counseling may interact with each client approximately two to three hours per week, a nontraditional model that has worked well with this population.

Compañeras de Apoyo ("Support Companions"), a peer support program, was developed to provide *Nueva Vida*'s new clients the opportunity to make connections with other Latina breast cancer survivors who understand the experiences and challenges in dealing with a cancer diagnosis. The program is volunteer based and includes Latina breast cancer survivors who have participated in the support groups for at least a year, and are at least one year past their cancer diagnosis and treatment. Typically, volunteers have completed their cancer treatment regimens and are now in remission. These peer support workers participate in a formal training session at least twice a year. Topics covered in the sessions include communication styles, the needs of a newly diagnosed person, ways to be respectful and nonintrusive, and basic counseling skills. The peer support workers are asked to engage in only two phone conversations with their support partner so that the volunteers do not become overwhelmed with the task. Additionally, peer support workers are not paired with women who have metastatic cancer, in order to protect the volunteers from the emotional burden associated with forming a close connection to a person with a terminal diagnosis. The organization does not have difficulty recruiting volunteers for the peer support program. In fact, women often volunteer because they believe that helping others will aid in their own personal healing process as well.

On one Saturday each month, the organization sponsors a psychoeducational general support group that is conducted in Spanish. Each group follows the same basic format: (a) introduction of support group participants; (b) presentation of a psychoeducational topic; (c) personal sharing and discussion of the group topic; (d) guest speaker regarding a self-care technique (e.g., Tai Chi); (e) group chorus of an inspirational song, "Gracias por la Vida" (Thank you for life); and (f) refreshments and socialization. Sample psychoeducational topics covered in past sessions include: Family, Friends, and Cancer Diagnosis; Sexuality and Breast Cancer; Spirituality and Breast Cancer; Alternative, Complementary Medicine and Breast Cancer; Myths about Breast Cancer; Advocacy and Breast Cancer; Emotional Reactions of Breast Cancer Diagnosis, Treatment, and Recovery; Coping with Pain; and Smiles and Laughter: A Positive Effect on the Cancer Experience. To assist with transportation issues, the meetings are held at a hospital that has a public bus stop on campus. The staff also offer rides to the clients, if needed.

Typical group therapy protocols require members to attend sessions on a regular basis for a set period of time and to disclose any plans to leave the group. However, because many of *Nueva Vida's* clients are low-income wage earners, this traditional approach to group therapy is not feasible for clients. The participating women often have limited flexibility with regard to their work schedules and family obligations. This means that, for a breast cancer survivor who works 12-hour shifts including weekends without opportunities for supplemental child care, committing to support group meetings more than once a month may be a considerable hardship. In lieu of attending each group meeting regularly, some women may only attend the group a few times a year, depending on their schedules.

On alternate Saturdays when the general support group is not held, the Mental Health Support Program hosts an Open House within *Nueva Vida*'s office suite. The Open House allows Latina breast cancer survivors and women at risk to visit *Nueva Vida*'s office and participate in an orientation meeting concerning the services provided, including the Mental Health Support Program. Moreover, a staff member provides a bilingual (Spanish/English) introduction to the written health education materials located on the bookshelves within the organization. The staff also offer a packet of handouts for clients to take home. Refreshments are served at the end of the meeting and participants are able to socialize with other Open House attendees, as well as the staff.

Recommendations for Infrastructure Building

As the only organization in the United States to provide comprehensive, culturally appropriate psychosocial services to Latina breast cancer survivors, *Nueva Vida* offers a model of care for those interested in assisting Latinas with cancer. The staff credits the holistic nature of their psychosocial services programs for the success of the organization as a source of support for Latinas. As *Nueva Vida* grew as an organization, it became evident that Latina breast cancer survivors' psychological and emotional well-being are inextricably linked with their access to medical treatment and their ability to support their family financially, a finding borne out in research as well (Ashing-Giwa et al. 2006; Ashing-Giwa and Lim 2010; Buki et al. 2008). The counselors in the Mental Health Services Program realized that they could not adequately treat Latina breast cancer survivors' psychological concerns without addressing their access to quality and affordable cancer early detection and treatment. By reaching out to meet the needs of Latinas beyond their intrapersonal concerns, the staff created an organization flexible enough to provide an integrated approach to mental health. They are able to refer women in need of medical interpreter services to the Navigation Support Program, uninsured women who need cancer treatment to the Access Program, and women battling depression to the Mental Health Support Program.

Nueva Vida's model of therapeutic service provision to Latina breast cancer survivors reflects an appreciation for the unique way the process of cancer survivorship (i.e., coping with psychological distress and adjusting to disruption of life roles, as well navigating the health care system) affects the Latino community and how socioeconomic status, immigration, and culture influence survivorship. The use of this knowledge is foundational in the development and implementation of culturally appropriate treatment protocols. Additionally, meeting unmet health care needs requires that service providers collaborate with other breast cancer programs at the county, state, and federal levels, national breast cancer organizations, local hospitals, and research institutions. For instance, *Nueva Vida*'s staff often refers Latina breast cancer survivors to a local hospital that provides mammograms for the uninsured. Women are also referred to research programs that offer free detection and treatment services for breast cancer survivors who are willing to participate in a clinical trial.

In addition to offering a broad range of psychosocial services, mental health service providers should allow for flexibility in their psychotherapy protocols to accommodate the cultural and social demands of Latina breast cancer survivors. Such accommodations may call for a diversion from traditional therapeutic models. For instance, group therapy participants typically commit to regular attendance at sessions based on a specific schedule. However, the *Nueva Vida* group facilitators realized that because many clients have inconsistent work schedules, regular attendance at support group meetings was not feasible for many survivors. Therefore, the organization offers an "open" therapy group, where regular attendance is not required and women can join the group as needed without causing an additional disruption in their lives. *Nueva Vida* also offers individual therapy as an alternative course of treatment for women who are experiencing psychological or emotional distress but cannot attend the support group regularly. Their individual therapy services are offered within the client's home or in an office at *Nueva Vida*, depending on the client's preference. Recognizing the many burdens on low-income women, counselors conduct telephone check-ins during the week to monitor the clients' status and convey a concern for their well-being.

The ongoing cultivation of multicultural competence among staff must underlie mental health service provision to Latina breast cancer survivors. Because Latina breast cancer survivors have come from diverse cultural, economic, and political backgrounds, these factors may have a strong influence on a client's course of psychotherapy. For instance, *Nueva Vida*'s staff recognizes that the socioeconomic and political conditions of their clients' countries of origin, as well as their cultural or spiritual beliefs, play an important role in the client's coping mechanisms and decision-making processes regarding health. The organization creates a supervision culture within the mental health program that encourages counselors to self-reflect on how their own sociocultural backgrounds and biases may affect their clinical work with clients and to use this increased awareness for professional growth.

Finally, given the instrumental role counselors play in any mental health services program, continual professional development of staff must be seen as a standard practice. *Nueva Vida* requires that all counselors within the Mental Health Support Program receive professional supervision and support while leading support groups. The organization also encourages self-care among counselors, given that dealing with difficult psychological issues such death and mortality may put the counselors at risk of becoming emotionally overwhelmed.

Conclusion

Breast cancer presents not only physical challenges for Latina breast cancer survivors, but also mental health concerns such as depression, negative body image, and inadequate social support. Unfortunately, the existing infrastructure has few resources available where breast cancer survivors can seek psychosocial services. Lack of health insurance, limited English proficiency, lower socioeconomic status, and difficulty in securing child care or transportation are just a few of the significant barriers for survivors' access to care.

Nueva Vida serves as a model of the potential that nonprofit organizations have to bridge the gap in psychosocial services in the Latina community. Nonprofit, community-based organizations must provide mental health services that are affordable, available in Spanish as well as English, and accommodate survivors' work and family obligations. We conclude this chapter with the hope that the information we have provided will assist other organizations as they develop infrastructures designed to address survivors' psychosocial needs in a culturally congruent and holistic manner.

References

Alfano, C., & Rowland, J. (2006). Recovery issues in cancer survivorship: A new challenge for supportive care. *Cancer Journal, 12*(5), 432–443.

Alferi, S., Carver, C., Antoni, M., Weiss, S., & Durán, R. (2001). An exploratory study of social support, distress, and life disruption among low-income Hispanic women under treatment for early stage breast cancer. *Health Psychology, 20*(1), 41–46. doi:10.1037//0278-6133.20.1.41

Altman, R. (1996). *The politics of breast cancer: Waking up, fighting back.* Boston, MA: Little, Brown.

American Cancer Society. (2009). *Cancer facts and figures for Hispanics.* Retrieved from http://www.cancer.org/Research/CancerFactsFigures/CancerFactsFiguresforHispanicsLatinos/cancer-facts-figures-for-hispanics-latinos-2009-2011

American Cancer Society. (2010, November). *Breast cancer.* Retrieved from http://www.cancer.org/Cancer/BreastCancer/DetailedGuide/index

Arias, E. (2010). United States life tables by Hispanic origin. *Vital & Health Statistics, 2*(152), 2010–1352.

Ashing-Giwa, K., & Lim, J. (2010). Exploring the association between functional strain and emotional well-being among a population-based sample of breast cancer survivors. *Psycho-Oncology, 19*(2), 150–159. doi:10.1002/pon.1517

Ashing-Giwa, K., Padilla, G., Bohorquez, D., Tejero, J., & Garcia, M. (2006). Understanding the breast cancer experience of Latina women. *Journal of Psychosocial Oncology, 24*(3), 19–52. doi:10.1300/J077v24n03_02

Ashing-Giwa, K. T., Padilla, G., Tejero, J., Kraemer, J., Wright, K., Coscarelli, A., …Hills, D. (2004). Understanding the breast cancer experience of women: A qualitative study of African American, Asian American, Latina and Caucasian cancer survivors. *Psycho-Oncology, 13*(6), 408–428. doi:10.1002/pon.750

Ashing-Giwa, K., Tejero, J., Kim, J., Padilla, V., & Hellemann, G. (2007). Examining predictive models of HRQOL in a population-based, multiethnic sample of women with breast carcinoma. *Quality of Life Research, 16*(3), 413–428. doi:10.1007/s11136-006-9138-4

Avis, N., Crawford, S., & Manuel, J. (2004). Psychosocial problems among younger women with breast cancer. *Psycho-Oncology, 13*(5), 295–308.

Badger, T., Braden, C., Mishel, M., & Longman, A. (2004). Depression burden, psychological adjustment, and quality of life in women with breast cancer: Patterns over time. *Research in Nursing & Health, 27*(1), 19–28. doi:10.1002/nur.20002

Bauer, K., Brown, M., Cress, R., Parise, C., & Caggiano, V. (2007). Descriptive analysis of estrogen receptor (er)negative, progesterone receptor (pr)-negative, and her2-negative invasive breast cancer, the so-called triple-negative phenotype: A population-based study from the California Cancer Registry. *Cancer, 109*(9), 1721–1728. doi:10.1002/cncr.22618

Beard, H., Al Ghatrif, M., Samper-Ternent, R., Gerst, K., & Markides, K. (2009). Trends in diabetes prevalence and diabetes-related complications in older Mexican Americans from 1993–1994 to 2004–2005. *Diabetes Care, 32*(12), 2212–2217. doi:10.2337/dc09-0938

Beckjord, E., & Compas, B. (2007). Sexual quality of life in women with newly diagnosed breast cancer. *Journal of Psychosocial Oncology, 25*(2), 19–36. doi:10.1300/8077v2502_02

Bower, J. (2008). Behavioral symptoms in patients with breast cancer and survivors. *Journal of Clinical Oncology, 26*(5), 768–777. doi:10.1200/JCO.2007.14.3248

Buki, L. P., & Grupski, A. (2010). *Identified gaps in our readiness to meet the psychosocial needs of Latina women with breast cancer.* Unpublished manuscript.

Buki, L. P., & Selem, M. (2009). Cancer screening and survivorship in Latino populations: A primer for psychologists. In F. A. Villarruel, G. Carlo, J. M. Grau, M. Azmitia, N. Cabrera, & T. J. Chahin (Eds.), *U.S. handbook of Latina/o psychology* (pp. 363–378). Thousand Oaks, CA: Sage.

Buki, L. P., Garcés, D. M., Hinestrosa, M. C., Kogan, L., Carrillo, I. Y., & French, B. (2008). Latina breast cancer survivors' lived experiences: Diagnosis, treatment, and beyond. *Cultural Diversity & Ethnic Minority Psychology, 14*(2), 163–167.

Burgess, C., Cornelius, V., Love, S., Graham, J., Richards, M., & Ramirez, A. (2005, February 4). Depression and anxiety in women with early breast cancer: Five-year observational cohort study. *British Medical Journal* (Compact ed.), *330*(7493), 702-705. doi: 10.1136/bmj.38343.670868.D3

Campesino, M., Ruiz, E., Glover, J., & Koithan, M. (2009). Counternarratives of Mexican-origin women with breast cancer. *ANS Advances in Nursing Science, 32*(2), E57–E67. doi:10.1097/ANS.0b013e3181a3b47c

Carver, C. S., Smith, R. G., Petronis, V. M., & Antoni, M. H. (2006). Quality of life among long-term survivors of breast cancer: Different types of antecedents predict different classes of outcomes. *Psycho-Oncology, 15*, 749–758. doi: 10.1002/pon.1006

Centers for Disease Control and Prevention. (2007). *HIV/AIDS surveillance report, 2007.* Atlanta, GA: U.S. Department of Health and Human Services, 1–63. Retrieved from http://www.cdc. gov/hiv/surveillance/resources/reports/2007report/

Christie, K., Meyerowitz, B., & Maly, R. (2009). Depression and sexual adjustment following breast cancer in low-income Hispanic and non-Hispanic white women. *Psycho-Oncology, 19*(10), 1069–1077. doi:10.1002/pon.1661

Cohen, S. (2004). Social relationships and health. *American Psychologist, 59*(8), 676–684.

Dausch, B. M., Compas, B. E., Beckjord, E., Luecken, L., Anderson-Hanley, C., Sherman, M., & Grossman, C. (2004). Rates and correlates of DSM-IV diagnoses in women newly diagnosed with breast cancer. *Journal of Clinical Psychology in Medical Settings, 11*(3), 159–169.

Dwight-Johnson, M., Ell, K., & Lee, P. (2005). Can collaborative care address the needs of low-income Latinas with comorbid depression and cancer? Results from a randomized pilot study. *Psychosomatics, 46*, 224–232.

Ell, K., Sanchez, K, Vourlekis, B., Lee, P., Dwight-Johnson, M., Lagomasino, I., … Russell, C. (2005). Depression, correlates of depression, and receipt of depression care among low-income women with breast or gynecologic cancer. *Journal of Clinical Oncology, 23*(13), 3052–3060. doi:10.1200/JCO.2005.08.041

Figueiredo, M., Fries, E., & Ingram, K. (2004). The role of disclosure patterns and unsupportive social interactions in the well-being of breast cancer patients. *Psycho-Oncology, 13*(2), 96–105. doi:10.1002/pon.717

Fisher, B., Anderson, S., Bryant, J., Margolese, R., Deutsch, M., Fisher, E., … Wolmark, N. (2002). Twenty-year follow-up of a randomized trial comparing total mastectomy, lumpectomy, and lumpectomy plus irradiation for the treatment of invasive breast cancer. *New England Journal of Medicine, 347*(16), 1233–1241.

Galván, N., Buki, L. P., & Garcés, D. M. (2009). Suddenly, a carriage appears: Social support needs of Latina breast cancer survivors. *Journal of Psychosocial Oncology, 27*, 361–382.

Ganz, P., Kwan, L., Stanton, A., Krupnick, J., Rowland, J., Meyerowitz, B., … Belin, T. (2004). Quality of life at the end of primary treatment of breast cancer: First results from the Moving Beyond Cancer randomized trial. *Journal of the National Cancer Institute, 96*(5), 376–387. doi:10.1093/jnci/djh060

Giedzinska, A., Meyerowitz, B., Ganz, P., & Rowland, J. (2004). Health-related quality of life in a multiethnic sample of breast cancer survivors. *Annals of Behavioral Medicine, 28*(1), 39–51.

Golden-Kreutz, D., & Andersen, B. (2004). Depressive symptoms after breast cancer surgery: Relationships with global, cancer-related, and life event stress. *Psycho-Oncology, 13*(3), 211–220. doi:10.1002/pon.736

Grieve, M. (2003). Nonprofit organizations in the Canadian breast cancer network. In K. L. Brock & K. G. Banting (Eds.), *The nonprofit sector in interesting times* (pp. 99–128). Montreal: McGill-Queen's University Press.

Institute of Medicine. (2002). *Unequal treatment: Confronting racial and ethnic disparities in health care.* Washington, DC: National Academies Press.

Institute of Medicine. (2004). *Health literacy: A prescription to end confusion.* Washington, DC: National Academies Press.

Institute of Medicine. (2005). *From cancer patient to cancer survivor: Lost in transition.* Washington, DC: National Academies Press.

Janz, N., Mujahid, M., Hawley, S., Griggs, J., Alderman, A., Hamilton, A., … Katz, S. (2009). Racial/ethnic differences in quality of life after diagnosis of breast cancer. *Journal of Cancer Survivorship, 3*(4), 212–222.

Living Beyond Breast Cancer. (n.d.). *About LBBC.* Retrieved May 2, 2007 from http://www.lbbc. org/mission-statement.asp

Livingston, G., Minushkin, S., & Cohn, D. (2008). Hispanics and health care in the United States: Access, information, and knowledge. Retrieved from Pew Hispanic Center website at http://pewhispanic.org/reports/report.php?ReportID=91

Love, A., Grabsch, B., Clarke, D., Bloch, S., & Kissane, D. (2004). Screening for depression in women with metastatic breast cancer: A comparison of the Beck Depression Inventory Short Form and the Hospital Anxiety and Depression Scale. *Australian & New Zealand Journal of Psychiatry, 38*(7), 526–531.

Metcalfe, K., Esplen, J., Goel, V., & Narod, S. (2004). Psychosocial functioning in women who have undergone bilateral prophylactic mastectomy. *Psycho-Oncology, 13*(1), 14–25.

Nápoles-Springer, A., Ortíz, C., Díaz-Méndez, M., & Pérez-Stable, E. (2007). Use of support groups among Latina breast cancer survivors. *Psycho-Oncology, 16*(3), S61–S62.

National Breast Cancer Coalition. (2006). *About NBCC and NBCCF.* Retrieved May 2, 2007 from http://www.natlbcc.org/bin/index.asp?strid=537&depid=1&btnid=0

Norman, S., Localio, A., Potashnik, S., Torpey, H., Kallan, M., Weber, A., … Solin, L. (2008). Lymphedema in breast cancer survivors: Incidence, degree, time course, treatment, and symptoms. *Journal of Clinical Oncology, 27*(3), 390–397. doi:10.1200/JCO.2008.17.9291

Nueva Vida. (n.d.). Retrieved September 10, 2007, from http://www.nueva-vida.org/index.htm

Parker, P., Baile, W., de Moor, C., & Cohen, L. (2003). Psychosocial and demographic predictors of quality of life in a large sample of cancer patients. *Psycho-Oncology, (12)*2, 183–193. doi:10.1002/pon.635

Paskett, E. D., & Stark, N. N. (2000). Lymphedema: Knowledge, treatment, and impact among breast cancer survivors. *Breast Journal, 6*(6), 373–378. doi:10.1046/j.1524-4741.2000.99072.x

Patel, T., Colon-Otero, G., Hume, C., Copland, J., & Perez, E. (2010). Breast cancer in Latinas: Gene expression, differential response to treatments, and differential toxicities in Latinas compared with other population groups. *The Oncologist, 15*(5), 466–475. doi:10.1634/theoncologist.2010-0004

Petronis, V., Carver, C., Antoni, M., & Weiss, S. (2003). Investment in body image and psychosocial well-being among women treated for early stage breast cancer: Partial replication and extension. *Psychology & Health, 1*(18), 1–13.

Pinquart, M., & Duberstein, P. (2010). Depression and cancer mortality: A meta-analysis. *Psychological Medicine, 40*(11), 1797–1810. doi:10.1017/S0033291709992285

Ramakrishnan, S. & Viramontes, C. (2006). *Civil inequalities: Immigrant volunteerism and community organizations in California.* San Francisco, CA: Public Policy Institute of California.

Sammarco, A., & Konecny, L. (2010). Quality of life, social support, and uncertainty among Latina and Caucasian breast cancer survivors: A comparative study. *Oncology Nursing Forum, 37*(1), 93–99.

Shavers, V., Harlan, L., & Stevens, J. (2003). Racial/ethnic variation in clinical presentation, treatment, and survival among breast cancer patients under age 35. *Cancer, 97*(1), 134–147.

Shelby, R. A., Taylor, K. L., Kerner, J. F., Coleman, E., & Blum, D. (2002). The role of community-based and philanthropic organizations in meeting cancer patient and caregiver needs. *CA: A Cancer Journal for Clinicians, 52,* 229–246.

The Sister Network, Inc. (n.d.). *History.* Retrieved May 2, 2007 from http://www.sistersnetwork-inc.org/about-us.asp

Spencer, S., Lehman, J., Wynings, C., Arena, P., Carver, C., Antoni, M., … Ironson, G. (1999). Concerns about breast cancer and relations to psychosocial well-being in a multiethnic sample of early-stage patients. *Health Psychology, 18*(2), 159–168.

Taylor, S., & Stanton, A. (2007). Coping resources, coping processes, and mental health. *Annual Review of Clinical Psychology, 3*(1), 377–401. doi:10.1146/annurev.clinpsy.3.022806.091520

Zakowski, S., Ramati, A., Morton, C., Johnson, P., & Flanigan, R. (2004). Written emotional disclosure buffers the effects of social constraints on distress among cancer patients. *Health Psychology, 23*(6), 555–563. doi:10.1037/0278-6133.23.6.555

Chapter 13
Lessons Learned from HIV Service Provision: Using a Targeted Behavioral Health Approach

Eduardo Morales

Abstract Approximately 1.1 million people are living with HIV/AIDS in the United States, including nearly 200,000 Latinos with 78% being Latino men who have sex with men. Governmental agencies do not always foster development and funding for Latinos and HIV/AIDS, especially for Latino men who have sex with men. The new Health Reform Act passed by congress in 2010 transforms the health system by incorporating behavioral health in an integrated and central man-ner. This paradigm shift necessitates a re-examination of existing organizational infra-structures. Mobilizing the community's social networks and resources is cen-tral for sustained prevention efforts. This chapter examines the use of social capi-tal theory in the execution of prevention and treatment programs. Efficacious and innovative social capital model and examples of interventions are presented and discussed.

According to the Kaiser Family Report (2009), there are approximately 1.1 mil-lion people living with HIV/AIDS in the United States, including nearly 200,000 Latinos. Because Latinos constitute the largest and fastest-growing ethnic minority group in the United States, the impact of HIV/AIDS in this community takes on increased importance. The negative impact of this epidemic is evident in Latinos' disproportionate burden of the disease. The prevalence of AIDS among Latinos increased by 26% between 2003 and 2007, compared to an 18% increase among non-Latino Whites (Kaiser Family Report 2009). Although the number of deaths among Latinos with AIDS declined between 2003 and 2007, non-Latino Blacks and non-Latino Whites experienced more significant decreases.

The challenge in the field of HIV centers on targeting high-risk groups relative to their prevalence and incidence regionally. For example, there are more Latinas with HIV on the East Coast than the West Coast; also, there have been almost no cases of new HIV infection of women and no babies born with HIV in San Francisco for the past five to eight years (San Francisco HIV Prevention Plan [SFHIV] n.d.).

E. Morales (✉)
Alliant International University, CA, USA
e-mail: dremorales@aol.com

In contrast, for most of the United States, the highest risk group among Latinos is men who have sex with men (MSM), a group that is hard to reach, not easily visible, has limited opportunities for outreach, and experiences numerous psychosocial stressors and prejudice due to their ethnicity and sexual orientation. Therefore, this chapter focuses mainly on reaching Latino men who are gay, bisexual, or MSM and related funding and service delivery challenges.

In the context of a changing health services environment, I discuss the challenges inherent in meeting the needs of this population as a prologue to innovation. Because the HIV epidemic has forced the health field to use media, social marketing strategies, advocacy, and various creative outreach, prevention, and funding efforts, an array of interventions has emerged that were never attempted before. Thus, I present specific models that foster the development of social networks and organizational infrastructure that have proved effective in reducing HIV infection rates among Latino gay and bisexual men. I begin my discussion by providing a statistical overview and explaining how the geographic distribution of HIV/AIDS for Latinos calls for a targeted outreach approach for hard-to-reach populations.

HIV/AIDS in Latinos: Statistics and Geographic Distribution

An examination of recent HIV and AIDS statistics brings to light several major trends (Centers for Disease Control and Prevention [CDC] 2010a). First, the proportion of Latinos living with HIV relative to the general population is increasing. In 2007, Latinos comprised 20% of individuals living with the infection, reflecting a 3% increase over the prior five to seven years (CDC 2010a). Second, the mode of transmission differs among women and men. Among Latina women diagnosed with AIDS in 2008, approximately 75% became infected through heterosexual contact, and 25% through IV drug use (CDC 2010a). Among Latino men diagnosed with AIDS in 2008, 63% became infected through male-to-male sexual contact; of those living with an AIDS diagnosis in 2007, 90% ($n=48,288$) were MSM (CDC 2010a). Third, the virus plagues populations of all ages. From 2001 to 2006, increases in diagnoses were observed for Latino MSM aged 13 to 24 years (CDC 2008, 2010a). In 2008, the largest proportion of new HIV diagnoses was among those aged 40 to 44 years. Another documented trend is that AIDS cases vary by place of birth. Among Latinos, those born in the United States accounted for 41% of estimated AIDS cases in 2007, followed by Latinos born in Mexico (23%) and Puerto Rico (20%) (Kaiser Family Report 2009).

Although AIDS cases among Latinos are reported throughout the country, the impact of the epidemic is not uniformly distributed. AIDS case rates per 100,000 among Latinos are highest in the eastern part of the United States, particularly in the northeast. In 2007, 10 states accounted for 88% of Latinos estimated to be living with AIDS. Among the states, New York, California, and Puerto Rico were at the top of the list, followed by Texas, Florida, New Jersey, Illinois, Connecticut, Pennsylvania, and Massachusetts. These 10 states also accounted for the majority of newly reported AIDS cases among Latinos (83% in 2007).

Latino MSM

The overrepresentation of MSM among Latino men and adolescents living with HIV/AIDS warrants attention. Some men have sex with men, but do not identify as gay or bisexual, even though their lifestyle and sexual activity may resemble those of someone who is openly gay. As a minority within a minority, Latino gay and bisexual men often find themselves trying to manage their lives by maneuvering among and balancing three different communities (Morales 1992, 1996, 1998). In their Latino community, they must engage with individuals who do not approve of their lifestyle. The lesbian-gay-bisexual-transgendered community offers individuals a way to express their sexual orientation freely, yet it might still expose them to the racist and micro-aggressive attitudes, beliefs, and behaviors of mainstream society. Moreover, family rejection, discrimination at work, and sexual objectification in the gay community, combined with anxiety, depression, and suicidal tendencies, are associated with engagement in riskier sexual situations (Díaz et al. 2001, 2004). In other words, HIV risk is an outcome of social discrimination. When the complexities of managing minority statuses are combined with a life-threatening and chronic disease like HIV, significant challenges ensue for the development of prevention and treatment services.

Major Challenges in Service Provision

A major obstacle for service provision is the lack of bilingual and bicultural clinicians with expertise in HIV/AIDS. Thus, service providers must rely on a select group of staff and interpreters to transcend language and cultural divides. Although pragmatic, such a strategy is not without limitations. The standards used to identify translators vary, the quality of the interaction is often questionable, and the few staff who are tasked with serving the population may feel isolated and find that the employment setting does not provide professional growth (Morales et al. 2008). In addition, specifically for Latino-led multiservice agencies, the need to channel resources toward advocacy and funding may limit their capacity to develop specialized HIV/AIDS services. Consequently, high-risk, hard-to-reach populations like Latino gay and bisexual men often do not get the support and resources needed from these organizations. In my experience of 30 years working with populations affected by HIV/AIDS, I have encountered numerous complaints from Latino gay and bisexual staff who perceive that HIV programs take a back seat to other programs and activities in the agency. Thus, given the critical role of funding in the development of infrastructure, in the following section I illustrate how our current funding mechanisms work against program development for Latinos living with HIV/AIDS.

Governmental Funding Barriers for Program Development

It is difficult to get a comprehensive picture of the funding available for Latinos and HIV. Most agencies within the United States Department of Health and Human Services post on their websites information about the grants they have funded, including a copy of an abstract of the project, amount awarded, and project contact information. In contrast, the CDC, an agency that provides significant funding for HIV/AIDS, does not post such information. To obtain this information from the CDC, one must submit a written inquiry, which is then processed and referred to the CDC's Freedom of Information Act Office. To call this a rather lengthy process is a massive understatement. To illustrate, this author submitted a request for information about who was funded, a summary of the project funded, and the amount of funding that targets Latino MSM in September of 2009. Twelve months later, I received a response from the CDC informing me that more time was needed to process the request.

The limited information available engenders concern. For example, in 2009 the CDC (2009a) provided more than US $4.8 million in funding to 14 agencies for capacity building in high-risk communities of color, with an average grant of US $347,143 per agency. Of these agencies, only one had a focus on Latinos. This agency, located in New York City, proposed to serve three high-risk Latino groups: intravenous drug users, women and children, and MSM. Thus, less than one-third of the funding given to 1 of 14 agencies was dedicated to programs for Latino MSM in all of the United States and Puerto Rico. Also in 2009, the CDC funded 133 agencies, for a total of more than US $42 million, to provide HIV prevention services, with an average of US $323,000 per agency. Only seven of the agencies funded (which accounted for less than 5.4% of the total US $42 million) had a focus on Latino populations, despite the fact that more than 20% of the HIV/AIDS cases are Latino and are considered top priority by the CDC. Moreover, only one of the seven agencies was located west of the Mississippi, where more than 65% of Latinos in the United States reside. Thus, about US $323,000 (0.77%) of the US $42 million was dedicated to serving more than 65% of Latinos in the United States (CDC 2010c). These funding patterns mean that the majority of Latino MSM or gay and bisexual men are left without direct CDC funding for the next 5 to 10 years, even as the number of HIV/AIDS cases in this population continues to increase (CDC 2010a).

Similarly, local and state governments have HIV prevention funding and a strategic plan that acknowledges the need to serve the Latino population, yet this does not guarantee that they will fund their priorities accordingly. Based on published trends (CDC 2010a), I have estimated that we can continue to expect an increase in AIDS cases among Latinos at the rate of about 0.5–1% per year for the next 5-year period.

By 2014 and 2015, when grant opportunities open up again for CDC direct funding, we can expect Latino MSM to represent 25% or more of the AIDS cases and at least 25% of the new HIV infections in the United States. At this rate, it will take at least 10 or more years to start even slowing down the rate of infection through aggressive HIV prevention efforts—assuming that by then there are ways to access populations, a trained workforce, and organizational infrastructures that can reach Latino MSM in the geographical regions that are most affected.

This lack of funding has the additional effect of diminishing the social capital and institutional infrastructures that serve the needs of Latinos. For example, as of August 2010, there remain only four agencies across the United States that provide HIV interventions for and by Latino gay and bisexual men. The scarce resources allocated to this problem, as well as the lack of transparency in funding information, foster a sense of mistrust of governmental agencies and their procedures. Historical issues of disenfranchisement of minorities, the resurrection of conspiracy theories related to fostering genocide of undesirable groups, and structural funding concerns all become formative and formidable barriers in executing behavioral interventions. The only recourse for these communities is to engage in very aggressive community organizing and advocacy to demand accountability and distribution of resources in accordance with established plans and priorities. Given the resources needed to deliver effective advocacy and the competing priorities of Latino agencies (such as immigration issues, general health care, educational achievement, and reduction of delinquency, violence, and gangs in the community), it is likely that Latinos will continue to be left out of the HIV prevention efforts, even as new infection rates and AIDS cases to continue to rise.

Addressing the Challenges and New Opportunities

The new Health Reform Act passed by Congress in 2010, H. R. 3962 (Affordable Health Care for America; available at http://www.opencongress.org/bill/111-h3962/show) fosters a transformation of the health care system that incorporates behavioral health in an integrated and central manner. To provide health care coverage for all, this new law relies on integrating behavioral services into primary medical care practices to reduce cost and enhance health through prevention. Thus, an opportunity exists to develop a system that incorporates interventions, prevention, and recovery. The integration of behavioral services into mainstream medical care is largely facilitated by the work already undertaken in the mental health field. Over the past decades, professionals in the field of mental health have developed theories and technologies focused on the treatment of mental illnesses as defined by the *Diagnostic and Statistical Manual* (American Psychiatric Association 2000). These developments have been applied to related areas in prevention, health promotion, psycho-education, substance abuse treatment, risk-reduction interventions, and self-help strategies, all part of the field now called *behavioral health* (Matarazzo 1980; Schwartz and Weiss 1978).

This paradigm shift in the health field necessitates a reexamination of existing organizational infrastructures. To address the cultural and linguistic needs of Latinos, community-based organizations have played a major role by increasing access through the provision of culturally sensitive services (see Chap. 12 in this volume). In many cases, these organizations created systems that mimic traditional health care models, due to external pressures to conform to organizational structures familiar to funding agencies. However, conforming to traditional models ultimately affects these organizations' vision and undermines community empowerment, a critical aspect of intervention directed at marginalized populations. Thus, organizations now have the opportunity to revisit their history, vision, and mission, and to redesign their organizational structures to achieve more active community engagement. With this new redirection, organizations can incorporate Latino cultural values into the organizations' design and structure, empowering Latinos in all of their diversity and identities.

Social Capital Development: Building Infrastructures from the Ground Up

In the field of HIV prevention, various interventions have demonstrated short-term effectiveness in reducing high-risk HIV behaviors for all targeted groups (CDC 2009c). In essence, a well-conceived intervention that is culturally and linguistically appropriate and well executed will effect a change in the rate of risky HIV behavior within a three-month window (Global HIV Prevention Working Group 2008). However, these behavior changes are lost over time if efforts directed at sustainability are not applied early. In fact, the sustainability of behavior changes over the long haul represents a major challenge in the prevention and management of HIV. Interventions that use the synergy of existing social support and the community's social networks—important forms of social capital—are effective in maintaining behavior changes (Latkin and Knowlton 2005).

According to the CDC, *social capital* refers to the fabric of a community as well as to the community's available pool of human resources (CDC 2009b). It includes the individual and communal time and energy that are available for such things as community improvement, social networking, civic engagement, personal recreation, and other activities that create social bonds between individuals and groups (CDC 2009b). Researchers have added to this definition by focusing on institutional networks (Bourdieu 1983), social interactive networks (Coleman 1990, 1994), and shared common values (Putnam 2000).

For the purposes of behavioral interventions, a more comprehensive definition of social capital is useful. The World Bank offers a definition of social capital that refers to the norms and networks that enable collective action. According to this definition, community empowerment and community driven development (CDD) are interrelated concepts. *Empowerment* is the process of increasing capacity to make choices and transform them into desired actions and outcomes, whereas CDD refers to giving control of decisions and resources to community groups (The World Bank n.d.).

Formal and informal networks are central to building social capital, and are defined as the personal relationships that include families, workplaces, neighborhoods, local associations, and a range of informal and formal meeting places. Without healthy interactions among these spheres, trust decays and serious social problems can begin to manifest. The various types of interactions foster different types of relationships, such as personal and familial bonding, bridging and partnering collaborations, and systems of linkages and contacts.

Essential Elements for Harnessing Social Capital in Behavioral Health

The essential elements for development of social capital have been noted by various writers in the literature (Bourdieu 1983; Coleman 1988; 1990, 1994; The World Bank n.d.). These elements can be grouped into two major areas: (a) building and engaging community-level social networks, and (b) building and engaging institutional networks. The first area includes the five elements necessary to build and engage social networks within a community, namely: (a) bonding intergenerationally for support across generations, (b) building bridges between neighbor and neighbor and creating linkages within the community, (c) cultivating social and behavioral expectations of the community, (d) building leadership within the community, and (e) providing effective advocacy for the community. The second area focuses on the four elements necessary to build institutional networks within a community: (a) generating sustainability through community capacity building, (b) advancing social policy, (c) developing comprehensive stakeholder investments, and (d) creating healthy places. These elements for the development of social capital in behavioral health are described in more detail in the next two sections.

Building and Engaging Community-level Social Networks

Intergenerational bonding for support across generations. Relationship building across generations in a community is critical for developing mentoring processes and for maintaining a sense of history. For Latinos, respect for elders and the use of titles such as *Don* and *Doña* accentuate the importance of elders, grandparents, and seniors. Similarly, elders learn from the younger generation as part of this mentoring collaboration so that the relationship is mutually beneficial. These are the hands across generations.

Building bridges and creating linkages. This element refers to the fostering of relationships between neighbors for reciprocal exchanges. Relationships are highly valued within Latino culture. The cultural concept of *familia* underscores the importance of interdependent networks with both the immediate and extended family, and highlights a social expectation of sensitivity to relationships. Closely related to this value are codes for culturally acceptable behavior, such as *respeto, simpatía,* and *personalismo.* By integrating these values throughout interventions, programs can be enhanced. Some Latino programs build on this concept, using program names like *mano a mano* (hand to hand).

Social and behavioral expectations. This element refers to the shared values, norms, and behavioral expectations that are encouraged by community members, and to the consequences for community members who do not meet these expectations.

Building leadership. Leadership-building efforts foster development of the educational pipeline through mentorship and formal training in leadership skills. Leadership may be built by participating in mentor programs, leadership institutes, traineeships, internships, and organizational leadership positions.

Effective advocacy. Advocacy efforts for MSM may take various forms, such as capacity building, social marketing, dissemination of messages using a range of mass media, public relations campaigns, promotion of community well-being, and attraction of resources to meet community needs. To this end, community members may receive media training on how to talk on radio programs, how to talk to news reporters, and how to write press releases. Other skills that are necessary for advocacy include the ability to mobilize stakeholders (e.g., organize people to advocate for a common interest) and use communication systems effectively (e.g., alerting stakeholders about breaking news, so that they can write letters and communicate with elected officials).

Advocacy efforts are effective in promoting accountability among social systems such as governmental departments, social policymakers, legislators, and health officials. These efforts are necessary because bureaucratic systems are too slow and cumbersome to correct errors in the implementation of laws and social policies. Thus, by engaging in advocacy, communities help ensure that adequate resources are allocated, policies are implemented, and monitoring systems are in place to address a given issue.

Institutional Network Building and Engagement

Generating sustainability through community capacity building. Sustainability is a critical component to ensure longevity and resilience of program efforts. *Sustainability* refers to efforts that maintain the activities of the agency through the ongoing development of leadership, economic resources, and frontline workers. Moreover, it refers to the organization's flexibility and ability to accommodate fluctuations in grant funding.

To successfully build the community's capacity for sustainability, five general elements require attention: (a) the provision of ongoing training and skill building for stakeholders in management and finance, (b) the development of program activities and business models that make use of social networks, (c) the use of Internet social networks, (d) ongoing program evaluation, and (e) the continued engagement of activities to protect, maintain, and promote social capital.

Advancing legal and social policy. These are the laws, strategic plans, and policies that formally direct, drive, and support norms, values, and cultures, such as no-smoking areas and drug-free zones.

Developing comprehensive stakeholder investments. This element focuses on involving a wide spectrum of organizations (e.g., businesses, churches, governmental entities, public safety departments, financial institutions, schools, universities) to contribute social capital to their community.

Creating healthy places. Healthy places are environments designed and built to improve the quality of life for all people who live, work, worship, learn, and play within their borders. The goal is for every person to choose among a variety of healthy, available, accessible, and affordable possibilities within the community (CDC 2010b).

Examples of Behavioral Health Interventions That Rely on Social Capital

This section describes two promising programs that make use of a community's existing social networks and capital. Programmatic efforts focus on engaging Latino gay men through social networks. Once engaged, the same networks are used to strengthen relations among members and foster greater outreach efforts, enhancing the social capital available in the community.

Mpowerment: Intervention for Building and Engaging Social Networks

The Mpowerment Project is a CDC-approved, evidence-based, community-level intervention based on an empowerment model. Developed by a team of researchers, this intervention focuses on building social capital through the use of the five previously noted elements for building and engaging social networks (Kahn et al. 2001; Kegeles et al. 1996, 1999; Mpowerment n.d.). A core group of 10 to 15 young gay men engage in various activities to promote sexual health. These young men are empowered to design activities that are fun, productive, and relevant. In the implementation of the activities, these men are expected to be attentive to issues of racial/ethnic, socioeconomic, and educational diversity. Some activities involve small teams going to locations frequented by young gay men to deliver informational literature on HIV, promote safer sex, and distribute condoms. Team members also connect with friends in their social networks to promote health messages through informal channels.

A special feature of Mpowerment is the establishment of *M-groups*, are peer-led discussion sessions, with 8 to 10 young gay men as participants, that last 2 to 3 hours. Topics discussed include safe sex practices, misconceptions about enjoying safer sex, and communication skills. By engaging in skill-building exercises, the men's self-efficacy for safe sex practices increases. Free condoms and lubricant are provided and participants are trained to conduct informal outreach to their friends. An ongoing publicity campaign attracts men to the project by word of mouth and through articles and advertisements. A community advisory board serves as a resource for the core group of organizers and staff by providing expertise for capacity building and for enhancing program activities.

Given the difficulties of reaching Latino gay and bisexual men through traditional organizational public health models, Mpowerment's strategy to harness the social capital of the community represents a promising alternative. The program has been successful at empowering participants, promoting pride, and helping men combat the social isolation that puts them at risk for HIV infection.

El Ambiente: *An HIV Prevention Program at AGUILAS*

AGUILAS is an acronym for *Asociación Gay Unida Impactando Latinos/Latinas A Superarse*, which translates to "Association of United Gays Impacting Latinos/ Latinas toward Self-Empowerment." Today, AGUILAS (a word that means *eagle* in Spanish) is a nonprofit organization and the largest gay Latino organization in northern California. One of its programs, *El Ambiente* (which refers to the climate or "ambience" present within a social group), is the subject of this example. *El Ambiente* is a multisession HIV prevention program. It uses group and individual interventions created by and for gay and bisexual Latino men. *El Ambiente* follows a process of engagement similar to Mpowerment's, but goes a step further by focusing on the role of organizational infrastructure in promoting behavior change.

Specifically, the goal of *El Ambiente* is to support individual self-empowerment to prevent men from engaging in unsafe sexual practices that increase the risk of HIV transmission. The intervention is grounded on published research about HIV prevention in Latino gay and bisexual men (Díaz et al. 1999; Morales 2009). *El Ambiente* is based on Freire's Empowerment Theory (Freire 1973, 1990) and an evolving theory called Contextual Community Prevention Theory (CCPT) (Morales 2009). Consistent with these conceptual frameworks, the process of program and intervention development begins by examining the context and environment of the target population. Specifically, contextual factors examined include: the resources available to members of the organization, the organizational infrastructure present across institutional sectors, community assets and limitations, the physical space and geographical location of the agency, the marketability of the efforts, and cultural factors (AGUILAS n.d.).

El Ambiente fosters a sense of community by facilitating peer support, implementing suggestions provided by participants, delivering bilingual services, and sustaining consistent communications with program participants. Programmatically, *El Ambiente* offers a variety of interventions that include individual counseling, discussion and skill-building group sessions, and outreach activities. Participants start with an initial orientation group session, *Cuerpo a Cuerpo* ("body to body"), developed by a team of Latino gay and bisexual psychologists (Díaz et al. 1999). Following this orientation, participants are invited to select discussion groups and skill-building workshops according to their interest. Individual counseling is available in Spanish or English. All of the groups and individual sessions are facilitated by a licensed psychologist or by a license-eligible clinician supervised by a licensed psychologist. Experts on a given topic (e.g., lawyers, dietitians) lead some workshops. In its activities, *El Ambiente* accounts for the multidimensional nature of culture by addressing issues such as acculturation, ethnic identity development, cultural value systems, and ethnic communication.

Participants are considered members of AGUILAS rather than clients. Thus, they are never discharged. Many participants leave the program or move away, and later return to continue participating in program activities. The result is the presence of an institution within the community that provides an active and dynamic context that has proved to be a powerful attraction for community members.

To ensure program sustainability, the organization engages in ongoing program evaluation, advocacy, fund raising, and development activities. Ongoing program evaluation is a critical process, and program outcomes are examined to further improve program interventions. Data show that *El Ambiente* is effective in assisting targeted individuals in reducing their risk of HIV infection or transmission (Morales 2009). According to the 2010 SFHIV, three new HIV infections are reported each day in San Francisco (SFHIV n.d.). Based on the data collected at *El Ambiente* from more than 200 participants, only three new infections were reported over an eight-year period, from 2002 to 2009.

Due to the success of this program, AGUILAS has received numerous honors and awards, which have elevated the visibility of the organization and increased the credibility of the agency and its efforts, thus making advocacy efforts easier. When budget cuts and decisions for funding are in their critical stages, noting the contributions and honors received by the agency underscores the value of the agency for the community at large.

Moving Forward

HIV has challenged health systems by creating a need to address many psychosocial and health factors simultaneously, and to do so with hard-to-reach populations. For Latinos, the epidemic is further complicated by the various Latino cultures, language, and health disparities. Future efforts must build on successful models that incorporate behavioral interventions and develop social capital. It is critical that these efforts empower Latino communities at risk, which are marginalized by society at large. Thus, it is important that future activities promote the development of a workforce pipeline to focus on HIV prevention, and that programs provide high-quality services that are culturally and linguistically appropriate for the population. With these elements in place, we will be able to build effective infrastructures that can successfully serve Latino communities.

References

AGUILAS. (n.d.). AGUILAS *El Ambiente* program. Retrieved from http://www.sfaguilas.org
American Psychiatric Association. (2000). Diagnostic and statistical manual of mental disorders (4th ed., text revision). Washington, DC: Author.
Bourdieu, P. (1983). Forms of capital. In J. C. Richards (ed.), *Handbook of theory and research for the sociology of education*. New York, NY: Greenwood Press.
Centers for Disease Control and Prevention (CDC). (2008, June 27). Trends in HIV/AIDS diagnoses among men who have sex with men—33 states, 2001–2006. *MMWR Weekly, 57*(25), 681–686. Retrieved from http://www.cdc.gov/mmwr/preview/mmwrhtml/mm5725a2.htm?s_cid=mm5725a2_e#fig2
Centers for Disease Control and Prevention (CDC). (2009a). *Organizations awarded CDC funds to provide capacity building assistance to improve the delivery and effectiveness of HIV prevention services for high-risk and/or racial/ethnic minority populations. Funding opportunity announcement PS09-906.* Retrieved from http://www.cdc.gov/hiv/topics/funding/ps09-906/awards.htm
Centers for Disease Control and Prevention (CDC). (2009b). *Healthy places: Social capital.* Retrieved from http://www.cdc.gov/healthyplaces/healthtopics/social.htm
Centers for Disease Control and Prevention (CDC). (2009c). *2009 compendium of evidence-based HIV prevention interventions.* Retrieved from http://www.cdc.gov/hiv/topics/research/prs/evidence-based-interventions.htm
Centers for Disease Control and Prevention (CDC). (2010a). Diagnoses of HIV infection and AIDS in the United States and dependent areas, 2008. *HIV Surveillance Report, 20.* Retrieved from http://www.cdc.gov/hiv/surveillance/resources/reports/2008report/index.htm
Centers for Disease Control and Prevention (CDC). (2010b). *Healthy places: About healthy places.* Retrieved from http://www.cdc.gov/healthyplaces/about.htm
Centers for Disease Control and Prevention (CDC). (2010c). CDC awards $42 million to community-based organizations to support HIV prevention efforts across the nation. *CDC NCHHSTP Newsroom.* Retrieved from http://www.cdc.gov/nchhstp/newsroom/cboaward.html complete listing on http://www.cdc.gov/nchhstp/newsroom/docs/CBO-Awards-List-08-03-10-508.pdf
Coleman, J. C. (1988). Social capital in the creation of human capital. *American Journal of Sociology, 94,* S95–S120.
Coleman, J. C. (1990, 1994). *Foundations of social theory.* Cambridge, MA: Harvard University Press.
Díaz, R. M., Ayala, G., & Bein, E. (2004). Sexual risk as an outcome of social oppression: Data from a probability sample of Latino gay men in three US cities. *Cultural Diversity & Ethnic Minority Psychology, 10*(3), 255–267.
Díaz, R. M., Ayala, G., Bein, E, Henne, J., & Marin, B. V. (2001). The impact of homophobia, poverty and racism on the mental health of gay and bisexual Latino men: Findings from 3 United States cities. *American Journal of Public Health, 91*(6), 927–932.
Díaz, R. M., Morales, E., Bein, E., Dilán, E., & Rodriguez, R. (1999). Predictors of sexual risk in Latino gay/bisexual men: The role of demographic, developmental, social cognitive and behavioral variables. *Hispanic Journal of the Behavioral Sciences, 21*(4), 480–501.
Freire, P. (1973). By learning they teach. *Convergence, 1.*
Freire, P. (1990). *Pedagogy of the oppressed.* New York, NY: Continuum.

Global HIV Prevention Working Group. (2008, August). *Behavior change and HIV prevention: Reconsiderations for the 21st century.* Retrieved from http://www.globalhivprevention.org/pdfs/PWG_behavior%20report_FINAL.pdf

Kahn, J. G., Kegeles, S. M., Hays, R., & Beltzer, N. (2001). Cost-effectiveness of the Mpowerment Project, a community-level intervention for young gay men. *Journal of Acquired Immune Deficiency Syndromes, 27*(5), 482–491.

Kaiser Family Report. (2009, September). *Fact Sheet: Latinos and HIV/AIDS—HIV/AIDS Policy.* Retrieved from http://www.kff.org/hivaids/upload/6007-07.pdf

Kegeles, S. M., Hays, R. B., & Coates, T. J. (1996). The Mpowerment Project: A community-level HIV prevention intervention for young gay men. *American Journal of Public Health, 86*(8), 1129–1136.

Kegeles, S. M., Hays, R. B., Pollack, L. M., & Coates, T. J. (1999). Mobilizing young gay and bisexual men for HIV prevention: a two-community study. *AIDS, 12,* 1753-1762.

Latkin, C. A., & Knowlton, A. R. (2005). Micro-social structural approaches to HIV prevention: A social ecological perspective. *AIDS Care, 17*(4 suppl. 1), 102–113.

Matarazzo, J. D. (1980). Behavioral health and behavioral medicine: Frontiers for a new health psychology. *American Psychologist, 35,* 807–817.

Morales, E. (1992). Counseling Latino gays and Latina lesbians. In F. Gutierrez & S. Dworkin (Eds.), *Counseling gay men and lesbians: Journey to the end of the rainbow.* Alexandria, VA: American Association for Counseling and Development.

Morales, E. (1996). Gender roles among Latino gay men. In Robert-Jay Green & Joan Laird (Eds.), *Lesbians and gays in couples and families: A handbook for therapists.* San Francisco, CA: Jossey-Bass.

Morales, E. (1998). Understanding and preventing HIV risk behavior: Safer sex and drug use. *Contemporary Psychology, 43*(3), 185–186.

Morales, E. (2009). Contextual Community Prevention Theory: Building interventions with community agency collaboration. *American Psychologist, 64*(8), 805–816.

Morales, E., Fuentes, M. A., Santos de Barona, M., Reynaga-Abiko, G., Gonzalez, S. M., Tazeau, Y. N., Gil-Kashiwabara, E., & Cardemil, E. (2008, November 16). Psychological testing by Latino/a psychologists for Latinos/as: National survey results. *Report from the NLPA Task Force on testing, measurements, and assessment of Latinas/os.*

Mpowerment. (n.d.). Retrieved September 6, 2010, from http://www.mpowerment.org/

Putnam, R. D. (2000). *Bowling alone. The collapse and revival of American community.* New York, NY: Simon & Schuster.

San Francisco HIV Prevention Plan (SFHIV). (n.d.). Retrieved September 6, 2010, from http://sfhiv.org/community.php

Schwartz, G. E., & Weiss, S. M. (1978). Behavioral medicine revisited: An amended definition. *Journal of Behavioral Medicine, 1,* 249–251.

The World Bank. (n.d.). Definitions. *PovertyNet.* Retrieved from http://web.worldbank.org/WBSITE/EXTERNAL/TOPICS/EXTPOVERTY/EXTEMPOWERMENT/0,,contentMDK:20267550~isCURL:Y~menuPK:543262~pagePK:148956~piPK:216618~theSitePK:486411,00.html

Chapter 14
Private Practice with Latinos: Brief Reflections and Suggestions

Lillian Comas-Díaz

Abstract The author reflects on the development of her private practice with Latinos. She examines the context of delivering clinical psychological services to this population. The author offers practical advice on how to develop and sustain a clinical practice for Latino clients.

Early in my life, I envisioned my professional identity as that of a scientist-practitioner. I thus began an academic career at the Yale University School of Medicine Department of Psychiatry. In that setting, I taught and supervised clinical psychology interns, as well as directed an inner-city mental health clinic. During this chapter of my life, I was able to preserve my "bicultural" professional identity as a scholar-scientist and clinician. The marriage of this "dual consciousness" has worked well for me. I later directed the university Hispanic clinic, a center offering both mental health and substance-abuse rehabilitation services. Such an experience has significantly enriched my clinical practice.

During my New Haven chapter, I sought supervision and training from several psychoanalysts, interpersonal psychotherapists, family clinicians, feminist therapists, community organizers, community mental health clinicians, and an array of other professionals, including folk healers. I was fortunate to arrive at a syncretism of all these diverse orientations. "*Todo suma, nada resta*" (everything adds up) became a way of being.

Continuing my professional journey, I moved from New Haven to Washington, D.C., to direct the Office of Ethnic Minority Affairs of the American Psychological Association (APA). This professional chapter helped to expand my political advocacy and commitment to solidarity, qualities that I later found useful in establishing a private practice. During this time, I collaborated with the APA Office of International Affairs in Psychology, an experience that proved beneficial to my clinical work with international individuals.

L. Comas-Díaz (✉)
Transcultural Mental Health Institute, The George Washington University Medical School,
Washington, DC, USA
e-mail: lilliancomasdiaz@gmail.com

What do these varied experiences have to do with being a psychologist in private practice? The answer is: *everything*.

The APA work was intensely exhilarating but demanding, leaving me no space for clinical work. I longed to return to clinical practice and at the conclusion of my APA life chapter, I co-founded the Transcultural Mental Health Institute, a setting for clinical and consultation services. The Institute co-founder, my husband Frederick M. Jacobsen, a physician with expertise in neuropsychiatry, infuses his practice with multiculturalism (he lived in Brazil, and is fluent in Portuguese and Spanish) combined with his ancestral background (Danish, British, German, and Cherokee). Having Fred as a colleague has been crucial for the development of our Institute. Although we practice in the same setting, we do not share clients, for legal and psychodynamic reasons (prevention of negative transference or becoming idealized parental objects among the latter).

Building a private practice from scratch was arduous. I began by offering education on diverse mental health topics to the multicultural community. Additionally, I worked part time in an inpatient hospital and did forensic work for lawyers representing Latinos. The forensic work was both regarding and challenging. Many Latinos face dire circumstances in the United States.

I resorted to multiple means to increase my visibility as a private practitioner. Because I am a media psychologist, I appeared on diverse Spanish-language media, including TV, radio, and print. Most of the Latinos in the United States maintain cultural ties through the Spanish-language media. Therefore, my media exposure gave me high visibility among the Latino community. The Spanish-language media baptized me as *Doctora* Lillian. I was able to use my academic-scientist identity to infuse a psychoeducational perspective into my media psychologist role.

During this period, an international adoption agency working with Latin American countries contacted me to perform psychological evaluations on prospective adopted parents. Given my proficiency in both Spanish and English, I was able to comply with the agency's requirement of writing two linguistic versions of the psychological report. Interestingly, years later I see some of the adopted children (now adults) whose parents I evaluated decades ago in my private practice.

As my practice grew, additional sources of referrals included other clinicians of color, as well as psychologists and therapists working with multicultural clients who needed a clinician for their clients' significant others. Word of mouth strengthened the building of my private practice. In fact, most of my referrals come by word of mouth. Because I tend to see clients in different phases of their lives, these clients eventually refer their relatives, friends, work colleagues, neighbors, and others to me. Certainly, my private practice reflects the power of familism: clients perceive me as a member of their extended family as well as a member of the communal *familia* Latina.

I have found the institution of church to be an interesting source of referral. One of my clinical expertise areas is working with victims of trauma—sexual, domestic, racial, political, and natural disaster, among others. Unfortunately, trauma is not a stranger to multicultural communities. The church of color represents a beacon of hope for many traumatized individuals. As a psychospiritual point of entry for many individuals, the church and its clergy refer those who suffer from trauma to clinicians for appropriate treatment.

In addition to my clinical work, I offer consultation on multicultural issues. Partly due to my international experience, I collaborate with international organizations based in Washington, D.C. Some of these organizations include embassies, schools, banks, and other international agencies. This type of work increases my professional network and generates additional referrals.

Today I continue to participate in multiple professional areas. For example, I am active in psychological associations, community agencies, cultural and arts associations, and in many other groups. These activities increase my visibility as a clinician and as a member of the community. Surprisingly, another professional activity—writing—has been a viable referral source. Along these lines, some individuals who have read some of my work and or who searched my name in the Internet come to me as prospective clients.

As you can see, I enjoy engaging in diverse professional activities. To manage my varied interests, I have streamlined how I run my practice. In other words, I have a "fee for service" clinical practice. Thus, I do not engage in administrative issues with third-party agencies. To balance this practice, I accommodate my commitment to social justice by using a sliding fee scale.

Based on my experience, let me offer you a series of suggestions that could help your clinical practice. Be mindful, however, to modify these suggestions to your particular clinical context:

- Enhance your clinical acumen. Include diverse perspectives in your theoretical orientation.
- Connect your practice with other parts of your life.
- Dare to heal with passion and compassion.
- Prioritize self-care. You cannot work effectively with others if you do not attend to your own well-being and that of your significant others.
- Seek supportive relations with psychologists and non-psychologists.
- Express yourself creatively. Creativity and healing go hand in hand.
- Increase your technological knowledge and capacity. Our society is becoming a digital global community.
- Learn about the business of running a private practice. After all, your clinical practice is a business.
- Culturally tailor your practice to the clientele you serve, but recognize the legal and ethical contexts of your clinical work.
- Foster abundance in your life as well as in your clients' lives.
- Include the promotion of financial health as part of your clients' well-being.
- Become critically conscious. That is, choose a multicultural or Latino social, cultural, or political cause to advocate for.
- Give psychology away—engage in community service.
- Rediscover who you are.

I conceptualize private practice as a service to my community as well as a liberating activity. In this context, liberation acquires multiple intersecting meanings. I am grounded as I foster liberation in my clients, their families, and their networks. In turn, this emancipatory clinical activity liberates me. It lets me orchestrate my "passion and compassion" in a meaningful way.

In these paragraphs, I endeavored to explain a bit how I developed the infrastructure for my private practice. I hope that your journey into clinical practice helps you arrive at a rewarding station in your life.

Epilogue
What Does Politics Have to Do with It? Policy and Mental Health Services Access for Latino Populations

Annie G. Toro

> *If we don't fight hard enough for the things we stand for, at some point we have to recognize that we don't really stand for them.*
> —Paul Wellstone, U.S. Senator from Minnesota (1944–2002)

Public policy formulation is frequently perceived as the sole responsibility of those working in Washington, DC. Making the connection between what happens in the nation's capital and how that affects the average citizen can be quite a stretch. And why should anyone be blamed for holding those views? Elected officials sound very similar during each election cycle, and what they say never stops us from going about our daily lives: taking our children to school, buying the groceries, going to work, paying the bills, and hoping to find some time to enjoy the presence of family and friends. At the same time, we all want to do something that matters and make our contribution to the world. We may volunteer, reduce the carbon footprint, donate to charities, or write a letter to a newspaper or city council. Still, I remain surprised by the number of people who cannot answer affirmatively the question "Do you know the name of your federal and state legislators?" The public elects its officials, who frequently make that clear in their speeches; therefore, their actions reflect our values. If you are one of the millions who would respond with a smile and a "no" to my question, this is a critical time for you to engage in the policy-making enterprise as both an informed citizen and a voting member of the polity. As the preceding chapters illustrate, the crucial role that Latinos will play in the future economy underscore the need to engage politically and promote the development of structures and services that support the well-being of this population.

For the purposes of this section, we are concerned with two key policy areas: (a) mental health service provision, and (b) immigration reform, which can influence access to health care services, as well as the social and psychological contexts in which immigrant and native-born Latinos live daily. Traditionally, mental health has not been a prominent theme in the legislative agenda, regardless of which political party has captured the congressional majority. Often it takes an elected official who

A. G. Toro (✉)
e-mail: annietoro@yahoo.es

has had a direct experience with mental illness health problems to appreciate the inadequacy of existing structures, generate a sense of urgency around these issues, and introduce new legislation. Similarly, immigration reform suffers from stagnation. Although everyone seems to agree that we need to change the status quo, discussions about the topic garner intense acrimony and polarization across political parties, resulting in near-total paralysis—to the detriment of those directly affected and broader society. Extremist convictions on both sides overshadow reasonable compromises. Thus, there is a great need to develop infrastructures that pave the way for increased access to quality mental health services for Latinos in the United States. How are we going to do this? The authors in this volume have presented an array of solutions. However, to realize these solutions, it is critical to consider the political climate and its influence on the processes and outcomes related to infrastructure building.

Political Context for Mental Health

Going back to efforts by the Clinton administration to achieve health reform in the early 1990s, the key to the policy-shift was an early decision made by the president and his advisers to include mental health and substance-abuse services in health care reform legislation. This decision led to the creation of Tipper Gore's mental health work group within the federal health care reform task force. No other area of benefits design was given such status (Koyanagi and Manes 1995). The mental health work group received guidance from health and mental health policy analysts as well as from national organizations and mental health economists. Some of the key lessons of the ensuing 1993–1994 debate on health care reform were that political organizing, built on a solid foundation of research and treatment experience, can triumph over issues of fear, apathy, and stigma, which are the three major rivals of nondiscriminatory mental health coverage (Koyanagi and Manes 1995). Specific factors that facilitated a focus on mental health include: (a) a significant shift in public attitudes about mental health care, due in part to the information received by the public about the brain and mental disorders during the decade prior to the health reform debate of the early 1990s; (b) research conducted as part of the movement toward evidence-based mental health treatment; (c) the increased awareness by large corporations and insurance companies that a greater focus on behavioral health care can keep down overall treatment costs; and (d) the trend toward greater advocacy efforts by consumers of mental health services and their families. With high-quality information about mental disorders and the effectiveness of treatment, key members of Congress, mental health groups, and advocates promoted the management of a comprehensive benefit as a cost-effective approach to coverage, successfully advancing their cause (Koyanagi and Manes 1995).

More recently, progress was made with the enactment in October 2008 of the long and hard-fought Paul Wellstone and Pete Domenici Mental Health Parity and Addiction Equity Act of 2008 (the Wellstone-Domenici Parity Act), which ends the health insurance benefits inequity between mental health/substance-use disorders and medical/surgical benefits for group health plans with more than 50 employees. (This law became effective on January 1, 2010.) There is promise, as well, of the changes that will come with the health reform legislation enacted in March 2010, the Patient Protection and Affordable Care Act (PPACA) (Pub. L. 111–148), which included significant provisions related to prevention and public health. For instance, the PPACA calls for the development of a national prevention, health promotion, and public health strategy, which will include the establishment of a national prevention council, the formation of an advisory group, and the creation of a fund ($ 15 billion over 10 years) to finance these important efforts. The law also establishes community transformation grants to promote community-based prevention initiatives aimed at addressing chronic disease and reducing health disparities (Foster 2010). Importantly, beginning in 2011, the law appropriates $ 12.5 billion over five years to expand services provided by both community health centers (CHCs) and the National Health Service Corps. Given that CHCs are one of the main sources of primary care in immigrant communities, and that the new appropriation is projected to double the number of patients served by the CHCs, it is likely that the health care infrastructure for medically underserved Latinos will strengthen in the coming years (Abascal 2010). By law, CHCs must be located in medically underserved communities or communities that are designated primary care shortage areas, or they must have as their target population communities that experience these circumstances. Now operating in more than 8,000 sites, both urban and rural, in every state and territory, and run by approximately 1,200 CHCs grantees, the centers are the medical home to approximately 20 million people in the United States. Regardless of ability to pay, the CHCs offer affordable, comprehensive, coordinated services, in facilities physically close to the patients who need it (Adashi et al. 2010; Foster 2010; Henry J. Kaiser Family Foundation 2009). Given the vital role of primary and preventive care in health promotion, it is encouraging that the aforementioned initiatives received support across political lines.

The real impact of the provisions in this new law, however, will depend on how the federal and state governments implement the PPACA, including citizenship verification requirements. This is why it is crucial for national, state, and local immigration advocates, as well as community-based organizations in immigrant communities, to be actively involved throughout the implementation process of the PPACA. In addition, it is imperative that professionals such as psychologists, social workers, physicians, public health experts, and nurses become involved during the implementation phase. Their expertise in research and practice with the Latino community should inform this critical policy agenda. Professionals can contribute their expertise through contacts with their local elected officials, federal agency administrators, relevant organizations, and community leaders.

Immigration Policy Reform

Immigration policy is a major controversial issue, and will likely remain so for many years given the projected continued influx of immigrants into the United States. This topic has traditionally elicited strong differences in ideology among politicians. On the one hand, there are advocates and policymakers across political affiliations who have been actively working to enact comprehensive federal immigration reform. These individuals have sought to end years of state and local laws, ordinances, and regulations that deprive immigrants of health services or erect obstacles to their access to mental health services. There are also many groups, as well as policymakers, actively working to deny benefits or constrain immigrants' ability to receive mental health and other essential health services. Given the many issues that remain unresolved at the policy level, immigrants are in a position of uncertainty, insecurity, anxiety, and fear. Moreover, they have limited access to much-needed mental health services. Among recent initiatives, the DREAM Act, currently making its way through Congress, could serve as an important step toward comprehensive immigration reform (Hollingshead 2010). The bill would allow certain young people—who were brought to the United States years ago as undocumented immigrant minors, who have been in the country continuously for at least five years prior to enactment of this legislation, and who are of good moral character—the opportunity to earn conditional permanent residency for six years. After this period, an immigrant student who complied with at least one of the requirements under the law would be eligible to apply for legal permanent resident status (National Immigration Law Center 2010).

Now, I would like to turn our attention to the needs of a unique immigrant group: Latino refugees, who come to the United States under trying political and social circumstances. In fact, nowhere are the health care needs of refugees more pronounced than in the area of mental health, given that they may have witnessed or have been victims of torture (Carlsten and Jackson 2003). Refugees are eligible for the same protections and benefits under the PPACA as U.S. citizens. The new law will give refugees access to affordable health coverage and protection against insurance practices that often deny coverage to individuals with preexisting conditions. Some of the provisions benefiting refugees under the new law include: (a) provision of the same benefits that exist in the larger insurance market, such as protections against lifetime benefit limits and rescissions; (b) new public and private health insurance coverage options beginning in 2014 (many refugees will qualify for premium tax credits to purchase coverage); (c) no dollar limits on coverage, and a maximum waiting period for health insurance coverage of 90 days, for plans beginning on or after September 2010 (Administration for Children and Families, Office of Refugee Resettlement 2010); (d) beginning in 2014, a ban on insurance companies' denial of coverage or charging higher premiums based on underlying health status; and (e) also effective in 2014, a requirement that states extend Medicaid coverage up to age 26 for young adults who spend their childhood and adolescence as wards of the state and who have since aged out of the foster care system, including those aging out of the Unaccompanied Refugee Minors program (Administration for Children and Families 2010).

Conclusion

A proper infrastructure for mental health services must address the factors that negatively influence Latinos' access to mental health services. When resources are limited and time is scarce, health comes second, and mental health services become a luxury for only the privileged ones. We, as a society, have a responsibility to ensure that health care, and specifically mental health, does not become an item of choice for those who need services but cannot afford them. It is our responsibility to continue educating and advocating for everyone in the United States to have access to mental health services, regardless of ability to pay, immigration status, lack of transportation, housing, or their knowledge of the English language, to name a few.

Our public policies have failed to address the gaps between what is available and what is needed. Public policies have also led to significant differences in the treatment of immigrants depending on their legal status in the United States. Despite these limitations, we must remember that a strong commitment exists among a number of policymakers across the political spectrum to fight for the rights of Latino immigrants and to make positive changes in Latino communities. Joining in these efforts as individuals and community members is necessary to empower more congressional leaders to support and expand these initiatives. At the same time, it is vital for all stakeholders (including you, dear reader) to continue efforts to eliminate mental health care disparities. Your efforts are critical if we are to make long-lasting, positive changes in the health of populations that have been largely marginalized and neglected by the health care system.

References

Abascal, M. C. (2010). Reform's mixed impact on immigrants: The new law's implications seem clear, but the indirect effects could be critical. *The American Prospect*. Available at http://www.prospect.org/cs/articles?article=reforms_mixed_impact_on_immigrants

Adashi, E. Y., Geiger, H. J., & Fine, M. D. (2010). Health care reform and primary care: The growing importance of the community health center. *New England Journal of Medicine, 362*, 22.

Administration for Children and Families. (2010). *Health care reform for refugees*. Available at http://www.acf.hhs.gov/programs/orr/whatsnew/health_reform_for_refugees.pdf

Administration for Children and Families, Office of Refugee Resettlement. (2010). *Who we serve*. Available at http://www.acf.hhs.gov/programs/orr/about/whoweserve.htm

Carlsten, C., & Jackson, C. (2003). Refugee and immigrant health care. Available at http://www.ethnomed.org/

Foster, J. (2010). Moving toward health equity: Health reform creates a foundation for eliminating disparities. *Families USA*. Available at http://www.familiesusa.org/assets/pdfs/health-reform/minority-health/moving-toward-health-equity.pdf

Henry J. Kaiser Family Foundation. (2009). Health reform and communities of color: How might it affect racial and ethnic health disparities? Available at www.kff.org

Hollingshead, E. (2010). Immigration reform: Harry Reid will bring the DREAM Act for a vote in 2010. *All247News*. Available at http://all247news.com/immigration-reform-harry-reid-will-bring-the-dream-act-for-a-vote-in-2010/2629/

Koyanagi, C., & Manes, J. (1995). What did the health care reform debate mean for mental health policy? *Health Affairs, 15*(3), 124-127.

National Immigration Law Center. (2010). Immigrant student adjustment/DREAM Act. Available at http://www.nilc.org/immlawpolicy/dream/index.htm

Index